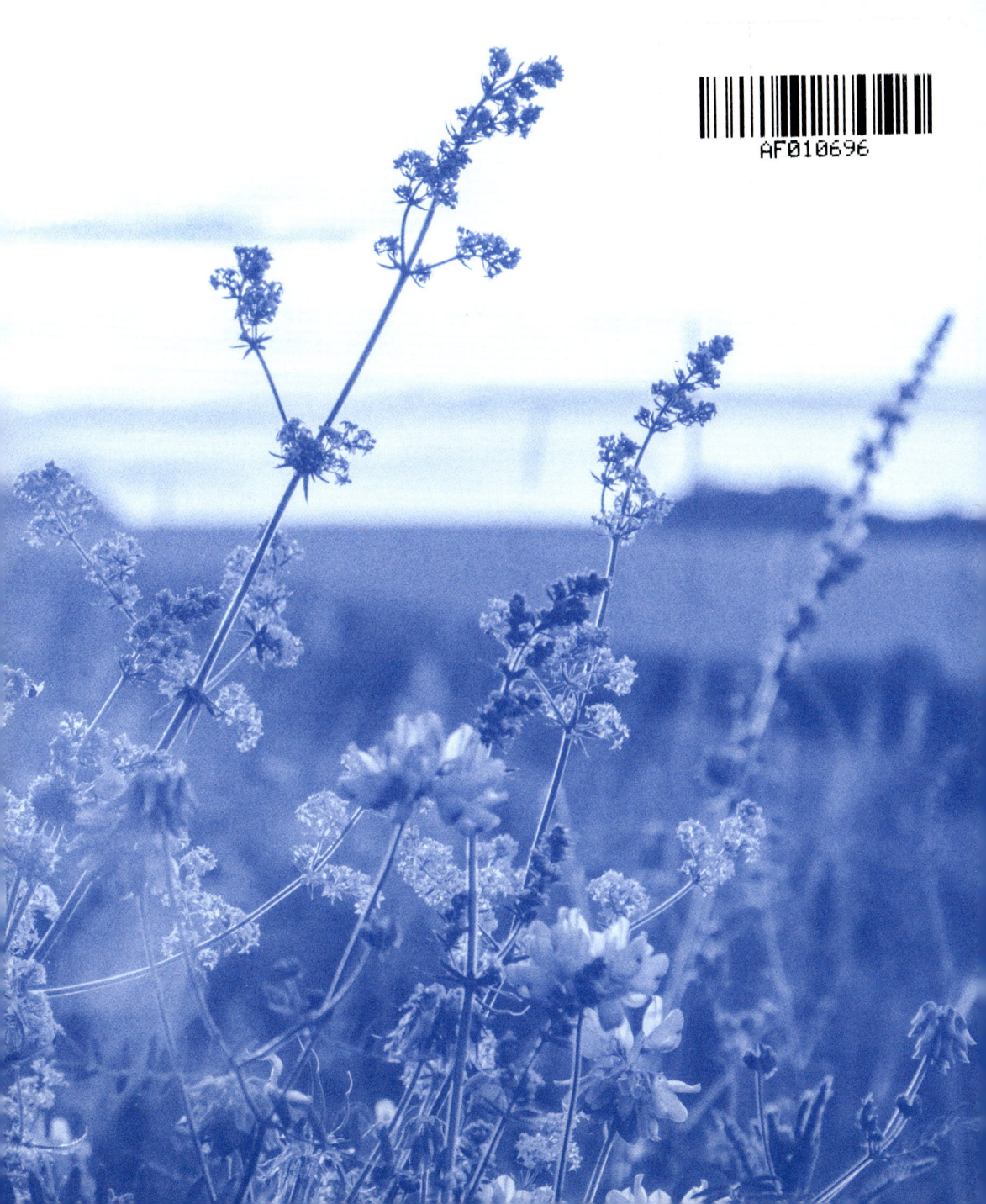

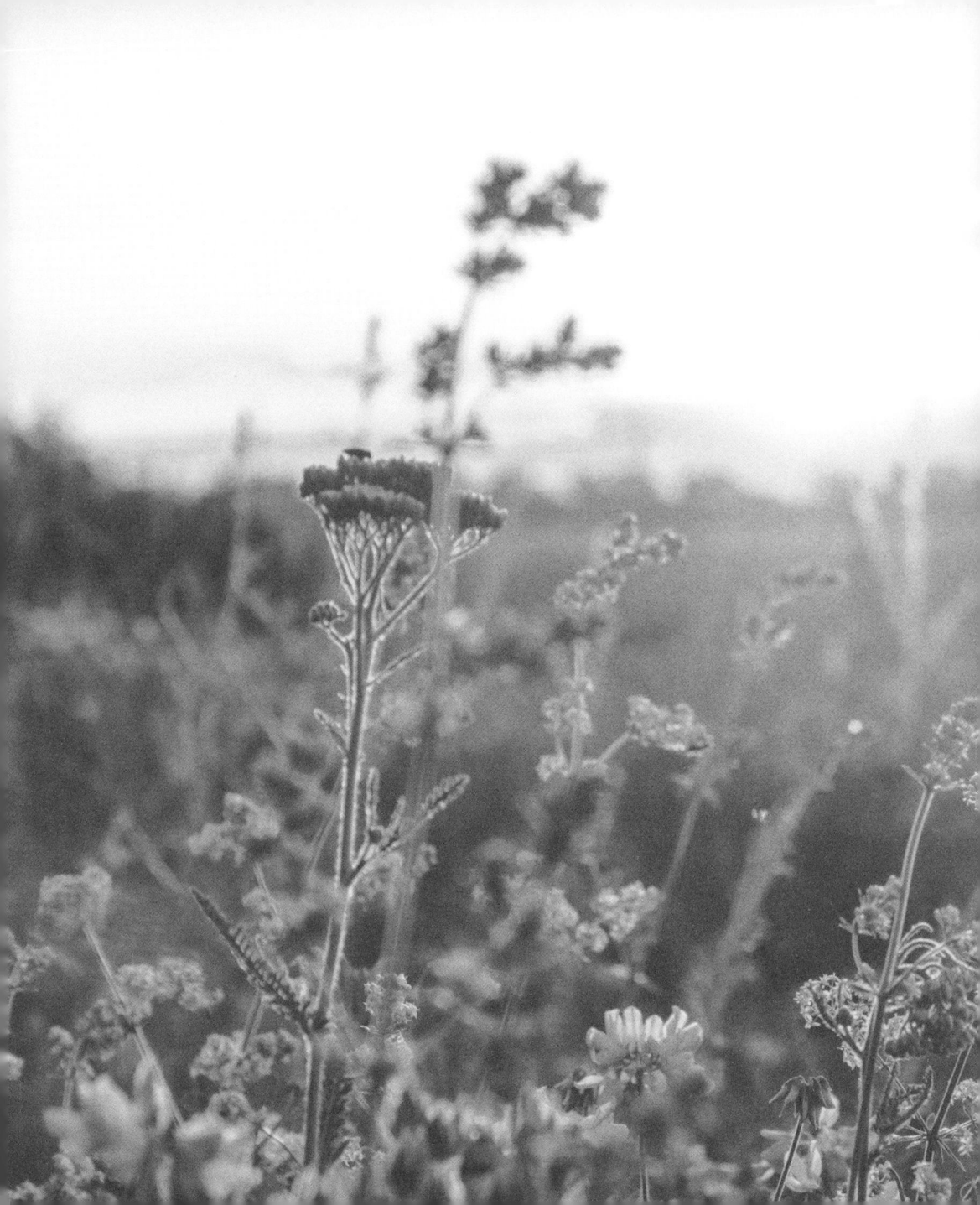

THE HEDGEROW APOTHECARY'S

FIELD GUIDE TO WILDFLOWERS

THE HEDGEROW APOTHECARY'S FIELD GUIDE TO WILDFLOWERS

Copyright © Christine Iverson, 2026

All rights reserved.

No part of this book may be reproduced by any means, nor transmitted, nor translated into a machine language, without the written permission of the publishers.

Christine Iverson has asserted their right to be identified as the author of this work in accordance with sections 77 and 78 of the Copyright, Designs and Patents Act 1988.

Condition of Sale
This book is sold subject to the condition that it shall not, by way of trade or otherwise, be lent, resold, hired out or otherwise circulated in any form of binding or cover other than that in which it is published and without a similar condition including this condition being imposed on the subsequent purchaser.

An Hachette UK Company
www.hachette.co.uk

Summersdale Publishers
Part of Octopus Publishing Group Limited
Carmelite House
50 Victoria Embankment
LONDON
EC4Y 0DZ
UK

This FSC® label means that materials and other controlled sources used for the product have been responsibly sourced

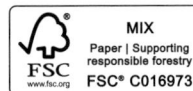

www.summersdale.com

The authorized representative in the EEA is Hachette Ireland, 8 Castlecourt Centre, Dublin 15, D15 XTP3, Ireland (email: info@hbgi.ie)

Printed and bound in China

ISBN: 978-1-83799-807-4
eISBN: 978-1-83799-808-1

Substantial discounts on bulk quantities of Summersdale books are available to corporations, professional associations and other organizations. For details contact general enquiries: telephone: +44 (0) 1243 771107 or email: enquiries@summersdale.com.

This book is NOT intended to provide medical advice. It is vital that you take personal responsibility for your own safety when using these remedies. Remedies made from some plants are best avoided during pregnancy and breastfeeding, and not recommended for babies, small children and people with certain medical conditions. Always do a patch test before putting things on your skin and hair in case of allergic reactions. Consult your doctor if you have any doubts and always do your research thoroughly.

THE HEDGEROW APOTHECARY'S

FIELD GUIDE TO WILDFLOWERS

RECIPES, REMEDIES AND FOLKLORE

CHRISTINE IVERSON

CONTENTS

7	About the Author	
8	Introduction	
9	Historic Herbalists	
12	Essential Wildflowers	
13	Growing Wildflowers in the Garden	
14	Growing Wildflowers in Pots	
15	Recipes and Remedies	
16	Preparing Flowers and Herbs	
18	Choosing the Right Carrier Oil	
20	How to Make Infused Carrier Oils	
22	Sterilizing Jars and Bottles	
23	Conversions and Measurements	
24	Bird's Foot Trefoil	
26	Bistort	
28	Bluebell	
30	Buttercup	
32	Coltsfoot	
34	Soothing Coltsfoot Balm	
36	Common Dodder	
38	Common Poppy	
40	Poppy Seed and Lemon Cake	
42	Corncockle	
44	Cornflower	
46	Wildflower-Seed Balls	
48	Cowslip	
50	Dandelion	
52	Dandelion-Flower Vinegar	
54	Devil's-Bit Scabious	
56	Dock	
58	Dock Root Upset Tummy Tea	
60	Early Purple Orchid	
62	Fairy Flax	
64	Fennel	
66	Foraged Fennel Fronds Pesto	
68	Fern	
70	Feverfew	
72	Fleabane	
74	Forget-Me-Not	
76	Foxglove	
78	Fumitory	
80	Green Alkanet	
82	Heather	
84	Hedge Woundwort	
86	Hemp Agrimony	
88	Herb Bennet	
90	Honesty	
92	Honeysuckle	
94	Honeysuckle and Wild Rose Lip Balm	
96	Lady's Bedstraw	
98	Lily-of-the-Valley	
100	Lords and Ladies	
102	Lungwort	
104	Milkwort	
106	Mugwort	
108	Navelwort	
110	Nettle	

112	Nettle Lotion Bar for Stiff Joints	152	Three-Cornered Leek	188	Wild Thyme-Infused Honey
114	Oxeye Daisy	154	Three-Cornered Leek and Cheese Scones	190	Woad
116	Oxeye Daisy Chest Rub	156	Toadflax	192	Wood Anemone
118	Pineapple Weed	158	Tormentil	194	Wood Betony
120	Pineapple Weed Posset	160	Traveller's Joy	196	Woody Nightshade
122	Primrose	162	Traveller's Joy Winter Wreath	198	Wormwood
124	Purple Loosestrife	164	Valerian	200	Yarrow
126	Ragwort	166	Water Mint	202	Yarrow and Plantain First-Aid Salve
128	Red Clover	168	Minty Mouthwash		
130	Red Clover Blossom Syrup	170	White Bryony	205	Final Thoughts
132	Rosebay Willowherb	172	Wild Carrot		
134	Rosebay Willowherb Jam	174	Wild Garlic		
136	Sea Holly	176	Wild Garlic Salt and Pepper Seasoning		
138	Shepherd's Purse	178	Wild Marjoram		
140	Silverweed	180	Soothing Marjoram and Rose Facial Compress		
142	Solomon's Seal	182	Wild Rose		
144	Spindle	184	Rosehip Under-Eye Oil		
146	Sundew	186	Wild Thyme		
148	Sweet Cicely				
150	Thistle				

In the Meadow – What in the Meadow?

In the meadow – what in the meadow?
Bluebells, buttercups, meadowsweet,
And fairy rings for the children's feet
*   In the meadow.*
In the garden – what in the garden?
Jacob's-ladder and Solomon's-seal,
And Love-lies-bleeding beside All-heal
*   In the garden.*

Christina Rossetti

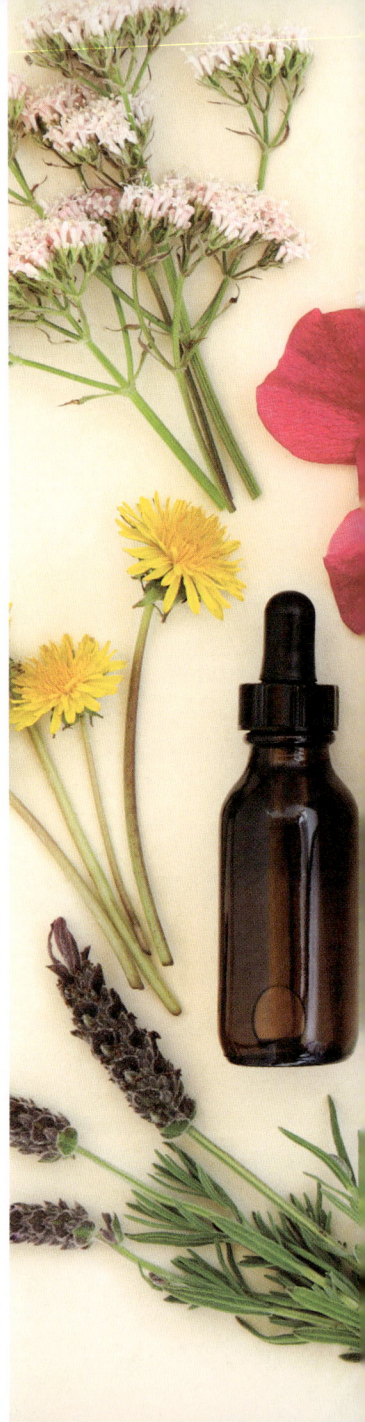

ABOUT THE AUTHOR

With a modest wildflower meadow in her small front garden, it was inevitable that Christine would be curious to research the history and superstition surrounding these beautiful plants. Living at the foot of the South Downs National Park, where there are lots of opportunities to seek out a huge diversity of native wildflowers, Christine's research uncovered a whole new world of fascinating recipes and remedies once used by our ancestors.

In 2019, the bestselling *Hedgerow Apothecary* was published by Summersdale, shortly to be followed by *The Garden Apothecary*, *The Hedgerow Apothecary Forager's Guide*, *The Herbal Apothecary*, *The Hedgerow Apothecary Forager's Card Deck* and now *The Hedgerow Apothecary's Field Guide to Wildflowers*.

Christine continues to get enormous pleasure from researching and writing about the plants all around us and likes to share her knowledge by giving talks to local horticultural societies and Women's Institutes.

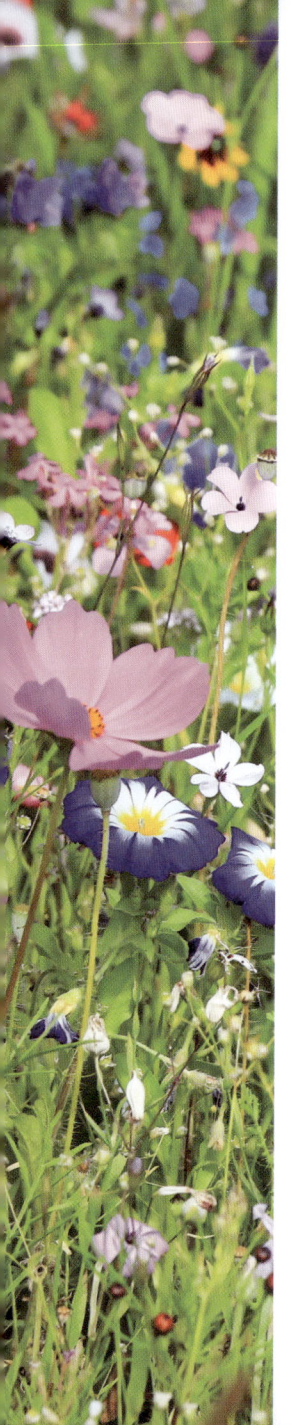

INTRODUCTION

How utterly delightful are wildflower meadows, continuously changing from one colour to another as the different species create a stunning patchwork from early spring through to late autumn? What better sight is there when driving through the British countryside? Stop, if you can, admire the beauty of nature and listen to the excited buzz as insects and bees flock to feed on all the native blooms.

Welcome to *The Hedgerow Apothecary's Field Guide to Wildflowers*, a guide to these natural treasures. Wonderful photographs and clear descriptions will give you the confidence to identify many of our very own native wild plants with a "look but don't pick" approach.

The variety of folklore and superstition attached to wildflowers is astounding and something that I always find a joy to research. The number of different folkloric names given to each plant gives us an insight into the humour of early Brits. Lords and ladies alone boasts over 60 different names – some of them slightly naughty – but it all helped with plant identification of the time.

I have thought carefully about which wildflowers we can harvest in small amounts and have created some exciting recipes and remedies using the more common plants, but please take only what you need. And remember, some plants can cause allergic reactions and can be fatal if ingested. Take lots of notes and photographs, be in the moment and take time to enjoy the simplicity of connecting with nature, but resist the temptation to touch unless you're 100 per cent certain of what you're picking.

Most important of all, take the time to explore nature. Studies show that spending time in green spaces can reduce stress, lower blood pressure, improve mood and well-being and help you sleep better. You'll soon start to notice the noises, smells and sights of the countryside and how it changes from season to season. Maybe do a little foraging or wildflower spotting – children love connecting with nature and you will too.

HISTORIC HERBALISTS

Throughout this book, I've quoted from several notable historic herbalists. The words of these trailblazers of their time make fascinating reading, but some of the information comes from as far back as the twelfth century and is included for your curiosity and amusement only. Medical knowledge has moved on a lot since the Middle Ages so don't be tempted to try any of the quoted remedies!

JOHN GERARD (1545–1612)

Born in Nantwich, Cheshire, John Gerard moved to London at the age of 17 as an apprentice barber surgeon. While studying, he began to grow plants in his Holborn garden and started to receive gifts of seeds and plants from around the world. In 1586, he established a physic garden – a herb garden with medicinal plants – and soon gained a reputation as a skilled herbalist. His most famous work, *The Herball, or, Generall Historie of Plantes* (1597), became the most circulated herbal guide in the seventeenth century despite the inclusion of some very dubious entries, such as the belief that mint could be used as an effective contraceptive, and wild parsnips, when eaten with wine, could protect deer from snake bites.

NICHOLAS CULPEPER (1616–1654)

After the death of his father, Culpeper was taken to live with his maternal grandparents in Isfield, East Sussex, where his grandmother introduced him to herbs and medicinal plants. From the age of 16, he studied at Cambridge, becoming apprenticed to an apothecary. Culpeper set up his own pharmacy in Spitalfields where he realized that ordinary working people could not afford the extortionate fees charged by practising physicians. He angrily stated that *"no man deserved to starve to pay an insulting, insolent physician"* and began gathering herbs from the countryside with which to treat patients free of charge – a move that didn't go down well with his contemporaries.

Despite opposition and even accusations of witchcraft, Culpeper continued working and served as a medic during the English Civil War. Unfortunately, he was shot in the chest on the battlefield; an injury he never fully recovered from. Culpeper's *Complete Herbal* was published in 1652, deliberately sold at a reasonable price and written in English instead of the more traditional Latin because he wanted it to be accessible for everyone.

MAUD GRIEVE (1858–1941)

Maud Grieve is probably one of the most important women of twentieth-century herbalism.

Before 1914, very few herbs were grown commercially in the UK, since it was cheaper to import them from overseas. During World War One, the shortages of herbs for medicine and food became a real issue. The Board of Agriculture actively encouraged farmers to grow key medicinal plants such as digitalis, henbane and goldenseal to make up for the shortfall.

Grieve was a founding member of The National Herb Growing Association, which provided seeds to the public and encouraged them to grow plants for the war effort.

Grieve posted out hundreds of packets of herb seeds along with pamphlets containing instructions on how to grow plants successfully and educating people on the medicinal benefits. These pamphlets were later expanded into *A Modern Herbal*, which her contemporaries considered to be "a marvellous piece of work".

During World War One, Grieve established the Whins Medicinal and Commercial Herb School and Farm in Buckinghamshire, where she ran three-year training courses, mostly for women, on plant identification, propagation, drying and harvesting.

THE PHYSICIANS OF MYDDFAI

The legend of the Physicians of Myddfai begins sometime in the twelfth century in a small village in Carmarthenshire, Wales and is the stuff of folklore.

Rhiwallon Feddyg (Rhiwallon the doctor) was thought to have mythical ancestry; his mother was believed to have been the Lady of the Lake who gave King Arthur his magical sword Excalibur at Avalon. She was credited with teaching her son the secrets of turning plants into effective herbal remedies.

Rhiwallon's knowledge of healing herbs gained him quite a reputation, and along with his three sons, Cadwgan, Gruffydd and Einion, he was soon invited to the Welsh court to treat the royal princes. They were known to have hundreds of remedies made from plants grown in the Myddfai area of Carmarthenshire.

Rhiwallon's remedies were written down in Welsh in *The Red Book of Hergest*, a medieval manuscript containing descriptions of surgery as well as herbal cures.

- **The antiviral and antioxidant properties of elderberries was well known even in the twelfth century:**
  "Take sage, rue, and berries of the elder tree, mallows and feverfew, put them in a mortar mixed with a little honey, white wine, or vinegar, pounding them well together."

- **A cure for boils:**
  "Take musk mallow, lard and earthworms; bruise together, and apply to the affected part."

- **To help a man to confess what he has done:**
  "Take a frog alive from the water, extract his tongue, and put him again in the water. Lay this same tongue upon the heart of a sleeping man, and he will confess his deeds in his sleep."

- **Recipe for a healing ointment:**
  "Take avens, violet, daisy, bugle, ribwort plantain, and feverfew; pound, and boil them well with fresh butter, and strain. Keep it, for it is useful."

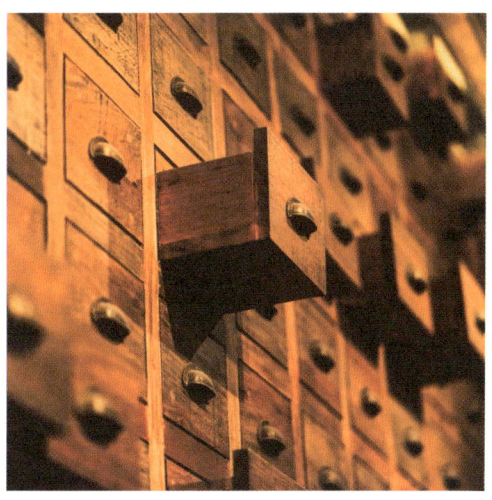

ESSENTIAL WILDFLOWERS

I was shocked to discover that in the UK we have lost over 97 per cent of our native wildflower meadows since the 1930s.

The Director of Kew Gardens Richard Deverell made a very strong statement: "British wildflowers are under threat and therefore so are the pollinators they feed. Not only is it heartbreaking to lose the beauty and colour these native flowers give the UK landscape, but the plight of pollinators has a very real impact on the food we eat ourselves."

Many of our pollinators, vital for our own food production, rely upon specific native flowers as both a source of food and a place to lay their eggs. A welcome side effect of increasing the numbers of wildflowers would be a boost in diversity, with greater numbers of insects and insect-eating wildlife such as hedgehogs, birds and mice.

Many wildflowers are protected and far too precious to pick, and we want to help them flourish for everyone to enjoy.

You may not live in the countryside or even have a garden, but you can still make a difference. A few pots of wildflowers or herbs on a veranda or patio will attract bees and butterflies. Also, try asking your local council not to cut or spray the grass verges quite so frequently; you'll be surprised at how quickly they flourish.

As gardeners, let's not be quite so tidy! Allow a few areas in your garden to grow a little wilder, leave a pile of logs untouched for insects to inhabit, plant pollinator-friendly plants, create a wildlife pond and, if you can, try not to use weed-killers and insecticides. Feed the birds and put up a few nest boxes – wild birds will be attracted into the garden and will be a delight to see.

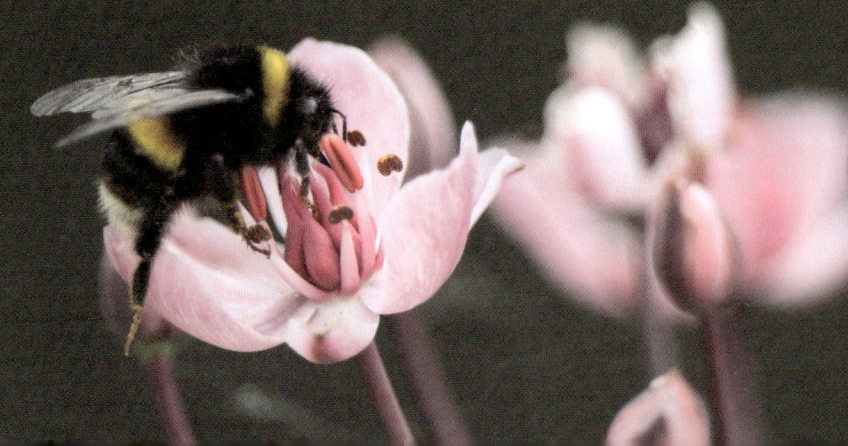

GROWING WILDFLOWERS IN THE GARDEN

No matter how big or small your garden, veranda or balcony, whether it's in town or country, you can still help a wide range of insects survive their ever-more challenging search for food.

Here are a few tips to help you create your own pollinator-friendly space.

CUT THE GRASS LESS OFTEN

Patches of long grass encourage different species to grow. You'll be amazed at the diversity of plants, insects, small mammals and birds that will be attracted by seed heads and flowers.

SOW SOME SEEDS

Pick an area that hasn't been fertilized or recently cultivated, since wildflower seeds establish best on poor soil.

Remove any weeds that may choke out your seeds and rake the seedbed to a fine powder.

Choose the right seeds for your soil type and location – seed merchants can advise you as to the best mix. Heavy clay soils should be sown in spring; other soil types in autumn.

Mixing your seeds with some fine sand or making seed balls (see page 46) helps you to distribute them more evenly, and you can see where they have landed.

Scatter seeds in all directions, rake lightly and water gently.

Wildflower turf and plug plants are available to buy, which will make an instant impact, but this is far more expensive than seeding the area yourself.

MAINTENANCE

Thistles, docks and nettles will need weeding out regularly.

Mow your wildflower patch at your highest setting once in July/early August and once in early autumn. Leave the cuttings on the soil for a couple of days to ensure that the seedheads have dropped their seeds, then gently rake over your patch and remove the cuttings into the compost.

Your wildflower meadow may take a year or so to establish and look beautiful, so be patient – it will be worth the wait and the bees and butterflies will love you for it.

GROWING WILDFLOWERS IN POTS

Growing wildflowers for nature in pots and containers can really help our struggling pollinators. No garden? No problem. Here's how:

CHOOSE YOUR CONTAINER

Pots bought from the garden centre are lovely, but can be expensive. As long as there are drainage holes in the bottom, you can upcycle practically any container that you have. Metal tins can work well as can old butler sinks or even plastic food tubs.

CHOOSE YOUR SEEDS

There are lots of pollinator-friendly varieties that will happily grow in containers but make sure that you pick native wildflowers or your local wildlife may not find them quite so attractive. If you're unsure what to choose, ask your local nursery for advice.

SOWING

Pop a few small stones or pieces of broken pottery into the bottom of your container to aid drainage.

Fill your pot with a 50:50 mix of garden soil and peat-free compost to ensure that the soil isn't too rich for wildflowers. Leave a gap of about 2.5 cm (1 in.) at the top for watering.

Sprinkle your seeds thinly on top then cover with 1 cm ($1/3$ in.) of your compost/soil mix.

Water gently so as not to disturb the seeds.

Place in a sunny spot and wait for the magic to happen.

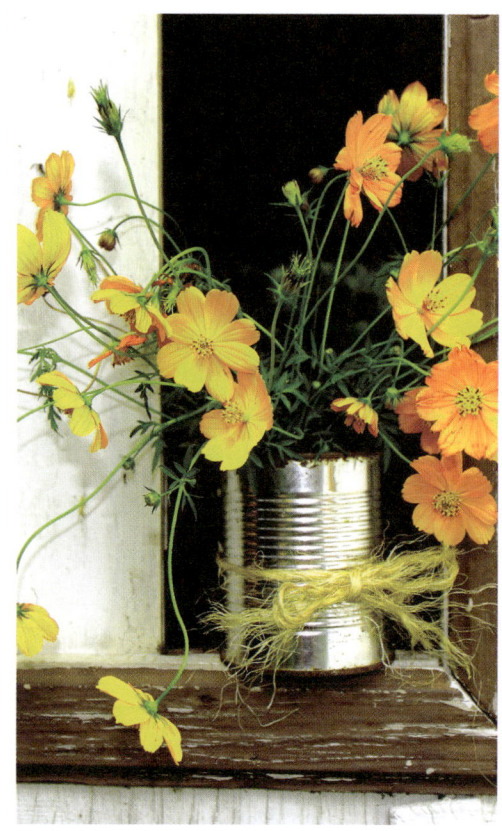

RECIPES AND REMEDIES

In this book you'll find some recipes and remedies using selected wildflowers. The following pages include everything you need to know to get going.

WILDFLOWER-SEED GATHERING ETIQUETTE

Many species of wildflower are protected. This means you are allowed to gather seeds in moderation and only for personal use – not for commercial gain. I like to carry a few little brown envelopes in my back pocket just in case I spot some interesting seed heads while out and about.

Under the Countryside Act 1981 it is illegal to dig up or uproot plants without the landowner's permission, you must not collect seeds from a site of special scientific interest (SSI) or a nature reserve, and you must not trespass.

Be mindful of where you are walking and try not to trample other plants. Collect ripe seed heads on a dry day and take only what you need.

KITCHEN ESSENTIALS

- A few large pans

- Sieve and colander

- Cotton muslin (or a clean cotton tea towel) for straining

- Pestle and mortar or food processor

- Jam jars and bottles of differing sizes, with well-fitting lids

- Labels

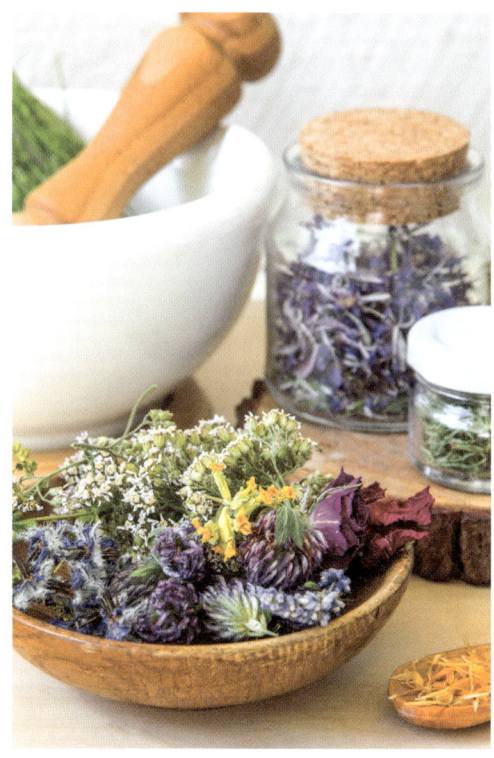

PREPARING FLOWERS AND HERBS

A common way to use fresh botanicals is to infuse them in carrier oils (see pages 20–21). It's important to prepare them properly before you do as excess moisture in the plants can turn the oil rancid, rendering it useless. You don't need equipment like dehydrators to prepare your herbs and flowers. I use a piece of chicken wire fashioned into a frame for drying flower heads and petals. Herbs and flowers don't have to be absolutely dry but do need to be "wilted" for a couple of hours to remove some of the moisture. Lay petals and leaves onto kitchen paper overnight – whole flower heads will take a little longer. Bunches of woody herbs can be hung up in cool airy places like outhouses or garden sheds, but avoid the cooking smells and smoke of the kitchen.

HERBS

Herbs are at their best before they begin to flower. Harvest them mid-morning on a dry day to preserve the herb's essential oils.

- Remove any old, dead or diseased leaves.

- There's no need to wash herbs if you grow them without pesticides. Give them a gentle shake to remove any insects.

- Tie the herbs into loose bundles with natural twine, hang upside down and put a brown paper bag over them to catch leaves as they dry.

- Keep them away from direct sunlight and leave for at least two weeks or until the leaves are crunchy. Check on them regularly and discard any that smell musty or have fluffy mould growing on them.

- Crumble the herbs with your fingers and store in an airtight container, where they will keep for about a year. Rubbing the dried herbs through a colander effectively removes any woody stalks and crumbles the leaves up finely.

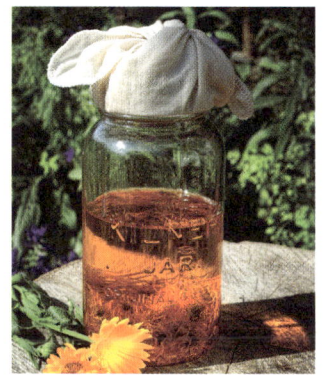
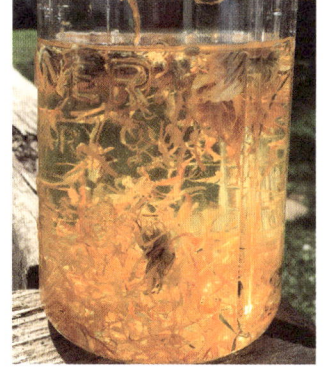
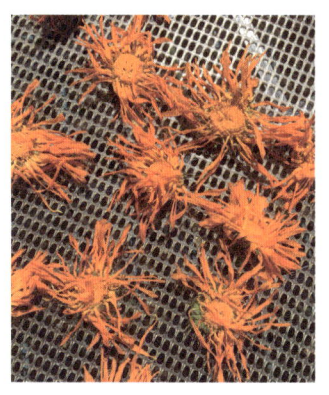

FLOWER HEADS AND PETALS

Harvest flower heads and petals mid-morning on a dry day when the flowers are looking their best. Avoid drying in direct sunlight as this can destroy the very health-giving properties that you wish to harness in your remedies. All you need for the drying process is a flat surface that allows air to circulate freely; chicken wire is perfect for this. Alternatively, hang up some muslin to create a flat hammock, or even use an old wire shelf from the oven. I place my chicken wire tray under the shade of a big old apple tree in the garden on a dry day, although if it's windy you might lose a few flowers. Remember to bring them back inside before nightfall otherwise the flowers will get damp with the morning dew.

- Lay baking paper over the wire of your drying surface, to prevent smaller petals falling through the gaps.

- Spread petals across the surface in a single layer, trying not to overlap them. They will dry quite quickly.

- Place flower heads far enough apart so they don't touch – these will take a while longer. They will shrivel and become crumbly as they dry. Place in a cool, airy place away from direct sunlight and turn them over occasionally.

- When they feel crunchy and crumble easily, store in an airtight container, label and date. Depending on the drying environment and type of flower they can take anything from two to four weeks to dry completely. Flower heads and petals will keep for up to a year.

CHOOSING THE RIGHT CARRIER OIL

There are a wide variety of plant-based carrier oils available on the market, all with different beneficial properties. These are used in homemade infused oils, lotions, massage oils and balms, and they also "carry" essential oils that need to be diluted before going onto the skin. You can use many of the oils that you have in your kitchen larder or there are a huge variety of sellers online; try to find one that is reputable and stocks good-quality oils – remember that this product will be absorbed into your skin and into your bloodstream.

Many oils are pressed from nuts, seeds and kernels. If you have any allergies, make sure you research thoroughly before using them and always do a patch test first.

TYPE OF OIL	PROPERTIES	HAIR/SCALP		SKIN	
		Oily	Dry	Oily	Dry
Almond	Moisturizing Antioxidant High in vitamin E Natural SPF Nourishing	✓	✓	✓	✓
Apricot kernel	Easily absorbed Antioxidant Anti-ageing Antiseptic High in vitamin A	X	✓	X	✓
Avocado	Soothing Hydrating Natural SPF Antioxidant Anti-inflammatory	X	✓	✓	✓

TYPE OF OIL	PROPERTIES	HAIR/SCALP		SKIN	
		Oily	Dry	Oily	Dry
Coconut	Easily available Antioxidant Anti-inflammatory Antimicrobial Anti-ageing Promotes hair growth	X	✓	X	✓
Grapeseed	High in vitamin E Easily absorbed Antibacterial Antioxidant Anti-dandruff	✓	✓	✓	✓
Jojoba	Antiseptic Hypoallergenic Hydrating Anti-inflammatory Anti-fungal Anti-acne Healing	✓	✓	✓	✓
Olive	Easily available Skin brightening Antioxidant Anti-ageing Collagen-boosting Cleansing	X	✓	✓	✓
Peach kernel	Easily absorbed High in vitamin E Hypoallergenic Good for older skin	X	✓	X	✓
Sunflower	Easily available Anti-inflammatory Moisturizing Easily absorbed	✓	✓	✓	✓

HOW TO MAKE INFUSED CARRIER OILS

Creating infused carrier oils is a lovely way to harness the properties of your garden flowers and herbs, and turn them into the wonderful lotions, balms and salves contained in this book.

SUN METHOD

Healers and apothecaries have used this traditional method for hundreds of years and, although it takes time and relies heavily on the appearance of the sun, this is definitely my preferred way. I just love to see jars of different-coloured botanical oils working their magic and infusing on my south-facing windowsill.

INGREDIENTS

Herbs or flowers (dried or fresh)

Carrier oil of your choice (see pages 18–19)

EQUIPMENT NEEDED

Glass jar

Muslin cloth

String or elastic band

METHOD

Fill the jar halfway with your plant material.

Cover with your chosen carrier oil, shaking to burst any bubbles. Ensure that all plant material is completely covered – anything sticking out could go mouldy.

Top with the muslin and secure with string or an elastic band.

Place on a sunny windowsill for at least two weeks until the oil has taken on some colour and scent.

Strain the oil through the muslin, squeezing to extract all the oil. Compost the plant material left behind.

Label and date – you might think that you'll remember which oil it is, but believe me, you won't!

Keep in a cool, dark place and use within a year.

QUICK INFUSION METHOD

This method is a lot quicker than relying on the sun, but may not extract as many beneficial oils as the traditional method. Be careful not to fry your plant material by heating the oil too much.

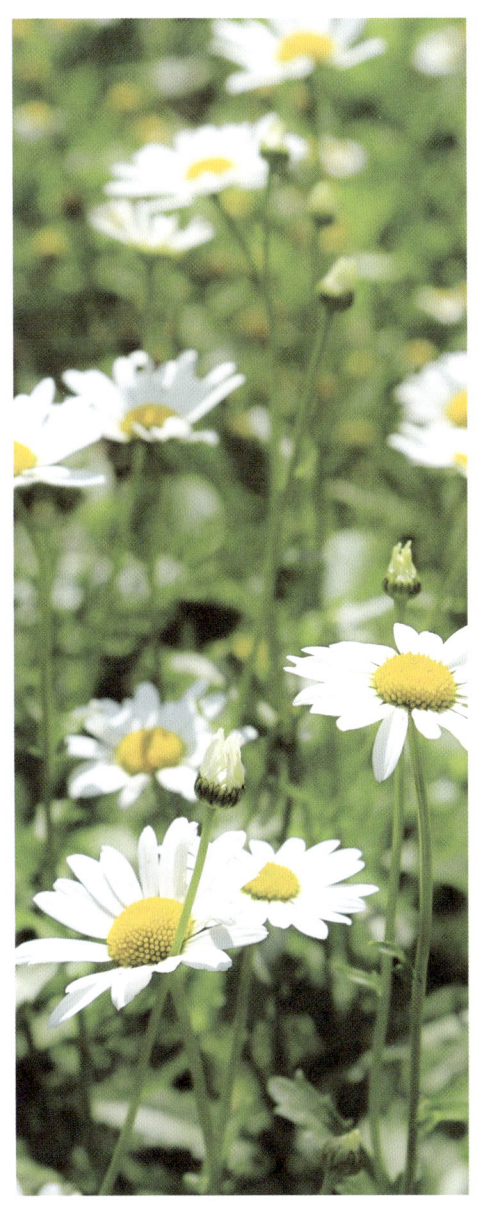

INGREDIENTS

Herbs or flowers (dried or freshly wilted)

Carrier oil of your choice (see pages 18–19)

Boiling water

EQUIPMENT NEEDED

Heatproof bowl

Saucepan

Strainer

Jar with lid

METHOD

Put the plant material and carrier oil into your heatproof bowl and suspend it over the pan of boiling water. Ensure the water doesn't touch the bottom of the bowl.

Simmer gently without a lid for 2 hours, checking the water level in the pan regularly.

Allow to cool, strain into the jar, label and date.

Keep in a cool, dark place and use within a year.

STERILIZING JARS AND BOTTLES

It's good practice to sterilize all your jars and bottles before use. This will extend the shelf life of your product by removing bacteria and germs.

- Wash jars and bottles in hot soapy water and rinse.

- Lay the jars in an oven preheated to 140°C (285°F) for 10–15 minutes until dry.

- Soak the lids in boiling water. Dry thoroughly with kitchen paper before use.

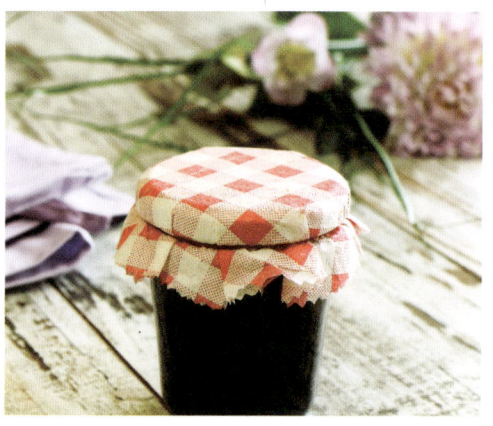
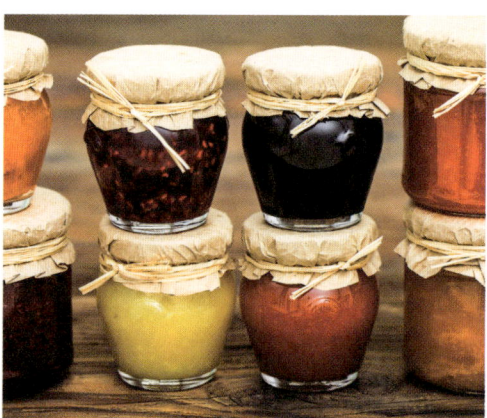

SETTING POINT FOR JAM

You'll need this when making the jam on page 134. Before beginning your jam-making, put a couple of small plates in the freezer. To test for setting point, take the pan off the heat and place a small blob onto one of the cold plates. Let it stand for a minute, then push the blob with your finger and you should see it wrinkle. If the jam is still liquid, pop it back on to boil for another 5 minutes and test again.

CONVERSIONS AND MEASUREMENTS

All the conversions in the tables below are approximations, which have been rounded up or down. When using a recipe, always stick to one unit of measurement and do not alternate between them.

LIQUID MEASUREMENTS

5 ml = 1 tsp
15 ml = 1 tbsp
30 ml = ⅛ cup
60 ml = ¼ cup
120 ml = ½ cup
240 ml = 1 cup
500 ml = 2¼ cups

DRIED INGREDIENT MEASUREMENTS

5 g = 1 tsp
15 g = 1 tbsp
30 g poppy seeds = ¼ cup
100 g caster sugar = ½ cup
300 g blackberries = 2 cups
400 g hazelnuts = 3 cups
450 g caster sugar = 2¼ cups

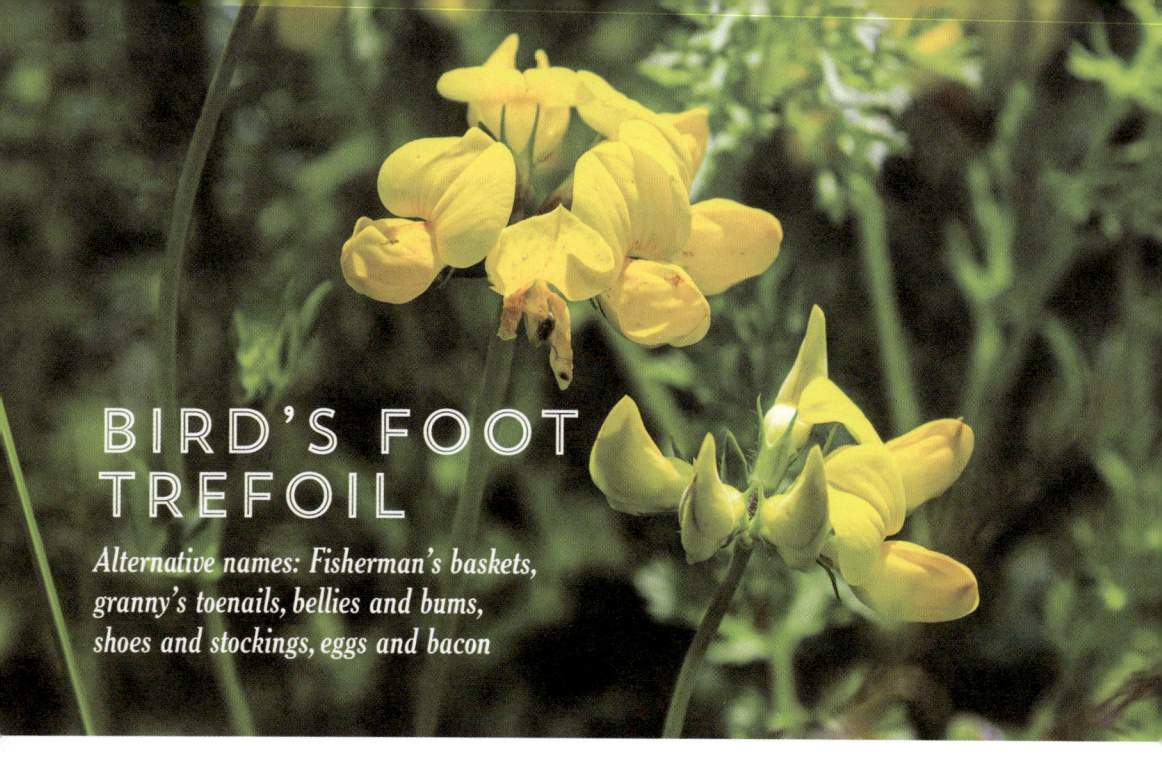

BIRD'S FOOT TREFOIL

Alternative names: Fisherman's baskets, granny's toenails, bellies and bums, shoes and stockings, eggs and bacon

HOW TO IDENTIFY: This attractive member of the pea family forms sprawling patches of bright yellow slipper-shaped flowers with a hint of red from May to September. Find it growing along roadside verges, well-drained grassland and rocky habitats. The leaves have five narrow oval leaflets covered in fine downy hair and the seedpods look distinctly like bird's claws, or – to quote a folk name – "granny's toenails".

HISTORY: Botanist John Gerard was the first to formally record the bird's foot trefoil in 1597, writing in his book *The Herball, or Generall Historie of Plantes* that it could be found "in the most fertill fields of England". Traditionally the bright yellow flowers were widely used as a pale yellow dye for woollen and cotton fabrics.

Bird's foot trefoil is an important food source for bees and the caterpillars of the wood white butterfly, the silver-studded blue butterfly and the common blue butterfly, all of which are listed as species of principal importance and are protected under the Countryside Act.

Bird's foot trefoil is a valuable crop for farmers since it can fix nitrogen from the air into the ground to help improve soil fertility and lessen the need for synthetic fertilizers.

FOLKLORE: In many cultures the plant was thought to have magical properties and was used to ward off evil spirits, cure ailments and bring good luck. In pagan times, to harness these magical powers of protection, it was woven into head wreaths along with other flowers to be worn during midsummer festivities.

In twentieth-century Scotland and Ireland, the plant had the nickname "no blame". Children would gather bird's foot trefoil from miles around, believing that it would prevent them from getting punished by their teacher.

It was used as a symbol of love and friendship and often given as a gift to express affection. However, according to the Victorian "language of flowers" (see page 43), which was used as a way of expressing feeling and sentiments through flowers, bird's foot trefoil was one of the few to represent a negative emotion as it also symbolized revenge – possibly because the plant contains trace amounts of cyanide.

FOLK MEDICINE: Culpeper describes bird's foot trefoil as having *"a drying, binding quality, and therefore very good to be used in wound drinks [...] bird's foot is found by experience to break the stone in the back or kidneys [...] and it wonderfully helpeth the ruptures, being taken inwardly, and outwardly applied to the place."*

In the nineteenth century, in the Outer Hebrides, an infusion of bird's foot trefoil was commonly used as an eyewash. Meanwhile, as recently as the 1960s in the West Country, the plant was still regularly used to staunch bleeding from the legs of horses.

Diluted infusions of bird's foot trefoil were traditionally prescribed for exhaustion, anxiety and insomnia in the Sannio region of Italy.

Bird's foot trefoil is toxic for dogs.

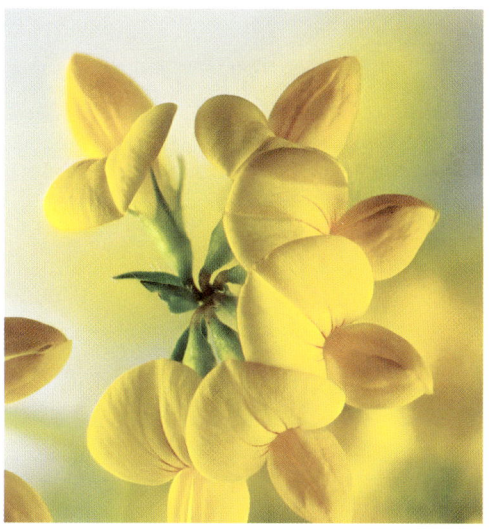

BISTORT

Alternative names: Snakeweed, dragon's wort, pudding dock, pink pokers, poor man's cabbage, twice writhen, Easter giant, Easter ledger

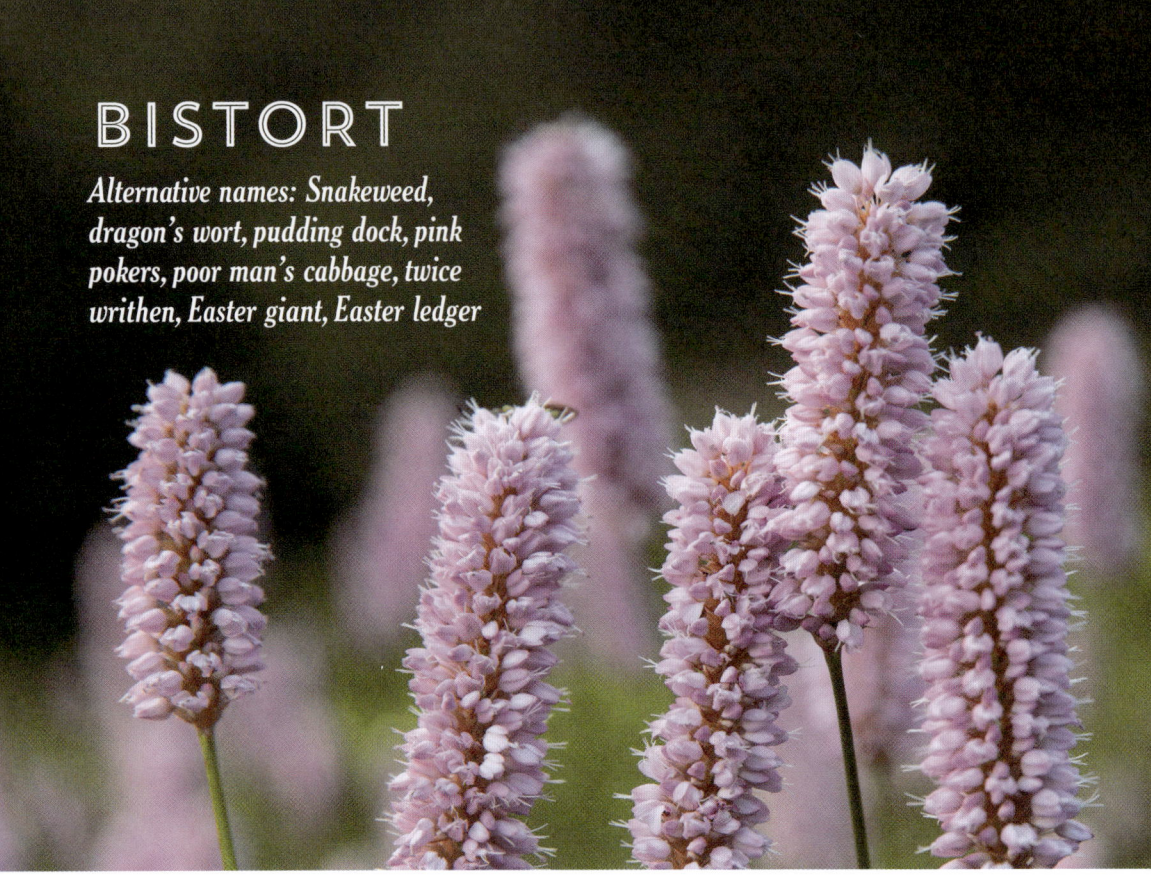

HOW TO IDENTIFY: Bistort is a member of the dock family that prefers to grow in damp places such as wet meadows and pastures and is most commonly found in the north of England. The striking pink poker-like flowers can be seen towering above the surrounding vegetation from June to August, with heart-shaped leaves that gradually decrease in size as they climb up the stem.

HISTORY: The name bistort comes from the Latin *bis* meaning twice and *torta* meaning twisted, as the plant has a thick, twisted root.

For hundreds of years, bistort was made into a savoury pudding known as Easter ledge pudding, traditionally eaten two weeks before Easter with spring lamb.

Easter ledge pudding's main ingredients were foraged leaves such as bistort, nettle and dandelion, which were boiled in a muslin bag with barley, oats and onions. Once cooked, an egg was added and it was formed into rounds to be fried in bacon fat. The pudding was considered to be a good tonic for the blood at a time of the year when food was in short supply.

FOLKLORE: Generally regarded as a plant of protection, an infusion of bistort sprinkled around your home will shield you and your family from evil spirits, witches and poltergeists.

Carrying a sprig or sachet of bistort would not only attract wealth but was also believed to be a powerful aid to conceiving a baby. It is a very welcome plant to give as a housewarming gift as it will ensure the safety and security of the new home.

Added to holy water, bistort has been used to banish earthbound spirits and is one of the herbs associated with exorcisms. Burning incense made from bistort and frankincense was believed to enhance psychic powers and aid divination.

FOLK MEDICINE: Culpeper used bistort for many ailments and recommends an infusion of bistort to *"wash any place bitten or stung by any venomous creature"*, or to *"wash any running sores or ulcers"*, and that *"the distilled water is very effectual to wash sores or cancers of the nose, or any other parts".* Of the root, *"taken in drink expelleth the venom of the plague, the small pox, measles, purples or any other infectious disease".*

A powder made from dried leaves was given to children to expel intestinal worms. Powdered root mixed into a paste with burnt allum, honey and pellitory of Spain inserted into any tooth cavities would ease the pain and stop infection from spreading. A gargle of the leaves and roots of bistort was believed to fix loose teeth, improve gum health of horses and people and ease sores in the mouth and throat.

Modern-day herbalists use bistort to treat digestive problems, ulcers, gum problems and piles, and as a laxative.

To be avoided during pregnancy and breastfeeding.

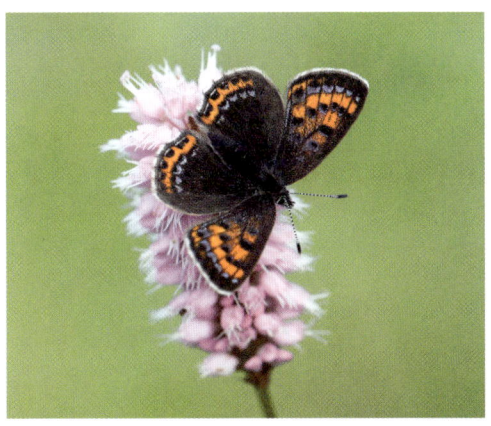

BLUEBELL

Alternative names: Nodding squill, wood bells, auld man's bells, dead man's bells, wild hyacinth

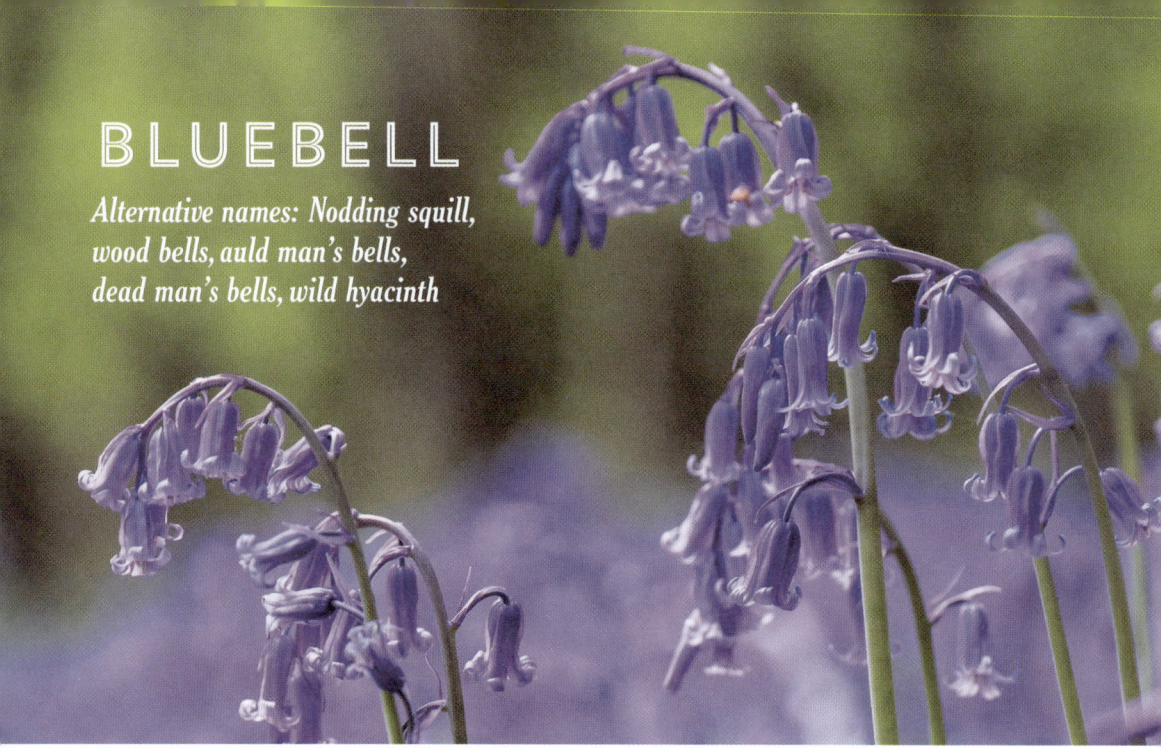

HOW TO IDENTIFY: The English bluebell is deep violet-blue in colour, has creamy white pollen and is bell-shaped with rolled-back tips. The flowers are almost always located on one side of the stem, causing them to droop over like a shepherd's crook. Sadly, in recent years, there has been an increase in the non-native Spanish bluebell, which has been imported to grow in domestic gardens. Spanish bluebells can cross pollinate with our native bluebells, diluting their purity. Spanish bluebells are paler, have much straighter stems and have little or no scent.

HISTORY: Bluebell woods have declined over the last century due to competition from other plants and the loss of suitable habitats; however, nearly 50 per cent of the world's bluebells can still be found in the UK. Because bluebells spread slowly, they're considered to be an indicator of ancient woodland sites.

During Victorian times, bluebell trains ran through the Chiltern Hills taking city-dwelling tourists on a wonderful journey to see the carpets of bluebells.

Apart from being a plant that delights us with its beauty, the sticky bluebell sap has been used by people in a variety of ways. Bronze Age hunters used bluebell sap to attach feathers to their arrows, bluebell bulbs were crushed to provide starch for the ruffs of Elizabethan and Victorian collars and sleeves, and sap was used to bind the spines of books as it is so toxic that it prevented insects from attacking the bindings.

FOLKLORE: Folklore tells us that a bluebell wood is an especially dangerous place for families as the faeries will use the bluebells to trap you and steal your children. At dawn the bells can be heard ringing to summon the faeries back from their slumbers in the woods, but if a human hears the bells, they will be visited by a malevolent faery and die soon after. Not surprisingly, it is considered bad luck to trample on bluebells as you will surely anger the faeries resting there.

Thankfully, not all the folklore about bluebells is quite so scary. Throughout the ages some have believed that by wearing a wreath made of the flowers, the wearer would be required to speak only the truth. Others thought that if you could turn one of the flowers inside out without tearing it, you would eventually win the heart of the one you love.

Placing a pouch of bluebells and mugwort under your pillow, meanwhile, was believed to prevent nightmares, while bluebells were planted on graves to give comfort to grieving relatives, since they represented rebirth. Finally, to dream of bluebells means that, unfortunately, you are married to a nagging spouse, but happily your relationship is also passionate.

Cunningham's *Encyclopedia of Magical Herbs* recommends that if you are in need of good fortune, place a bluebell in your shoe while saying:

> *"Bluebell, bluebell, bring me some luck before tomorrow night."*

FOLK MEDICINE: Herbalists would recommend bluebells to help prevent nightmares, and they were used as a remedy for leprosy, spider bites and tuberculosis.

However, beware: the bluebell is highly poisonous. In the UK, wild bluebells are protected by law with fines of up to £5,000 per bulb if you are caught digging them up.

Do not ingest any part of the plant.

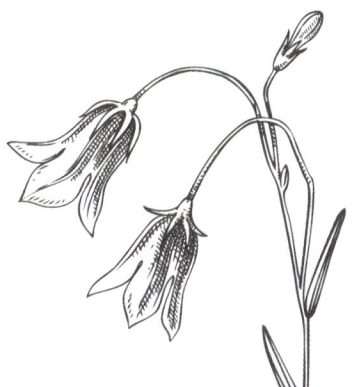

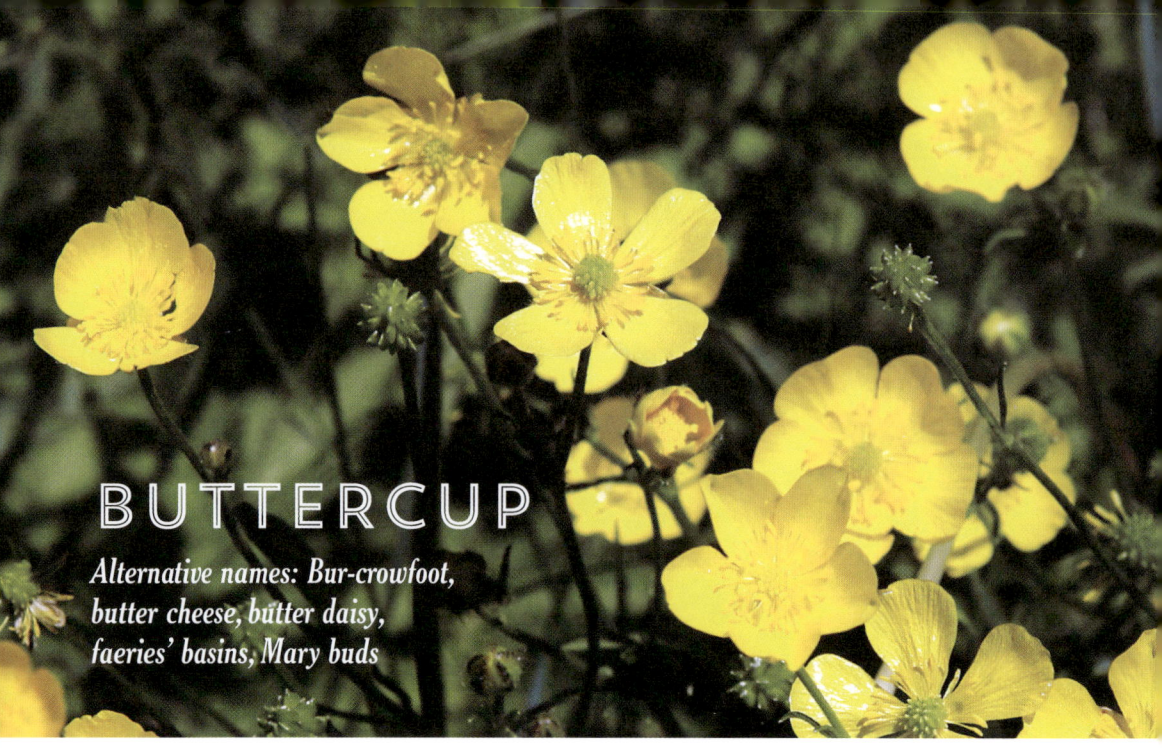

BUTTERCUP

Alternative names: Bur-crowfoot, butter cheese, butter daisy, faeries' basins, Mary buds

HOW TO IDENTIFY: Buttercups are easily identified with their bright yellow five-petalled glossy flowers. You will never see just one; they come in swathes that cover meadows, grasslands and woodland boundaries with their sunshiny brilliance from April to October. Meadow buttercups have rounded leaves divided into five or seven sections and can grow up to 1-m (3-ft) tall.

HISTORY: The first recorded mention of buttercups, or as he referred to them, *"crowfoot",* was in 1597 by Gerard.

There are over 1,700 species of buttercup, which even Culpeper considered too many to detail: *"Abundant are the sorts of this herb, and to describe them all would tire the patience of Socrates himself."*

FOLKLORE: If your chin turned yellow when a buttercup was placed underneath, it was a sure indication that you liked butter. The origins of this tradition, which survives to this day, seem to be the belief that cows ate buttercups thus giving butter its golden colour. However, in truth, cattle actively avoid eating the plant because of its bitter taste. Perhaps garlands of buttercups, placed around the necks of cattle at midsummer to bless the milk, gave butter its golden colour?

Buttercups were also known by the name of "crazies" in rural areas. In 1876 one countrywoman warned children to *"throw those nasty flowers away, for the smell will make you crazy!"* Conversely the Latin scholar Apuleius Platonicus recommended to *"hang the plant in a bag around the neck when the moon is on the wane, and you will be restored to sanity".*

Another story tells of an Irish miser who collected so much gold that his house was full. Walking across a meadow one day, with yet another sack of gold, he was approached by faeries who asked him if they could have just one gold coin to make a roof for the circular house they had been building. In return they promised him good luck forever. The miser shouted at the faeries and shooed them away. To teach him a lesson the faeries cut a hole in his sack of gold. As it tumbled out across the countryside it was transformed into buttercups, setting the whole meadow ablaze with golden flowers.

FOLK MEDICINE: The sap of the buttercup is caustic and causes painful blistering of the skin. This was used by beggars and wounded army veterans who would rub the sap into their sores to make them look worse, to gain sympathy and money from passersby.

Treated with caution, buttercups did have some medicinal uses. In Ireland, the plant was used to treat tuberculosis, mumps and heartburn as well as being combined with garlic to create an effective repellent for midges.

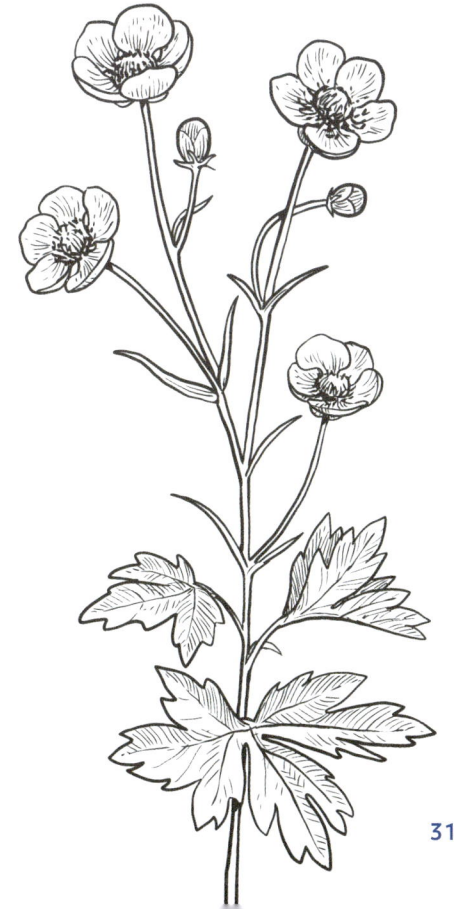

COLTSFOOT

Alternative names: Horse hoof, coughwort, sweep's brushes, son-before-father, baccy plant, yellow stars

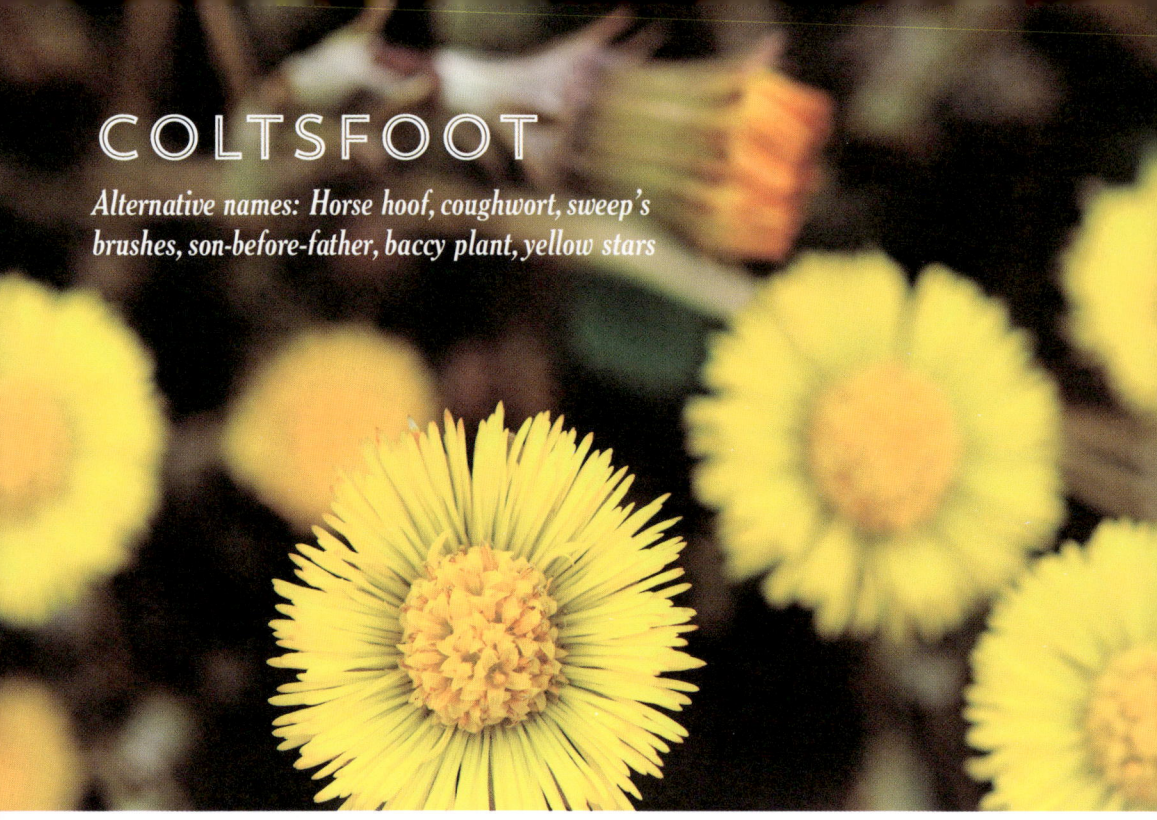

HOW TO IDENTIFY: This common creeping perennial can be found growing profusely on damp waste ground, roadside verges and around the edges of fields. With sunshine-yellow daisy-like flowers appearing as early as February, these colourful blooms could be mistaken for dandelions. However, coltsfoot is easily identified by its stalk that resembles overlapping scales and its distinctive hairy hoof-shaped leaves, which, unusually, appear after the flowering stems have gone.

HISTORY: Historically a coltsfoot flower was painted on the door of every eighteenth-century apothecary shop in Paris, indicating that this was the place to come if you needed to buy herbs and remedies.

It was also associated with coal: where coltsfoot grew in abundance, it was believed that coal would be discovered underneath the ground.

As for a different kind of rock, Stockley's confectioners in Lancashire have been making "coltsfoot rock" since 1918 for its reputed medicinal benefits. You can still buy it today.

Fast-forward to World War Two, and the smoking of dried coltsfoot was widely used as a tobacco substitute by European soldiers.

Goldfinches line their nests with the soft, hairy down of coltsfoot. Finally, it can be collected onto a cloth and used as tinder to help start a fire.

FOLKLORE: Coltsfoot has long been used for its magical properties to attract wealth and prosperity. Including it in talismans or charm bags will supposedly enable you to manifest material benefits or financial opportunities. It can also be incorporated into love spells to attract and nurture love in your life, strengthen relationships and reignite passion!

Peeling away the thin layer of soft tissue on a new leaf exposes a shiny mirror-like surface which, with the right charm, will reveal your future spouse to you.

FOLK MEDICINE: Coltsfoot has been used for many centuries to treat coughs, bronchitis, colds and other ailments affecting respiration. Wrapping a patient with a blanket soaked in coltsfoot solution was believed to cure whooping cough, while Cornish tin miners regularly smoked the dried leaves to protect themselves against lung diseases.

The "doctrine of signatures" was a medieval belief that each plant was put on this earth to heal man and that it resembled the part of the body that it could help, for example walnuts for brain health, tomatoes for heart health and so on. The leaves of the coltsfoot plant were said to resemble lungs and therefore could be used to help with any lung complaint such as coughing.

Culpeper wrote of coltsfoot, *"The fresh leaves, or juice, or a syrup made thereof, is good for a hot, dry cough, for wheezings and shortness of breath. The dry leaves are best for those that have the thin rheums [joint pain] and distillations upon their lungs, causing a cough, for which the dried leaves taken as tobacco or the root is very good."*

Traditionally used as a balm or poultice, coltsfoot was applied to the skin to ease inflammation and eczema.

Do not ingest any part of the plant.

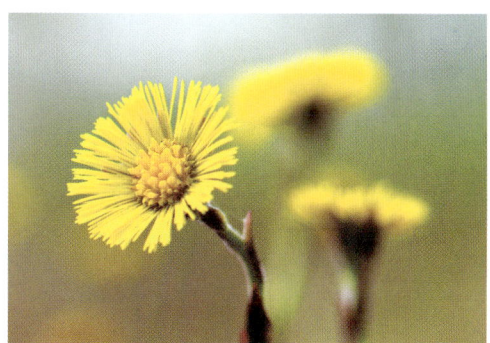

SOOTHING COLTSFOOT BALM

Coltsfoot is thought to encourage the growth of new skin cells, helping to push out toxins and fight free radical damage caused by pollution, ultraviolet radiation and pesticides. It has natural moisturizing, anti-inflammatory and antibacterial properties which can benefit acne-prone skin as well as containing silica to make the skin softer and improve elasticity. This balm can be used topically to soothe rashes, bites, scabs, sunburn, pimples and spots and as an everyday moisturizer. Lavender and tea tree essential oils are added to the recipe for their anti-inflammatory and antiseptic properties which can promote healing and calm damaged skin.

Always try to use organic ingredients where possible so that your skin can benefit from the maximum goodness of this wonderful plant.

Makes approx. 120 ml

INGREDIENTS

14 g natural beeswax (or 7 g of soy or candelilla wax for a vegan alternative)

28 g organic shea butter

28 g organic coconut oil

90 ml coltsfoot-infused carrier oil (see pages 20-21 for how to infuse oils)

5 drops lavender essential oil

5 drops tea tree essential oil

EQUIPMENT NEEDED

Heatproof bowl

Saucepan

Small jars or tins with lids (see page 22)

METHOD

Place a heatproof bowl over a pan of boiling water. Gently melt the beeswax, shea butter, coconut oil and coltsfoot-infused oil in the bowl.

Once melted, take off the heat and stir in the essential oils.

Pour into sterilized jars or tins and allow to cool completely before popping on the lids.

Keeps for about six months or longer if refrigerated.

Not recommended for anyone with a history of liver disease. Always do a patch test before using.

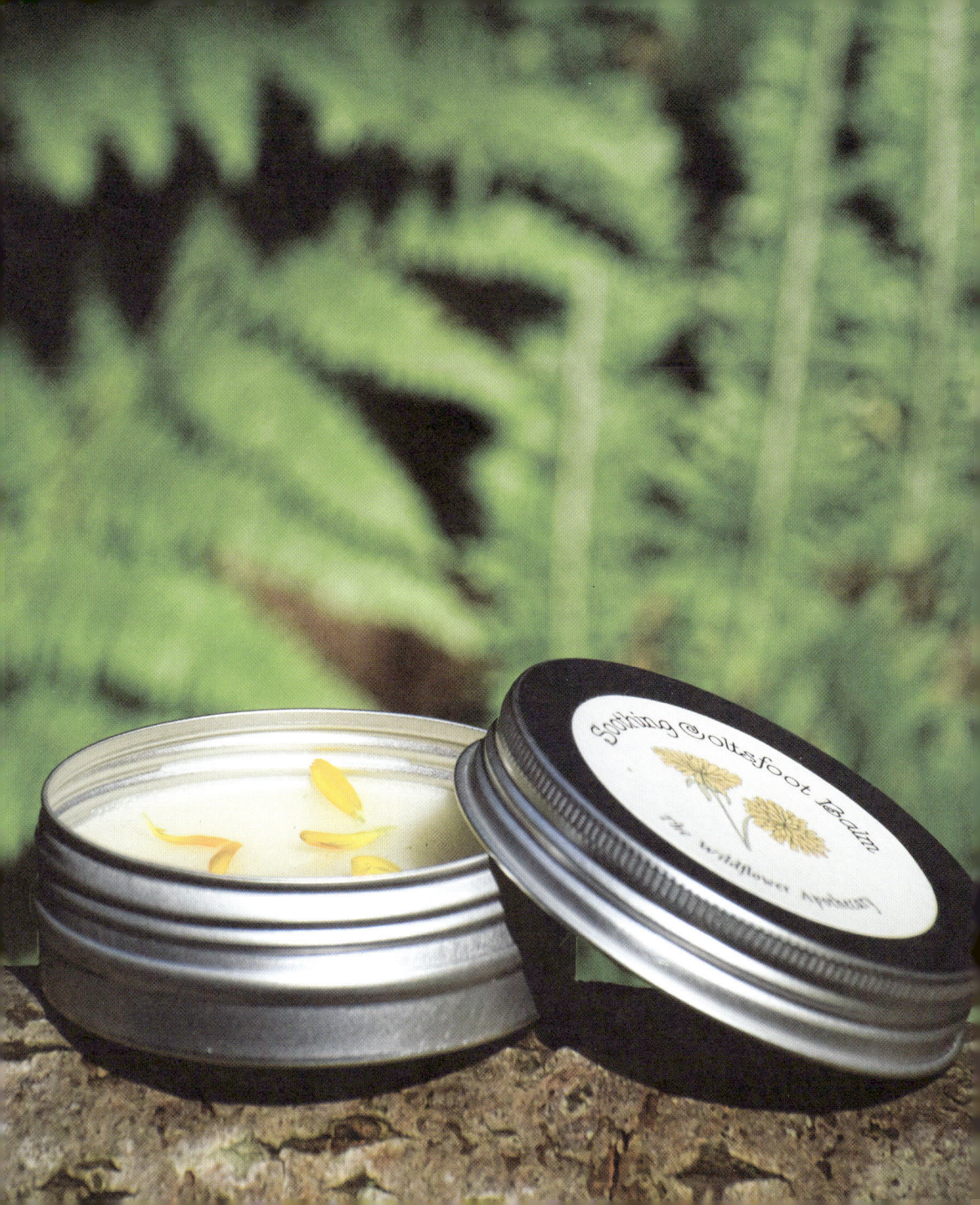

COMMON DODDER

Alternative names: Adder's cotton, devil's guts, faery hair, lady's laces, strangle-tare, witch's hair, angel's hair

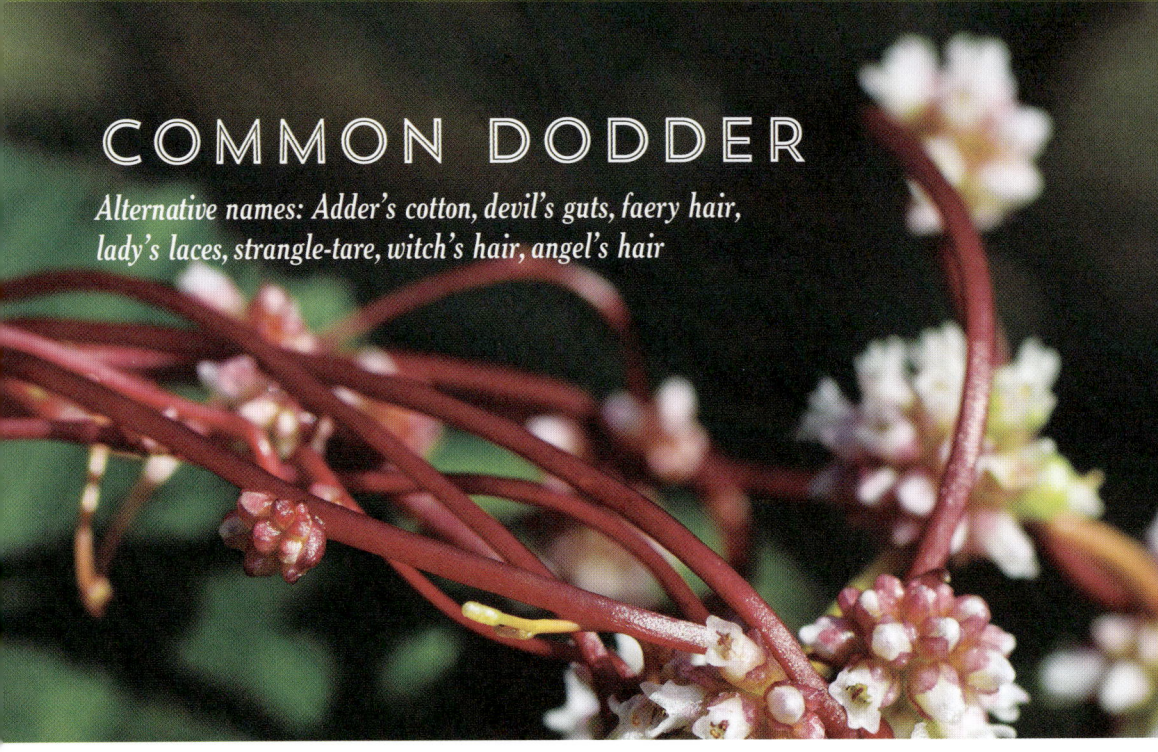

HOW TO IDENTIFY: A member of the bindweed family with small pink flowers, common dodder scrambles over the top of other plants like pink spaghetti. Dodder is a parasitic plant; it takes nutrients from its host plant by attaching itself with suckers while twisting itself anti-clockwise around its victim. You are most likely to spot dodder in flower on chalky downlands from July to September.

HISTORY: Common dodder posed a huge risk to crops by strangling agricultural land until the nineteenth century, when changes in farming practices meant the loss of its preferred habitat.

Improved methods of seed cleaning during the Industrial Revolution also minimized the accidental contamination by dodder seed into animal feed which would pass through cattle and be dispersed onto arable land.

Common dodder is now classified as "vulnerable" on the Great Britain Red List, meaning that it is considered scarce.

FOLKLORE: If you are lucky enough to see dodder under the light of the full moon you will see it glisten like "angel hair" or "faery hair" and understand immediately how it was given some of its wonderful common names.

In Jamaican folklore, dodder is known as the "love weed". If you are in love with someone who really doesn't like you, rub dodder all over your body but concentrate particularly on the back of your neck. The next time you see the object of your affections you should clap your hands then face your palms upwards while saying *"by Saint Peter, James and Paul"*, and they will instantly fall in love with you. Also in Jamaica, if you believe that you have been taken over by a bad spirit, some dodder mashed together with death-weed, laundry blue, asafoetida, salt and vinegar rubbed all over your body will protect you.

Dodder seems to particularly have been used in love divination. Doubting your partner's love? Pick some dodder and throw it over your shoulder back onto its host plant. If the dodder reattaches itself to its host, then your love is true. If not, then your partner hasn't been honest about their feelings.

In Christian mythology, clover is considered to be a plant that represents good. The devil, wanting to harm clover, created dodder to strangle it and remove it from the world.

FOLK MEDICINE: Gerard tells us that *"The nature of this herb changeth and altereth, according to the nature and quality of the herbs whereupon it groweth."* If found growing on thyme, dodder could *"taketh away old headaches, the falling sickness, madness that cometh of melancholy"*, whereas if it grew on flax it *"openeth the stoppings of the liver, the bladder, the gall, the milt, the kidneys and veins, and purgeth both by siege and urine choleric humours."*

If found growing on brambles, dodder was considered good for jaundice and fever, and on nettles it could aid the production of urine. What a clever and adaptable plant dodder is!

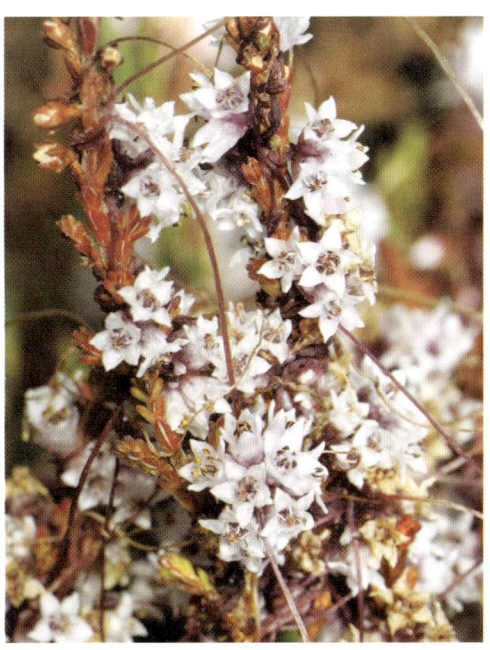

COMMON POPPY

Alternative names: Corn poppy, cock's comb, old woman's petticoat, wart flower, field poppy

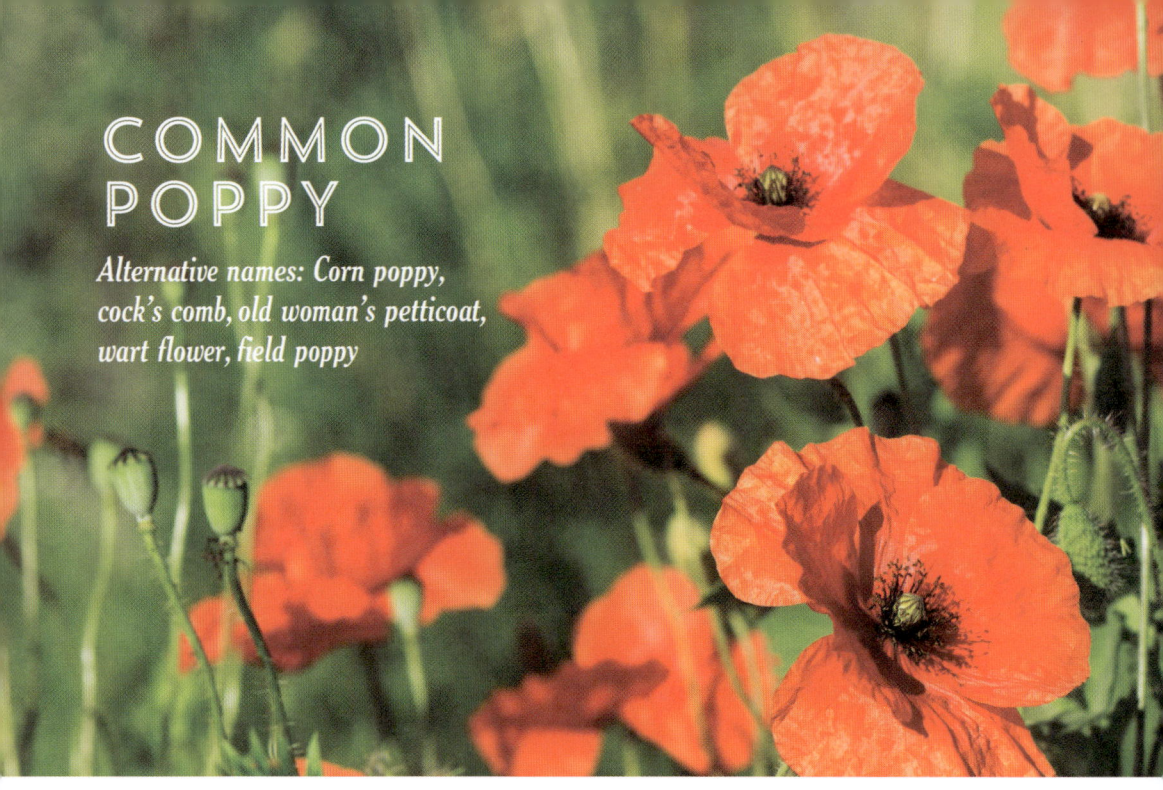

HOW TO IDENTIFY: Common poppies like to grow in land or fields that have been disturbed after a long period of neglect. Ploughing can bring seeds that have lain dormant for many years to the surface, allowing them to germinate. The paper-thin scarlet flowers appear between June and August sitting on top of tall, hairy stems.

HISTORY: The common corn poppy has become a very powerful symbol of Remembrance Day. Ground that was churned up on the battlefields of France disturbed the sleeping poppy seeds, enabling them to begin to bloom in abundance. The flowers were also seen growing on the graves of the fallen.

Inspired by the death of a friend on the battlefield, Canadian physician Lieutenant-Colonel John McCrae wrote his powerfully poignant poem "In Flanders Fields" during World War One.

"In Flanders Fields the poppies blow,
Between the crosses, row on row,
That mark our place; and in the sky,

*The larks still bravely singing, fly.
Scarce heard amid the guns below,
We are the dead. Short days ago
We lived, felt dawn, saw sunset glow,
Loved and were loved, and now we lie
In Flanders Fields."*

FOLKLORE: It seems that the poppy has always been associated with warnings of injury or harm. Pick or smell a poppy flower and you could quite possibly be struck by lightning, become blind or, rather worryingly, wake up covered in warts. Maybe these particular superstitions were concocted to stop children from trampling over precious cornfields where poppies once flourished. It was also considered bad luck to bring the flowers into your home since they would bring illness.

Despite the poppy's bleak historical associations, poppy petals could be used in the popular pastime of love divination. According to the Victorian language of flowers (see page 43), if you place a poppy petal in your left palm, strike it with your right palm and there is no sound, unfortunately there is no love either:

"By a prophetic poppy leaf, I found. Your changed affection, for it gave no sound, though in my hand struck hollow as it lay, but quickly withered, like your love, away."

To dream of your future partner, scatter poppy seeds behind you on St Andrew's Day (30 November). For fertility, wear a necklace of poppy seed heads – be careful though, because poppy seeds placed in the shoes of a new bride will render her infertile.

And if you are unfortunate enough to be chased by a demon, poppy seeds thrown in its path will distract it long enough for you to escape, as demons feel compelled to count things. The seeds are also recommended for keeping vampires away.

FOLK MEDICINE: Athletes in ancient Greece drank a concoction of wine, honey and poppy seeds to improve their health and give them strength. The petals and seeds are known to have mild sedative properties and were used to good effect by both land army girls and exhausted mothers during World War Two.

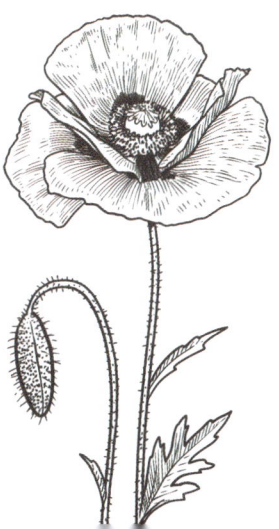

POPPY SEED AND LEMON CAKE

I'm not going to tell you that eating cake has health benefits, but this is a delicious recipe to share with friends and will certainly give you some feel-good energy that comes from pleasant company and eating cake.

Poppy seeds are a good source of protein, fibre, magnesium, calcium, iron and zinc, and they also support bone health. Lemon, as well as tasting great, is a source of vitamin C and antioxidants.

Serves one to 12 (depending on if you plan to share!)

INGREDIENTS

200 g caster sugar

200 g butter

3 free-range eggs, beaten

Zest of 2 unwaxed lemons

Splash of milk

200 g plain flour (gluten-free works well)

100 g ground almonds

2 tsp baking powder

½ tsp salt

3 level tbsp poppy seeds, plus 1 tsp for the topping

Juice of 2 lemons

1 tbsp granulated sugar

EQUIPMENT NEEDED

Scales

Mixing bowl

Citrus juicer

Zester/fine grater

Electric whisk (or wooden spoon)

A 23-cm round loose-bottomed cake tin, buttered and lined with greaseproof paper

Spatula

Skewer

METHOD

Preheat the oven to 180°C (350°F).

Using an electric whisk, beat together the sugar and butter until light and fluffy.

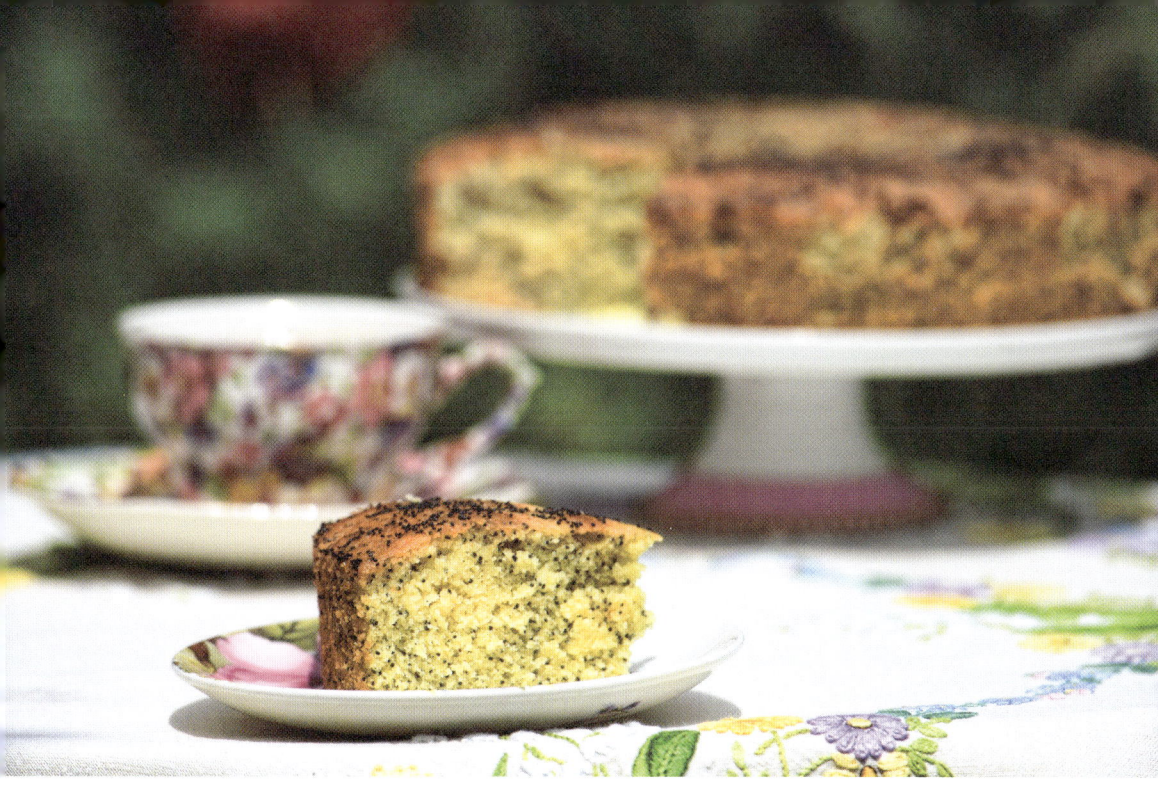

Beat in the eggs a little at a time, add the lemon zest and milk and combine.

Add the flour, ground almonds, baking powder, salt and poppy seeds and mix carefully using a spatula.

Lastly add the juice of one lemon and stir.

Pour into your prepared tin and level the top.

Bake for 40–45 minutes or until the cake is golden brown and a skewer inserted into the middle comes out clean.

Mix the remaining lemon juice with the granulated sugar and a teaspoon of poppy seeds. Pour over the top of the cake while it is still warm.

Allow to cool.

Enjoy!

Contains nuts.

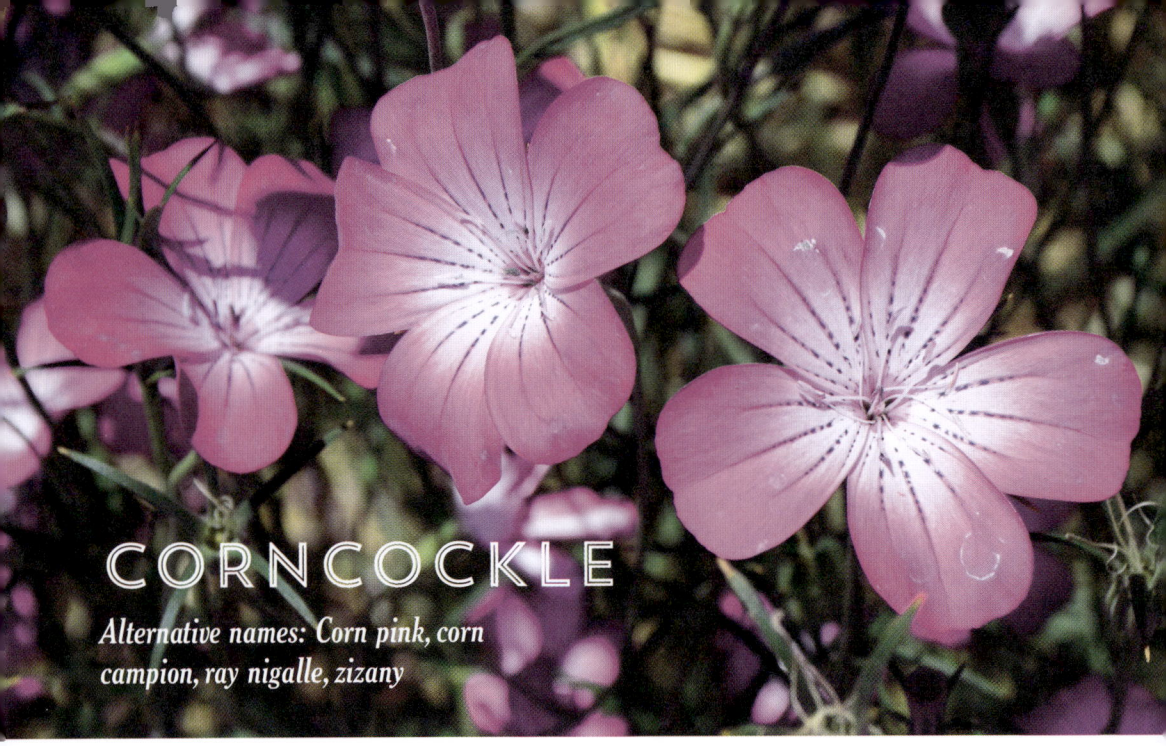

CORNCOCKLE

Alternative names: Corn pink, corn campion, ray nigalle, zizany

HOW TO IDENTIFY: This lovely summer flowering annual can reach 1 m (3 ft) tall and is topped with striking trumpet-shaped purple-pink flowers on single stems. Leaves are soft, long and hairy and spaced out along the tall stem. Corncockles flower from June to August and grow best in full sun on well-drained soil in field margins, waste ground and disturbed soil.

HISTORY: It is believed that corncockle seeds were first brought to Europe by unsuspecting Iron Age farmers some 2,400 years ago as a contaminant hidden in grain. This caused a huge problem as corncockle seeds are toxic and were being harvested alongside corn and rye to be made into bread. Loaves contaminated with corncockle seeds would taste bitter and consuming it could cause headaches, nausea, delirium, convulsions and even death.

Eating corncockle-contaminated bread was common until farming methods improved in the nineteenth century. Agricultural machines like the threshing griddle improved the purity of the seed as well as modern weed-killing techniques, leading to the rapid decline of the corncockle.

FOLKLORE: In Victorian times it was popular for suitors in Britain and America to send bouquets of flowers to communicate messages, in a fashion known as floriography or the language of flowers. Corncockles are listed to denote gentility, charm and daintiness.

Every plant had a hidden meaning and this method of communicating your feelings became so popular that a floral dictionary was needed just to decode the message contained within. How you carried or wore a certain flower could also denote a different meaning, changing it from a compliment to an insult. Greetings cards and picture postcards could be sent with these popular messages. This custom only died out after the outbreak of World War One in 1914, when it became unfashionable and insensitive against the backdrop of so many lives tragically lost.

FOLK MEDICINE: In the twelfth century a group of herbalists called the Physicians of Myddfai lived and worked in a small village in Carmarthenshire, Wales (see page 11). They concocted their own remedy for pneumonia:

"Let a medicine be prepared, by digesting the following herbs in wheat ale or red wine: madder, sharp dock, anise, agrimony, daisy, round birthwort, meadow sweet, yellow goat's beard, heath, water avens, woodruff, crake berry, the corn cockle, caraway, and such other herbs as will seem good to the physician." Quite a list!

John Gerard recommended to *"giveth the seed parched and beaten to a powder to be drunk against yellow jaundice"*. He gave a stark warning about the dangers of ingesting the seed in bread: *"Some ignorant people have used the seed hereof [...] what hurt it doth among the corn, the spoil unto the bread as well in colour, taste and unwholesomeness..."*

Historically, corncockles have been used to treat constipation, abscesses, tumours, warts and oedema (fluid retention), as a diuretic (to increase urination), an expectorant (to promote coughing) and to rid the body of parasitic worms.

Do not ingest any part of the plant.

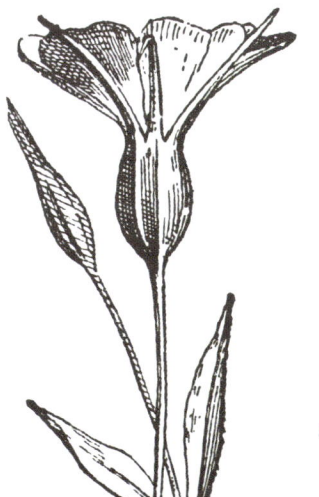

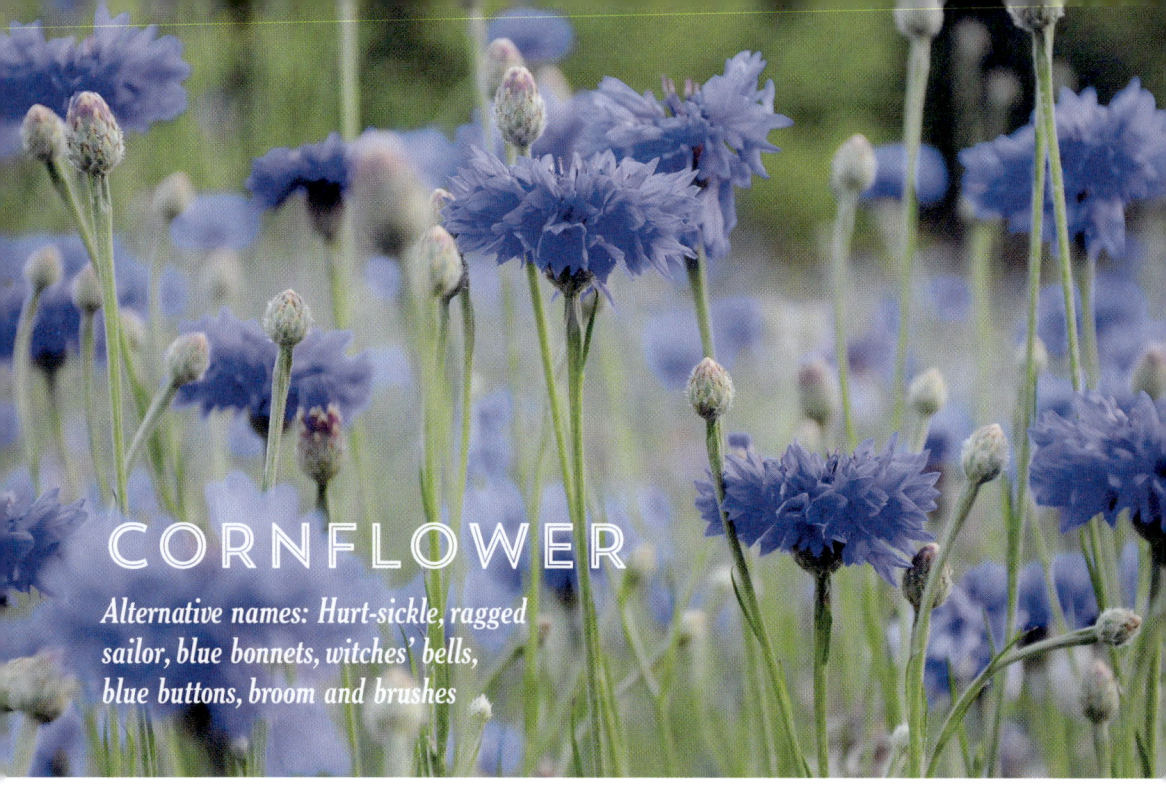

CORNFLOWER

Alternative names: Hurt-sickle, ragged sailor, blue bonnets, witches' bells, blue buttons, broom and brushes

HOW TO IDENTIFY: A member of the daisy family, the cornflower is recognized by its striking blue colour and star-like petals. Its stems and leaves are long and pointy and it grows to approximately 0.8 m (2½ ft) tall. Cornflowers can be seen in bloom from late June to early autumn, until the first frost.

HISTORY: Floral collars were worn by the ancient Egyptians who believed they represented new life and fertility. Cornflowers, olive leaves and poppies were found in terracotta storage jars in the tomb of Tutankhamun and, amazingly, were still identifiable after 3,000 years.

Considered to be a nuisance growing among the corn in arable fields in Europe, sadly cornflowers were almost completely wiped out in the 1970s by the overuse of agricultural pesticides. Thankfully they have since been rescued from obscurity by becoming a firm cottage garden favourite.

In France, cornflowers are worn for remembrance on Armistice Day in much the same way as poppies are worn in the UK.

FOLKLORE: Cornflowers are used in folk magic for fertility and abundance, placed by doors and in cupboards to prevent negative energy from entering and worn as a charm to attract love. Rolling in a field full of cornflowers was believed to attract youth, happiness, beauty and suitors. Young men wore cornflowers when they were in love. Unfortunately, if their love was not reciprocated, the beautiful blue colour would gradually fade away.

Victorian spinsters wore cornflowers on their clothing to indicate that they were single and looking for love, which gave the flowers the nickname "bachelor's buttons". However, if a spinster hid a cornflower underneath her apron, any man that she desired could be hers.

In other lore, people covered their eyes with cornflowers in the belief that their sight would be strengthened, with the added benefit that the flowers could enable them to see faeries. Finally, the flower would be burned by the Celts while saying a prayer of protection if a storm was known to be imminent.

FOLK MEDICINE: Cornflowers were reputed to stop a nosebleed, but only if picked on Corpus Christi Sunday (the first Sunday 60 days after Easter).

Historically they were used as a remedy for fever, plagues and poison. Culpeper advises:

> *"The powder or dried leaves of the cornflower is given with good success to those that are bruised by a fall, or have a broken vein inwardly [...] The seed or leaves taken in wine is very good against the plague, and all infectious diseases [...] The juice dropped in the eyes takes away the heat and inflammation in them."*

Eau de Casse Lunettes was a popular French eyewash made from cornflower petals to combat infection and cataracts. Apparently, it was particularly effective on blue eyes. A distillation of petals was also believed to soothe tired eyes.

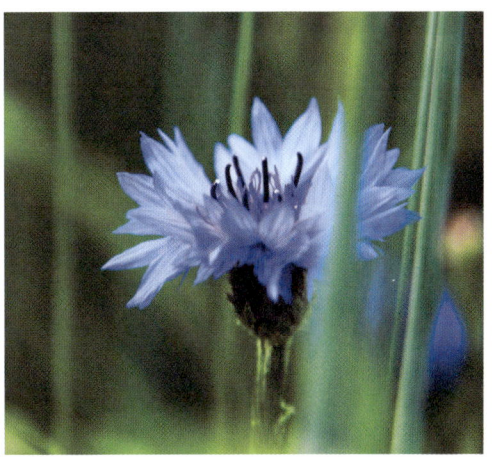

WILDFLOWER-SEED BALLS

This is a super activity to do with children, who will love creating their very own flower patch to attract wildlife. Although it is illegal to pick or uproot wildflowers in the UK, you are allowed to gather a small number of seeds for your own use. Seed balls are only for use in your garden as it is important not to introduce varieties into the countryside that don't naturally belong, since they may cause damage to wildlife.

If you can't find all the seeds that you would like, there are many native wildflower mixes readily available to buy.

Makes approx. six to eight balls

YOU WILL NEED

Native wildflower or garden seeds, such as cornflower, bird's foot trefoil, knapweed, red clover, lady's bedstraw and any other seeds that you find in your garden

100 g peat-free compost

20 g plain flour

Water

METHOD

Pour your seeds onto a shallow plate.

In a bowl, mix together the compost and flour with enough water to make a sticky dough.

Shape the compost mixture into tacky balls and squeeze it between your fingers to help it stick together.

Roll the balls around in your seeds until they are completely covered and leave to dry for a day or two.

TIPS

Scatter your seedballs in a sunny spot in spring or autumn. Try to make sure that they fall on bare earth.

Keep watered if the weather is dry.

These will grow just as well in a pot on a patio.

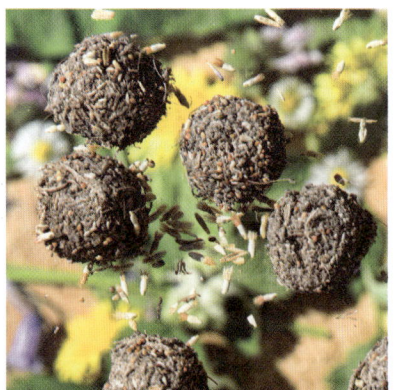

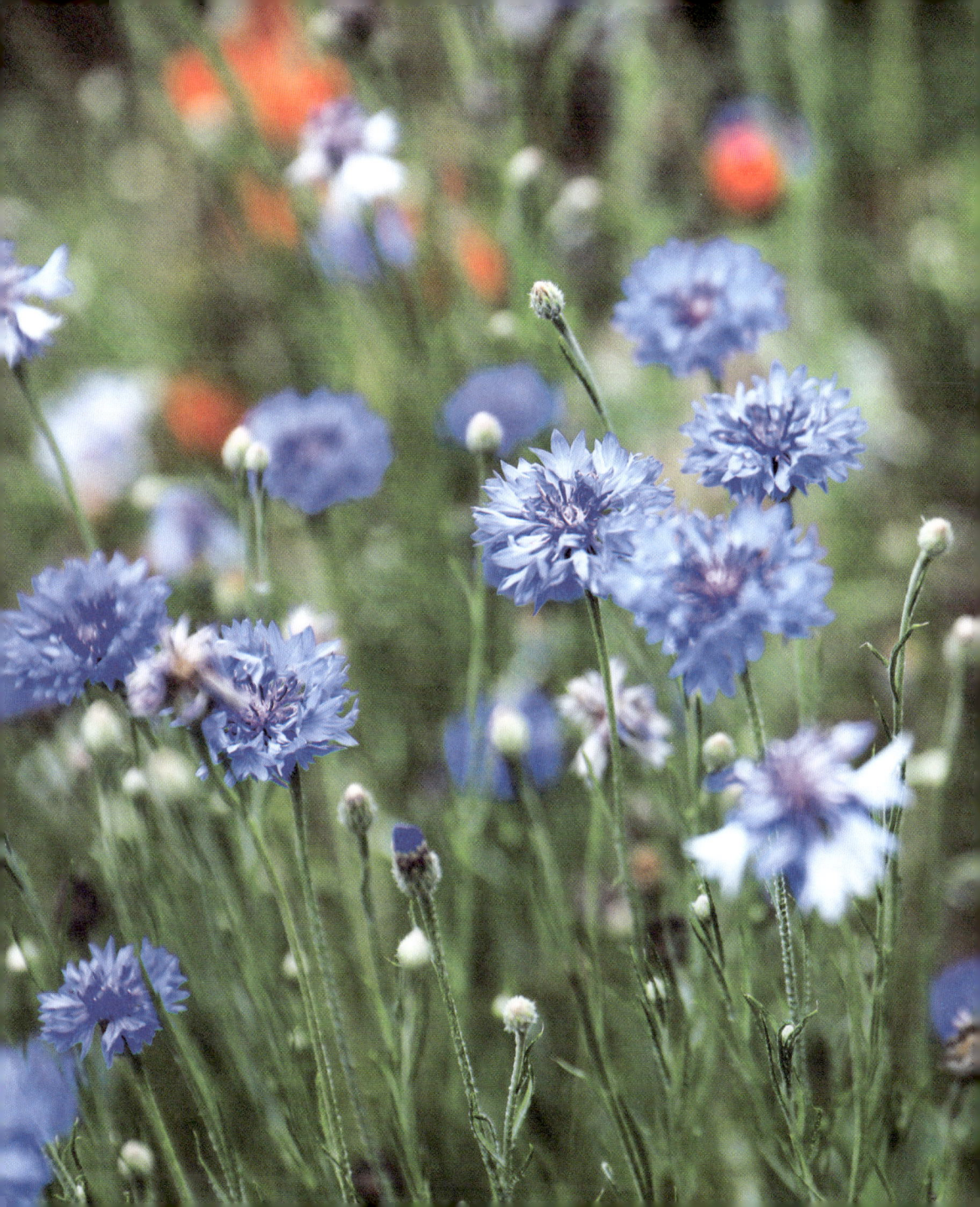

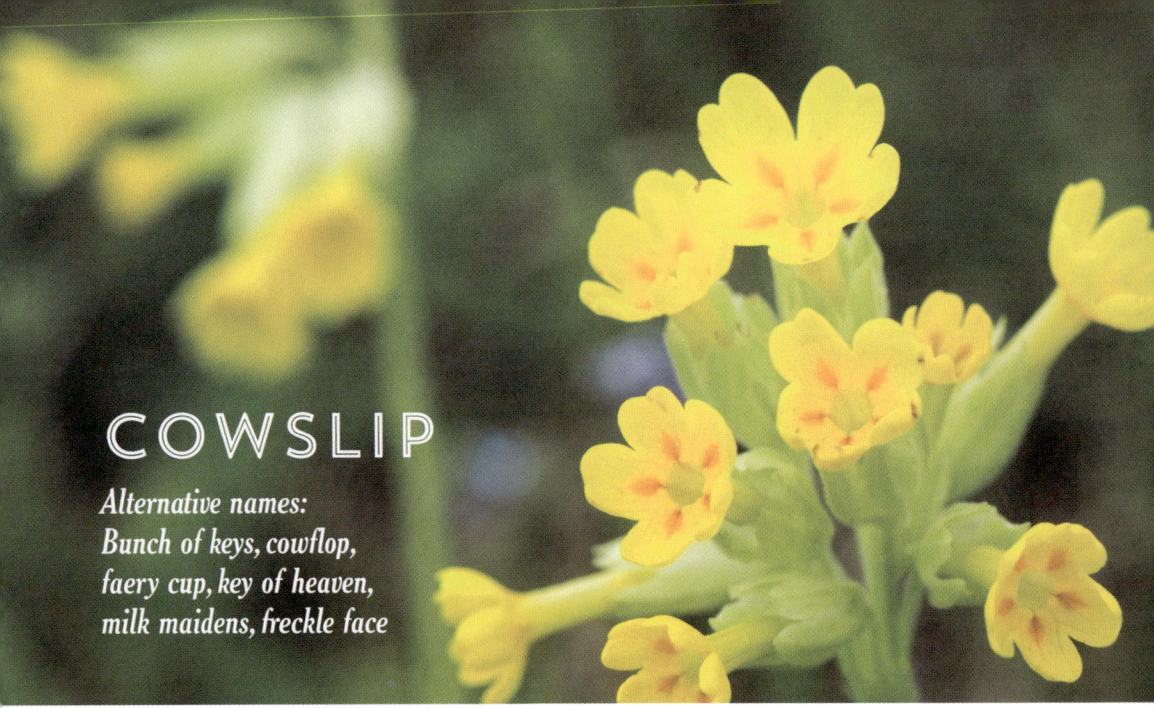

COWSLIP

Alternative names:
Bunch of keys, cowflop,
faery cup, key of heaven,
milk maidens, freckle face

HOW TO IDENTIFY: Cowslip leaves create a dark green wrinkled rosette close to the ground. Tube-like lemon flowers each with five peachy-coloured dots appear in clusters at the end of upright green stems from April to May.

Once a common sight in our hedgerows and meadows, cowslips have sadly now become rare due to continual loss of suitable habitats and the use of pesticides. For the best chance to locate some cowslips look in woodlands and grasslands, preferably where the soil is chalky.

Cowslips must have been prolific in the seventeenth century, for Culpeper dismisses them as *"so well known, that I will neither trouble myself or the reader with a description of them."*

HISTORY: Early Brits noticed that cowslips tended to grow in and among where a cow had "slupped" and cowslip is believed to have meant "cowpat".

Meanwhile, cowslip wine was regularly brewed by country people, although you would need to forage a "peck" of flowers which equates to just over 9 litres in volume.

Cowslips even get a mention in *A Midsummer Night's Dream:*

*"The cowslips tall her pensioners be;
In their gold coats spots you see;
Those be rubies, fairy favours;
In those freckles live their savours.
I must go seek some dewdrops here,
And hang a pearl in every cowslip's ear."*

FOLKLORE: Up until the beginning of the twentieth century, young country girls would craft "tissty-tossties", or balls of cowslips, to determine their future husbands. In her 1908 book, *Children and Gardens*, garden designer Gertrude Jekyll documented how they were made:

"You prepare the flowers by cutting the stalks just under the heads, and stretch a bit of very fine string by tying it to the backs of two chairs [...] Then you take the prepared flowers one by one and make them ride along the string, heads downwards. When there are as many on the string as you think will be enough to make a ball, you press them up together as they will go, bring up the two ends and tie them."

Anyone else confused? These balls would be tossed in the air while reciting names or occupations of potential suitors. As the last flower fell from the ball, your future partner would be revealed.

Other lore included washing your face with milk infused with cowslips to draw your beloved closer to you. Conversely, placing a cowslip under your doormat would deter visitors. Lastly, cowslips planted upside down on Good Friday were predicted to produce red flowers.

FOLK MEDICINE: Culpeper's answer to ageing was to make an ointment from cowslip flowers since it *"taketh away spots and wrinkles of the skin, sun-burning, and freckles, and adds beauty exceedingly"*.

He also praised the virtues of cowslip root as it could *"ease the pain in the back and bladder, and open the passage of urine"*.

Cowslip wine was taken as a mild treatment for insomnia, headaches and forgetfulness, while eating the flowers was believed to support brain health.

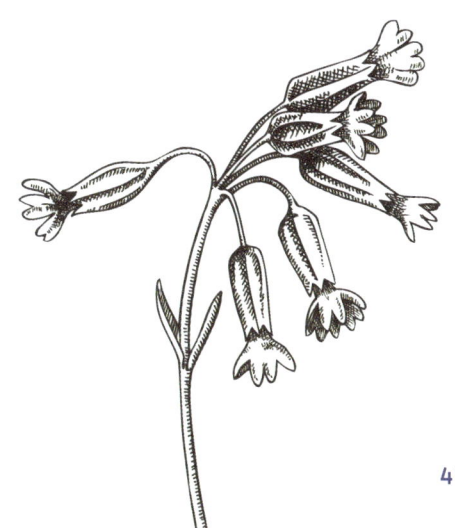

DANDELION

Alternative names: Clock flower, mess-a-bed, tiddle bed, old man's clock, shepherd's clock, time teller

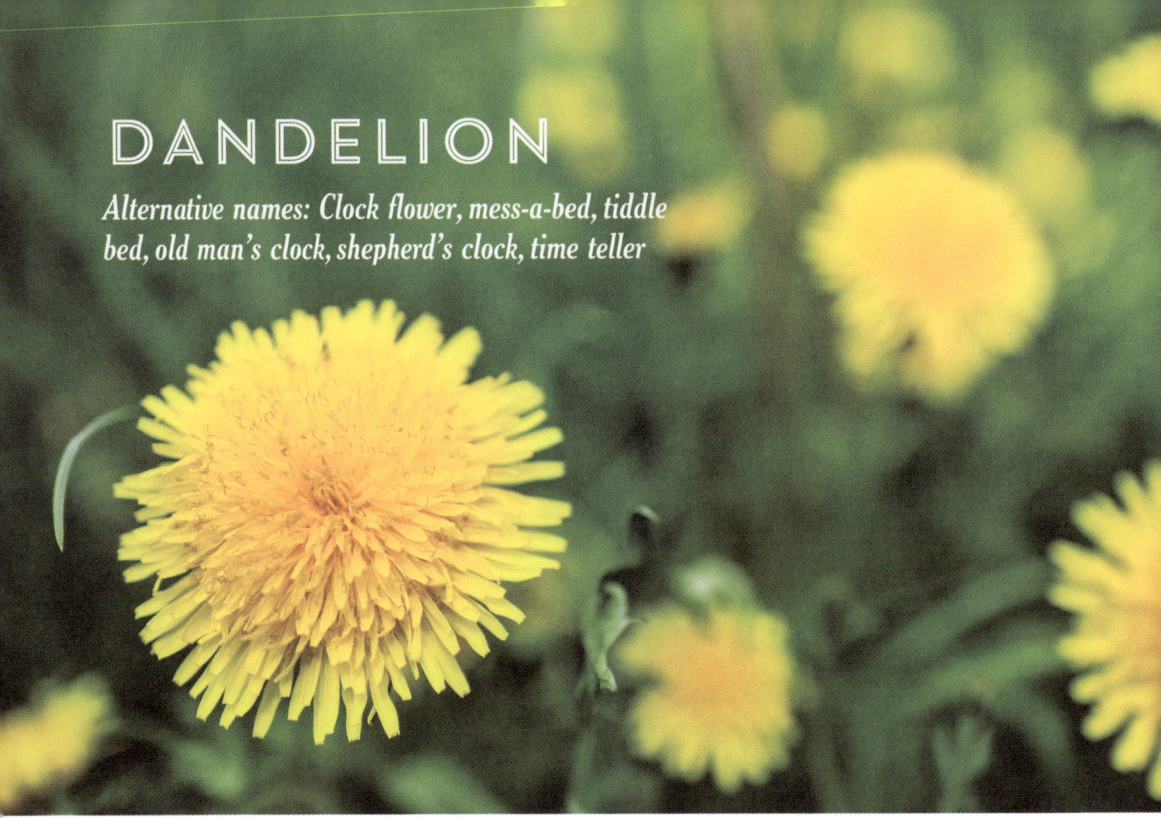

HOW TO IDENTIFY: Dandelions are probably the most familiar of our native wildflowers as you can see them growing practically everywhere. The beautiful golden yellow flowers shine like little suns early in spring, before turning into fluffy dandelion clocks later in the season.

The leaves are very distinctive with "lion's tooth" edges – the word dandelion originates from the French *dent-de-lion*. The stem is smooth and hollow and will ooze a milky sap once broken open.

HISTORY: Dandelions are regarded as a nuisance nowadays by many keen gardeners, but not so long ago it was possible to make a decent living from digging up the roots for use in herbal medicine. As recently as the 1930s, teams of "root diggers" would benefit local farmers by ridding their fields of dandelions. These roots were so sought-after for their medicinal properties that a special "green herb" rate was charged for sending them to London by train. A root digger could earn as much as 3 d (3 pence) per pound (454 g) in weight for washed roots and 1 d per pound in weight for unwashed roots.

Dandelion roots were also dried and ground coarsely to be used as a coffee substitute during World War Two.

FOLKLORE: The childhood joy of gently blowing the seeds off a dandelion head not only helps you to tell the time, but also reveals how much you are loved. Blow off all the seeds in one go and you are loved with a passion; however, if some seeds remain, unfortunately your partner has some doubts. If lots of seeds remain it might be best to look elsewhere for love. Blow the seeds in the direction of an absent lover to send a message to them.

To give yourself the best chance with all these superstitions, I recommend that you choose a sunny day and a dry, ripe seed head.

If all that wasn't enough, the dandelion globe can indicate the weather too. In fine sunny weather, the globe is round and fluffy; if rain is on its way, the globe shuts like an umbrella until the risk of rain has passed.

FOLK MEDICINE: An important and commonly used spring tonic, dandelion was regarded as a very powerful cure for many ailments including jaundice and kidney complaints. So effective were dandelion's diuretic properties that children were warned not to touch or pick it as they would most certainly wet the bed that night.

According to Culpeper, *"it openeth the passages of the urine in both young and old"* and is *"very effectual for obstructions of the liver, gall or spleen".*

The Physicians of Myddfai, meanwhile, recommended dandelion for the treatment of intermittent fevers: *"Take dandelion and fumitory, infused in water, the first thing in the morning."*

Topically, the plant was also used to treat warts. The milky sap from the stem was rubbed onto warts and allowed to dry; this was repeated until the wart had shrivelled away.

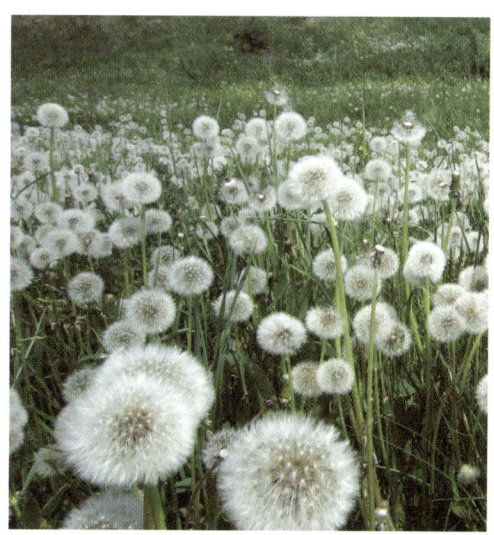

DANDELION-FLOWER VINEGAR

Like most herb vinegars, this one is very easy to make using ingredients that you probably already have in your kitchen. The bitterness of dandelion makes it a great herb to help digestion, detox the liver and calm an upset stomach. Vinegar is high in antioxidants and can be especially beneficial to your health if you use organic apple cider vinegar with all its marvellous properties.

Be sure to collect your dandelion flowers on a dry day away from roadsides, pesticides and pet waste. I like to collect mine from my own garden.

Makes 500 ml

INGREDIENTS

Enough dandelion flowers to loosely fill a 500-ml jar – if you have the patience, remove all the petals for use and compost the green calyx as this can be bitter

Approx. 500 ml organic apple cider vinegar or white wine vinegar

EQUIPMENT NEEDED

500 ml glass jar with lid

METHOD

Cover the dandelions in the jar with vinegar.

Pop on the lid.

Leave in a cool place to infuse for at least a fortnight or as long as six weeks. The longer it infuses, the more effective it will be.

Give it an occasional stir.

Strain out the flowers and the vinegar is ready to use.

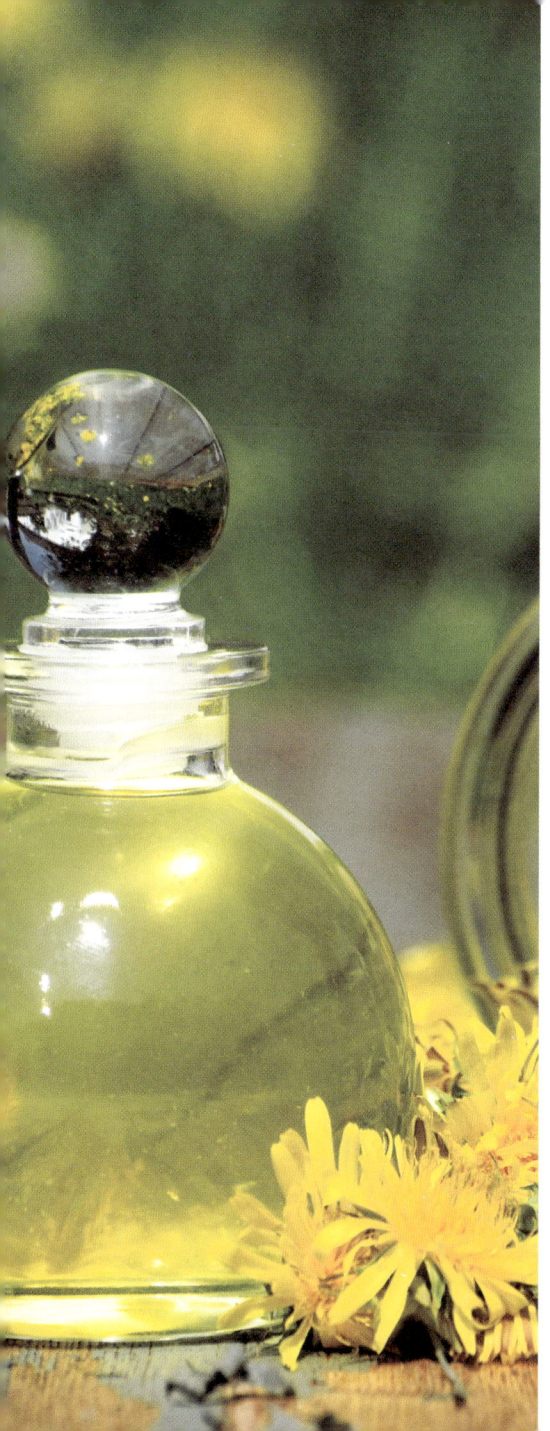

HOW TO USE

French dressing: Put 2 tbsp dandelion-flower vinegar, 6 tbsp olive oil, ¼ clove finely minced garlic and 1 tsp Dijon mustard into a jam jar, pop on a lid and shake well.

Marinade for vegetables, meat or fish: Combine together 3 tbsp dandelion-flower vinegar, 6 tbsp olive oil, 2 cloves finely chopped garlic, 1 tsp freshly ground black pepper and a small bunch of chopped herbs of your choice. Stir through your meat or vegetables and allow to sit for at least an hour.

Forager's salad: There are plenty of edible leaves and flowers to forage for your wild salad such as young dandelion leaves, garlic mustard, chickweed and wood sorrel, but make sure you know that what you're picking is safe to eat. Dress with dandelion-flower vinegar dressing.

Other uses: Dilute your dandelion vinegar 1:1 with water as a rinse for your hair to make it super shiny. Remember to rinse it off with water afterwards.

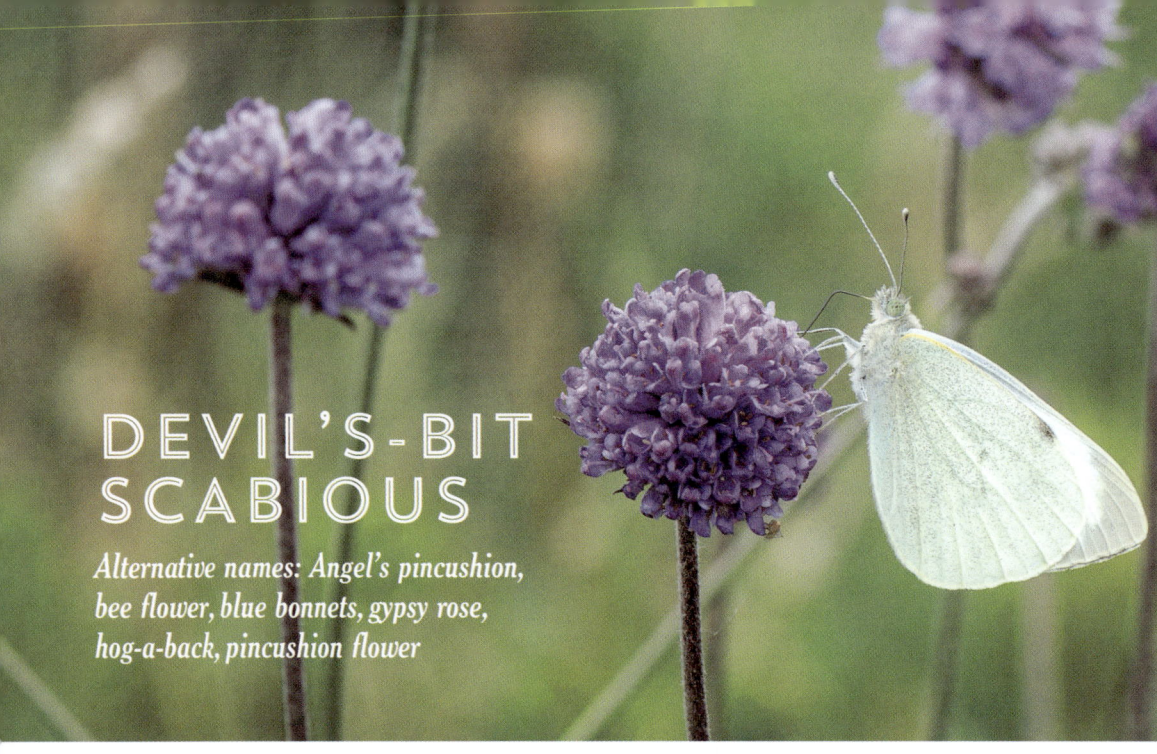

DEVIL'S-BIT SCABIOUS

Alternative names: Angel's pincushion, bee flower, blue bonnets, gypsy rose, hog-a-back, pincushion flower

HOW TO IDENTIFY: Found in damp meadows, field edges and marshes from July to October, devil's-bit scabious has a single pale purple or sometimes pink pincushion-like flower on the end of a tall stalk. Its leaves are long and oval, becoming broader towards the middle, and it can grow up to 1 m (3 ft) tall.

HISTORY: The plant's common name relates to its short, black root. Folklore tells us this was bitten off in the Garden of Eden by the devil, who was angry that the plant could cure man of ailments that he had worked so hard to create. Thankfully he did not succeed in destroying the plant, but we are cautioned not to touch the stumpy roots as they are contaminated by the devil's breath.

Another version of the story relates that a young Dutch girl sold her soul to the devil in exchange for him curing her dying father. Local villagers considered her to be a saint for being so selfless. This infuriated the devil, who retaliated by making her blind. To prevent the villagers from using the plant to cure her, he bit off a large piece of the root, leaving just a stump in its place.

Throughout history, the flowers have been much-valued by pollinators. Devil's-bit scabious is the larvae food plant for the very rare marsh fritillary butterfly and the narrow-bordered bee hawk moth, both of which have priority conservation status.

FOLKLORE: On the Hebridean island of Colonsay, children would twist the root of the devil's-bit and then let it go. If the root moved on its own, the person holding it possessed magical powers. An ancient Celtic spell to summon faery folk consisted of chanting an incantation while holding the plant, which in Scotland was known as a *"curl-doddy"*:

> *"Curl-doddy do my biddin*
> *Soop my house and hool*
> *my midden [toilet]."*

The faery folk would then carry out any domestic chores that you wished.

A piece of the plant worn around the neck was believed to offer protection from witches and evil spirits; however, beware picking devil's-bit if you live in Cornwall – the devil will appear at your bedside!

FOLK MEDICINE: Culpeper discovered that the plant had many uses:

> *"The root (all that the devil hath left of it) boiled in wine and drunk was very powerful against the plague and all pestilential diseases and fevers and poison and bites of venomous creatures […] the root powdered and taken in drink expels worms […] very effectual as a gargle for swollen throat and tonsils."*

The last part of its name derives from the Latin word *scabere* meaning "scratch", indicating that it was valuable in soothing many skin conditions such as eczema, dandruff, bruises and even the sores caused by the bubonic plague.

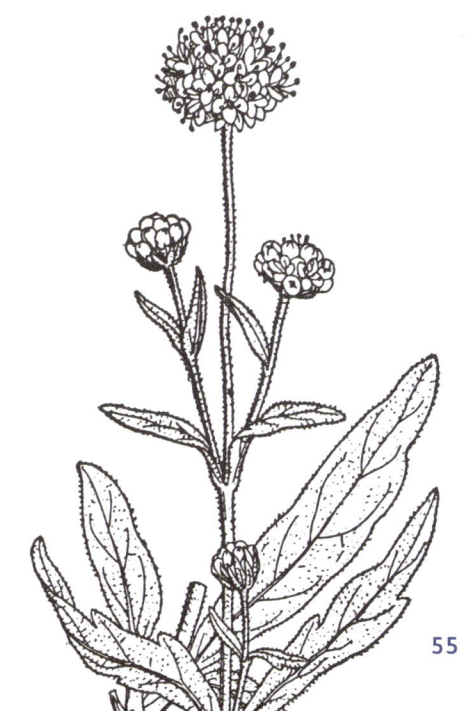

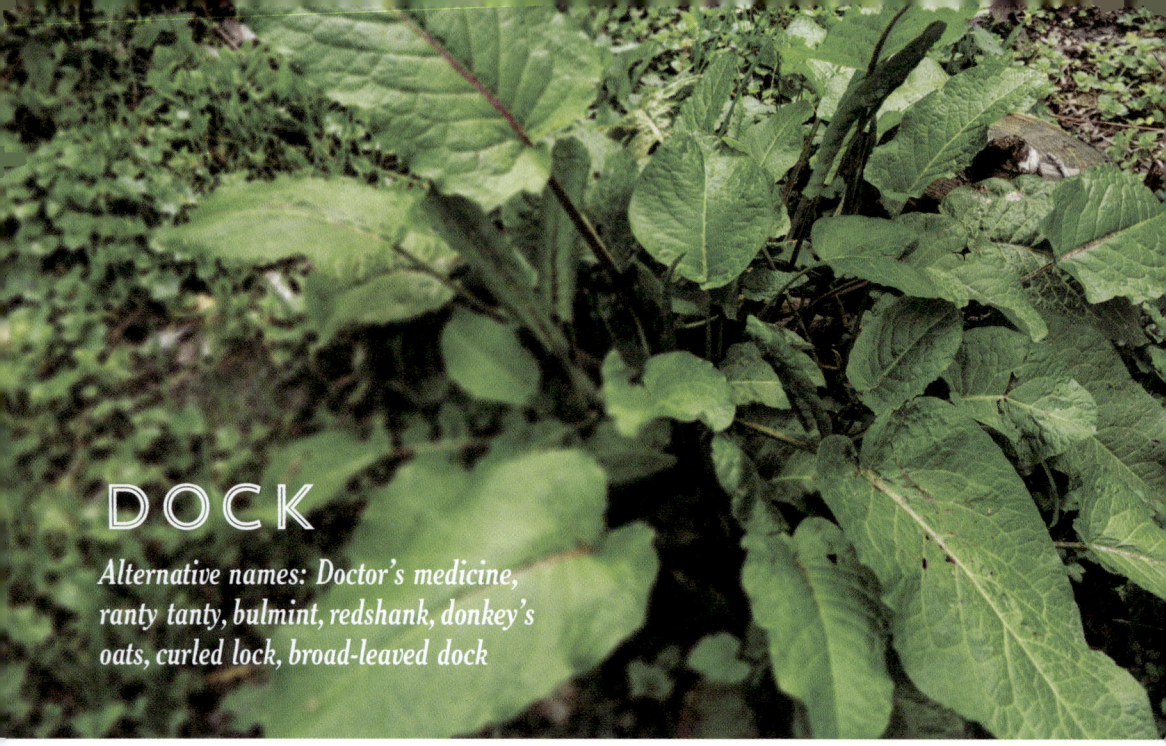

DOCK

Alternative names: Doctor's medicine, ranty tanty, bulmint, redshank, donkey's oats, curled lock, broad-leaved dock

HOW TO IDENTIFY: This vigorous and widespread perennial has large, oval leaves with slightly wavy edges growing in a rosette formation. New leaves appear in the spring followed by clusters of reddish-brown flowers on a tall stem from June to September. Dock can be found growing in gardens, fields and hedgerows. Seeds can lie dormant in the soil for up to 50 years and will germinate if the soil is disturbed, much to the annoyance of gardeners.

HISTORY: Dock was of much value to early Brits. When times were hard and food was scarce, dock leaves were a nutritious addition to the traditional pottage (a thick soup or stew made with whatever was available).

Cattle farmers allowed their herds to feed on dock leaves as the tannins present helped to prevent bloat, a disease involving a build-up of gas that can be life-threatening for cows.

Due to the size, strength and pliable quality of the leaves, farmers' wives would wrap their precious homemade cheese and butter in them to keep the produce cool on the way to market. Similarly, pouches of tobacco were lined with dock leaves to prevent the contents from drying out too much.

FOLKLORE: To attract personal wealth, put dock seeds into a charm bag with two gold coins and carry it with you. Sprinkling the seeds around your business or washing the floors, doors and windows with dock tea will surely bring in more customers.

Burning an entire dock plant is said to help you move on after a relationship, but for best results you must scatter the burnt ashes at a crossroads at the time of a new moon.

FOLK MEDICINE: If you've ever rubbed nettle stings with a dock leaf to ease the pain then you are repeating something that humans have done for hundreds of years. This custom was widespread as long ago as the ninth century, when it was recommended as a remedy in *The Anglo-Saxon Chronicles*.

In his poem "Troilus and Criseyde", the fourteenth-century chronicler Geoffrey Chaucer quotes a snippet of an old charm that was recited while rubbing a dock leaf on a nettle sting: *"Netle in, dokke out."*

In Cornwall, the charm went, *"Dock leaf, dock leaf, you go in; sting nettle, sting nettle, you come out."*

For a very different purpose, to aid women wishing to become pregnant, seventeenth-century botanist William Coles wrote in his book *The Art of Simpling* that *"The seeds of docke tyed to thye left arme of a woman doe help barrennesse."*

A hugely versatile plant, the roots were also prized. Dock roots were boiled and the liquid used to ease dermatitis, relieve the itchiness of insect bites, scalds and blisters, and drunk to purify the blood and cure boils.

Documenting its many applications, Culpeper writes that dock *"cleanseth the blood and strengthens the liver. The seed [...] is helpful for those that do spit blood [...] The roots boiled in vinegar helpeth the itch, scabs and breaking out of the skin."*

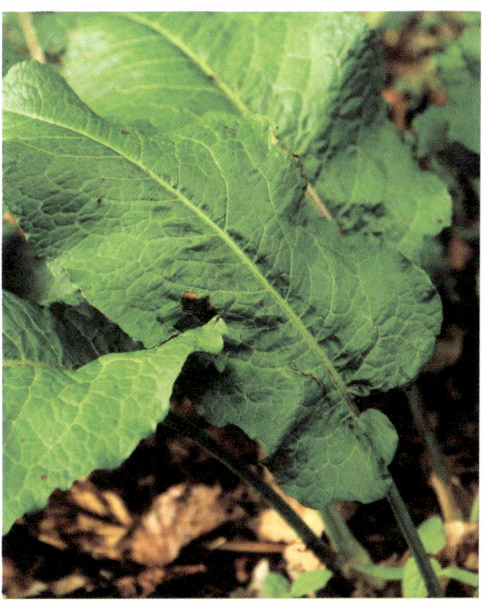

DOCK ROOT UPSET TUMMY TEA

Dock is classified as a "bitter herb" – bitters stimulate the production of saliva, bile and digestive enzymes which help to absorb and digest the food we eat. The occasional use of dock root upset tummy tea can help to ease the symptoms of acid reflux, indigestion and constipation and soothe the digestive tract without upsetting the natural balance of gut bacteria.

The addition of dandelion root can help to flush toxins and aid digestion; fennel seeds are known to reduce bloating and gas; while orange zest keeps your digestive system running smoothly as well as adding flavour.

It is illegal in the UK to dig up roots from the wild without the landowner's permission, however dock is so widespread you will easily be able to find it in your own or a neighbour's garden. Failing that, dried dock root and all other ingredients are widely available online.

Roots are best dug up in the autumn when the plant is dormant. Avoid areas that have been sprayed with pesticides or frequented by dog walkers.

Makes two to three cups

INGREDIENTS

4 tbsp dock root, peeled, washed and freshly grated (or 2 tbsp dried)

2 tbsp dandelion root, peeled, washed and freshly grated (or 1 tbsp dried)

½ tsp fennel seeds

Zest of ½ organic orange

Raw honey or maple syrup to taste

METHOD

Place all the ingredients, apart from the honey or maple syrup, into a teapot.

Pour over 500 ml of boiling water.

Allow to steep for 10–15 minutes.

Sweeten with honey or maple syrup to taste.

Dock root is not recommended for prolonged use.

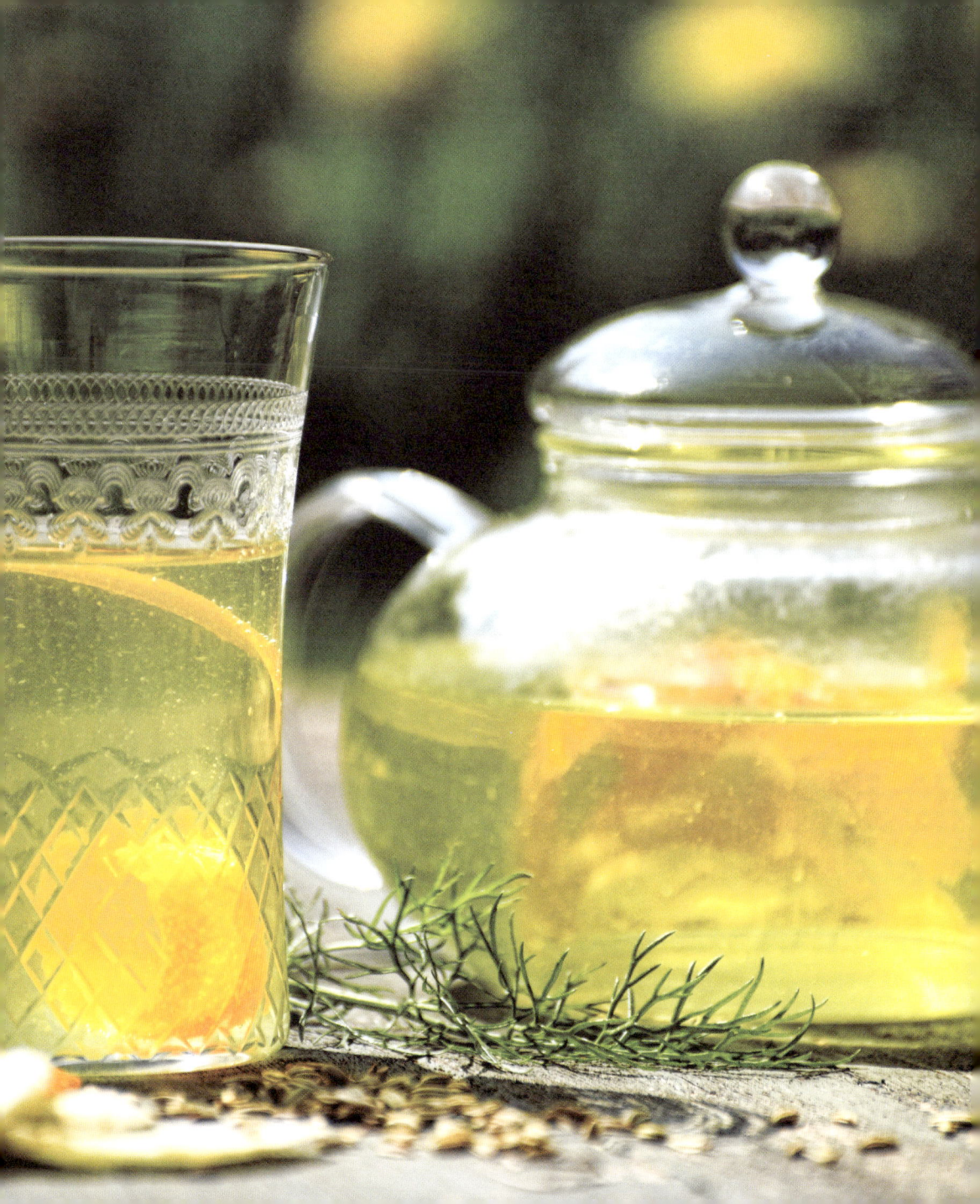

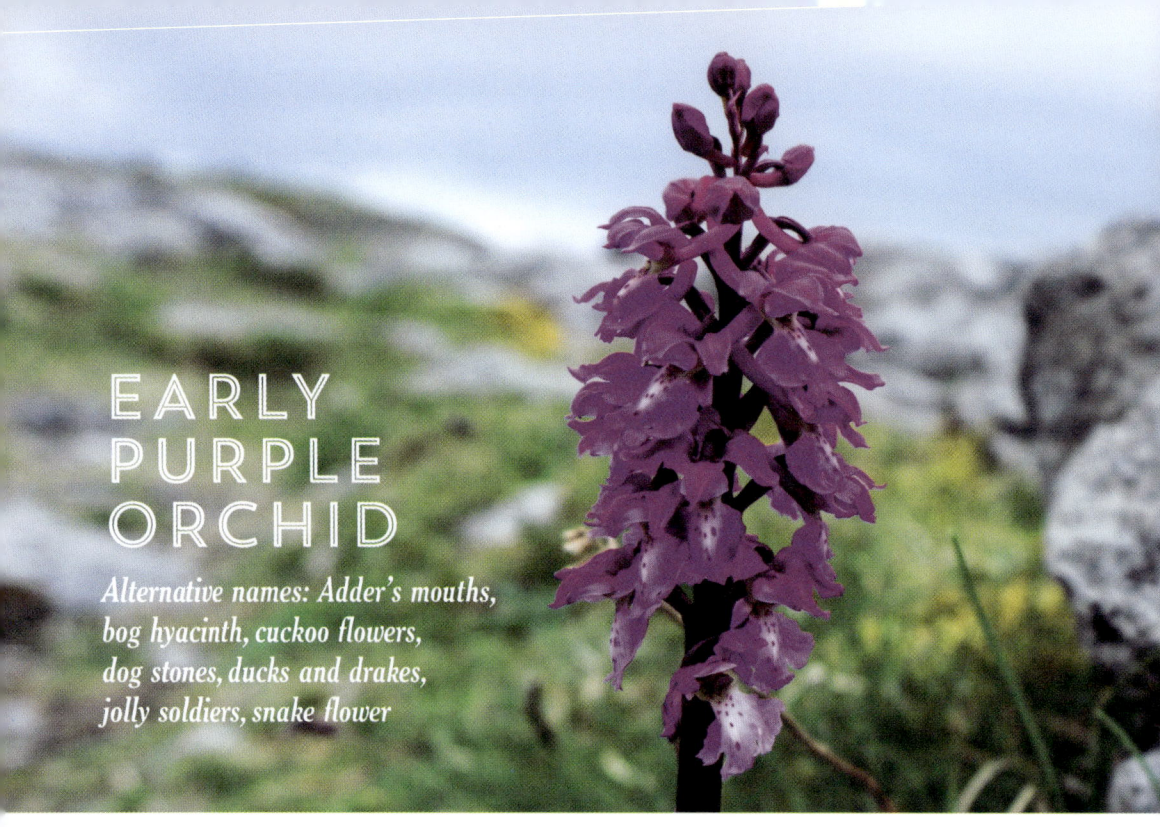

EARLY PURPLE ORCHID

Alternative names: Adder's mouths, bog hyacinth, cuckoo flowers, dog stones, ducks and drakes, jolly soldiers, snake flower

HOW TO IDENTIFY: Early purple orchids are often one of the first orchids to appear in spring. You may be able to spot them in non-acidic soil from April to June flowering in woodlands, grasslands and hedgerows and dotted in and among the bluebells. The tall flower spike can grow up to 60 cm (2 ft) and is covered in pinkish-purple flowers arranged in a dense cone-shaped cluster. Leaves, which appear from January onwards, are glossy and green with dark spots.

HISTORY: In the seventeenth and eighteenth centuries, saloop (or salep), made from dried orchid tubers, was a popular drink in English coffee houses. Tea and coffee were very expensive at this time and saloop was a nutritious and cheaper alternative for the working poor.

An eighteenth-century recipe written by Nathan Bailey tells us how to make saloop:

"Put an ounce of saloop or salep into a quart of water; set it on the fire, stirring

it till it is as thick as chocolate, and then put to it orange-flower water, rose-water or sack; or you may add a little juice of lemon and sugar. This is good for weak and consumptive people."

Captain Cook was believed to have taken saloop on voyages with him as a cheap, nourishing breakfast to help sailors who became ill while at sea.

By the nineteenth century, tea and coffee had become much more affordable and it seems that saloop went out of fashion mainly because it was considered to be a beverage for the "lower classes".

FOLKLORE: Early purple orchid is also known as "Gethsemane" (the biblical garden of Jesus's betrayal) as it was believed that the plant grew at the foot of the cross where Christ's blood dripped onto it, causing the distinctive dark spots on the leaves.

Early purple orchids have two orb-shaped tubers of different sizes under the ground thought to resemble male testicles, which led to them being used in love charms, aphrodisiacs and aids to conception. If the man wished to have a male child, he would eat the larger of the two tubers; if a female child was desired, the woman should eat the smaller tuber. A talisman containing the tuber was sure to attract love, while placing it under your pillow ensured that you would dream of your future spouse.

FOLK MEDICINE: In the medieval period doctors and apothecaries often treated their patients in accordance with "the doctrine of signatures" – the theory that a plant bears a physical resemblance to the part of the body that it cures. It follows then that orchid tubers were favoured to treat infertility problems in men.

As well as recommending the use of the tubers as an aphrodisiac, Culpeper tells us that *"they are held to kill worms in children; as also, being bruised and applied to the place, to heal the King's evil [a type of tuberculosis]."*

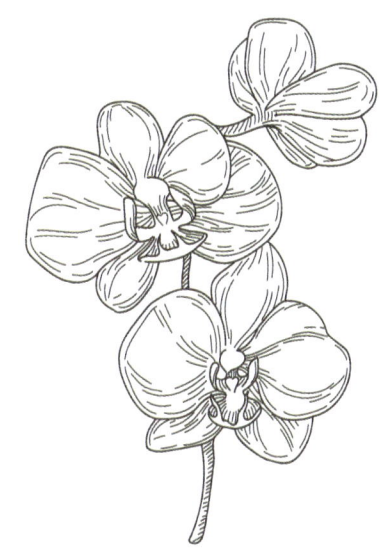

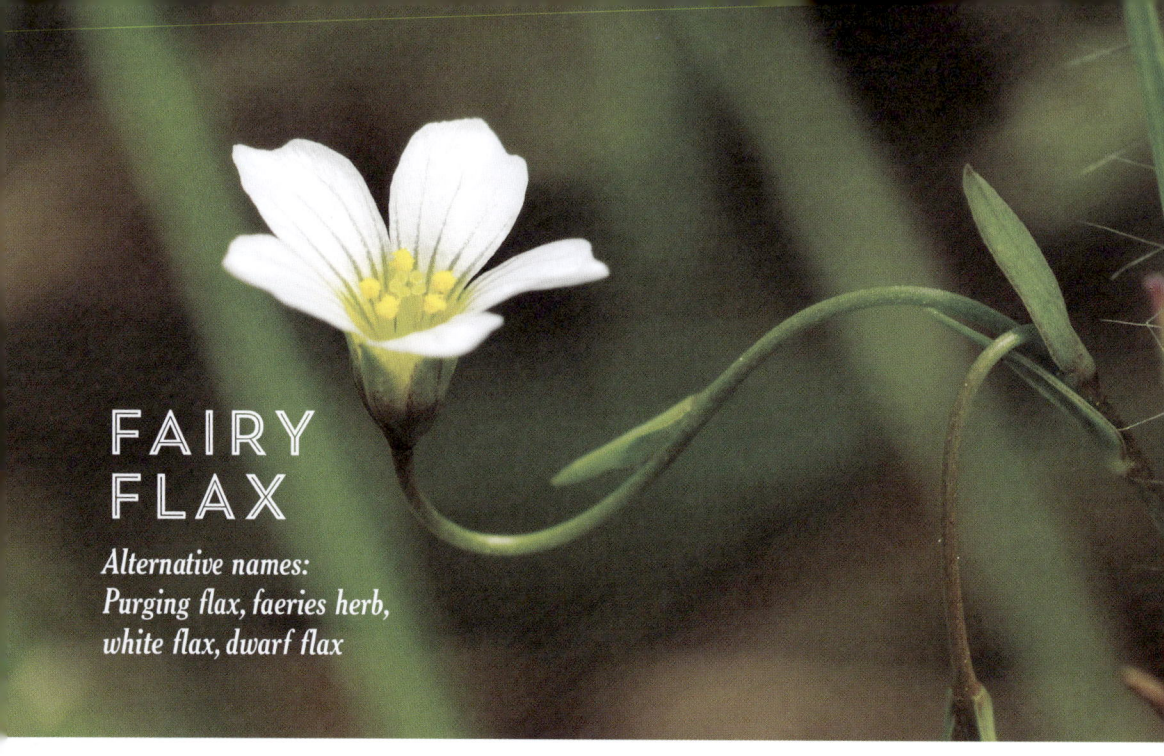

FAIRY FLAX

Alternative names:
Purging flax, faeries herb,
white flax, dwarf flax

HOW TO IDENTIFY: Flowering between May and September, fairy flax can be found in meadows, grassland and wasteland all over the UK. This small, scraggly plant can often get lost among other more dominant vegetation – its tiny white flowers struggle to be seen on the end of thin, wiry stems. What they lack in size, however, the star-like five-petalled blooms more than make up for in pretty daintiness.

HISTORY: Fairy flax fibres are much finer and softer than traditional flax and have been used all over northern Europe for centuries to weave into delicate soft textiles.

The plant also produces a natural rich blue dye, the use of which declined in favour of indigo as a huge amount of plant material was needed to make the dye and it became unsustainable.

Fairy flax is an important host for several species of butterfly larvae including one of the rarest and most endangered in the UK, the wood white butterfly, whose numbers have declined by over 80 per cent in the last 50 years.

FOLKLORE: As the name suggests, fairy flax was very much associated with the world of the fae. According to Irish folk tales, faeries adored the delicately fine fabric that could be woven from strands of fairy flax and were believed to fashion it into their teeny tiny clothing.

The flowers were believed to harbour magical powers: if you picked them, you would surely bring bad luck and misfortune upon yourself. Contrarily, wearing a garland woven out of the flowers was believed to bring good luck – but surely you had to pick them first?

FOLK MEDICINE: Much written about in Celtic literature, fairy flax was believed to be invaluable when a mother was struggling to deliver her baby. A folk tale written in the 1900s by Mary MacMillan of Uist in the Outer Hebrides relates that a hunter's wife was struggling with labour *"though the smooth fairy flax was under her foot".*

A little further south in Barra, we are told of a more successful outcome of using fairy flax on the feet: *"The child came into the world without toil or trouble to its mother."*

With a Latin name of *Linum catharticum* that translates as "flax purging", fairy flax was long used as a purging herb to treat constipation and as an emetic. However, it needed to be used with caution as too much could cause fatal poisoning.

Maud Grieve had recommendations when using fairy flax: *"As a laxative it is preferred to senna, though the action is very similar. It is generally taken combined with a carmative herb, such as peppermint."*

She continues: *"The dried herb has been found very useful in muscular rheumatism and catarrhal affections, the infusion of 1 oz in a pint of boiling water being taken in wineglassful doses. In liver complaints and jaundice, it has been employed with benefit."*

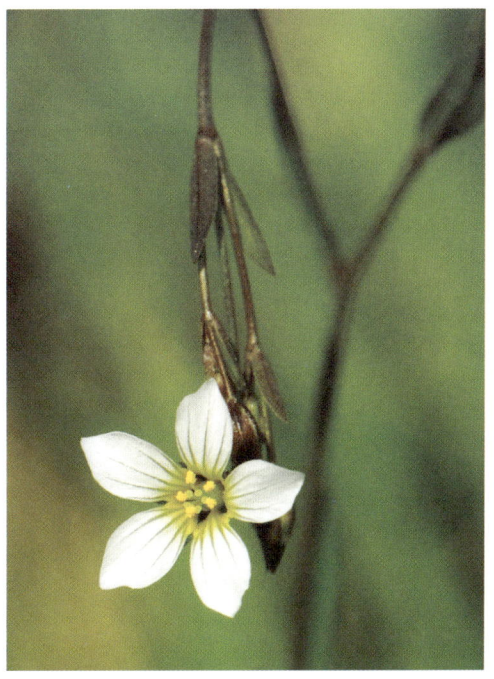

FENNEL

*Alternative names:
Spingel, sweet fennel,
wild fennel, finkle*

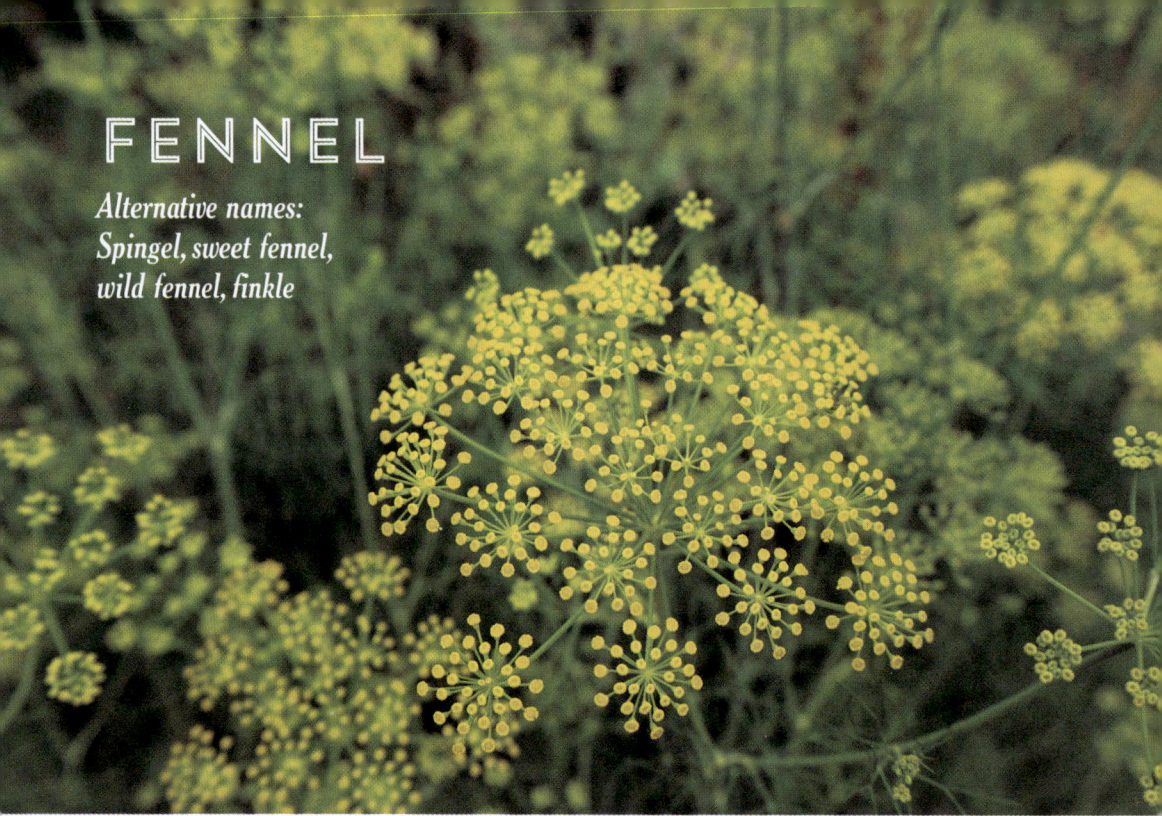

HOW TO IDENTIFY: Fennel is a tall and elegant member of the carrot family with very fine, feathery leaves, yellow umbel flowers and small, elongated seeds with a distinctive scent of aniseed. Wild fennel prefers a sunny location with well-drained soil and can be found in fields and meadows from spring to early autumn. Wild fennel differs from the cultivated variety of Florence fennel with which we are familiar; the bulb of the wild fennel is inedible but you can eat the fronds, pollen and seed.

HISTORY: Wild fennel was introduced to the UK by the Romans over 2,000 years ago, and was prized for its many medicinal and culinary uses.

Sixteenth-century Puritans referred to fennel seeds as "meeting house seeds" as they were chewed to help stave off hunger and keep children quiet during very long sermons – probably the most fun that Puritans allowed themselves to have!

Fennel also has insect-repelling properties and was, and still is, tucked into horses' bridles to keep flies away and used in dog kennels to deter fleas.

The fragrant fronds have stood the test of time: infant colic was treated with fennel tea as early as the third century BCE and twenty-first-century babies are still given gripe water containing fennel to ease trapped wind.

FOLKLORE: Fennel and St John's wort were hung around windows and doors at midsummer as protection against witches. As an extra precaution, some fennel seeds were put into keyholes to prevent ghosts from entering the home.

Fennel paste was rubbed into cows' udders in an attempt to protect the milk from being bewitched. For humans, fennel juice rubbed into your calf muscles – and a small piece placed in your shoes – would help to keep away ticks when you went walking in woodland.

It was considered unlucky to grow your own fennel and much safer to somehow acquire it: *"Sow fennel, sow trouble."*

FOLK MEDICINE: The Greeks and Romans drank fennel tea in the belief that it would suppress their appetites and help them lose weight. Fennel tea was also prescribed by William Coles, who recommended it *"for those that are grown fat, to abate their unwieldiness and cause them to grow more gaunt and lank."*

Culpeper wrote that *"the leaves or seed, boiled in barley water and drank, are good for nurses, to increase their milk, and make it more wholesome for the child."*

If you were unfortunate enough to have been bitten by a snake or eaten something that you shouldn't, *"the seed boiled in wine and drank, is good for those that are bit with serpents or have eat poisonous herbs or mushrooms".*

Finally, the tenth-century *Leechbook of Bald* counsels that, *"Against mental vacancy and against folly; put into ale bishopwort, lupins, betony, fennel, nepte, water agrimony, cockle, marche, then let the man drink".*

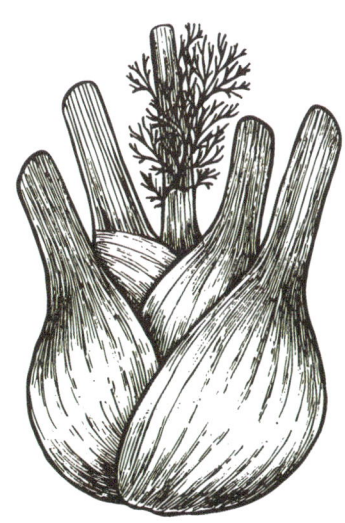

FORAGED FENNEL FRONDS PESTO

If you are unable to find and safely identify wild fennel, many farm shops and market gardens grow Florence fennel complete with fronds, or maybe talk to your local allotment association who could help. Fennel fronds have a very delicate aniseed flavour so will not overpower the other ingredients in this pesto recipe.

Serves four

INGREDIENTS

100 g walnuts, almonds, pine nuts or cashews

Two good handfuls fennel fronds, roughly chopped

Juice of one lemon

1 garlic clove, chopped

100 g grated Parmesan cheese, or vegetarian hard cheese (If you wish to make this recipe plant-based, replace the cheese with 3 tbsp nutritional yeast)

Approx. 100 ml olive oil

Sea salt and freshly ground black pepper to taste

METHOD

Place a dry frying pan over a medium heat and toast the nuts until they are aromatic and golden brown.

Add the nuts to a food processor or pestle and mortar with the fennel, lemon, garlic, Parmesan (or alternative) and most of the olive oil.

Blitz or pound to a rough paste.

Add salt and pepper to taste, and more olive oil if needed.

Stir fennel pesto through freshly cooked pasta, serve with salmon or even pop it on a pizza.

Will keep for about five days in the fridge or 12 months in the freezer.

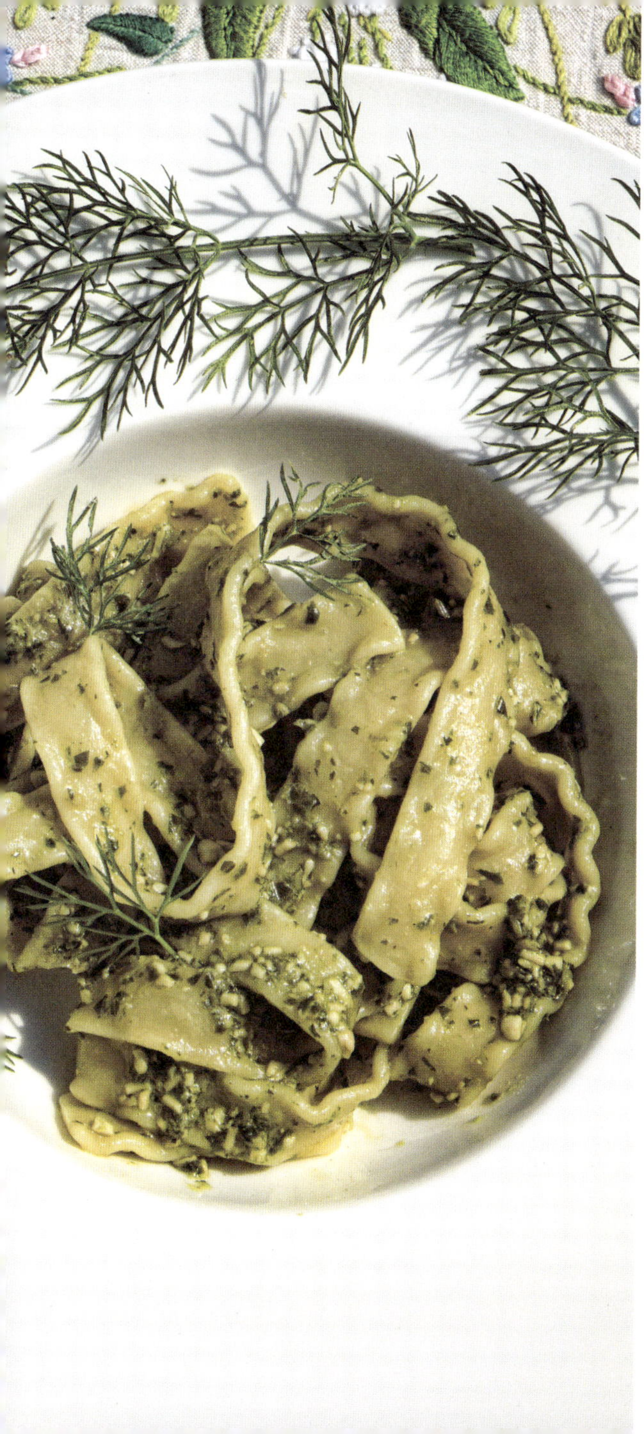

Fennel fronds can be added to roasted vegetables, soups, sauces and dressings. To make delightful herbal ice cubes, boil water several times to ensure that your ice cubes are crystal clear, allow to cool, pour into an ice cube tray and submerge some fennel fronds, herbs or edible flowers within, then freeze.

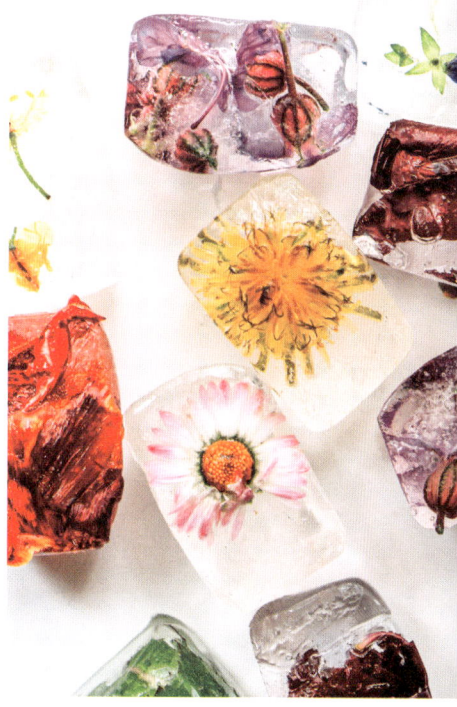

FERN

Alternative names: Common bracken, brake fern, pasture brake, eagle fern, devil's brushes

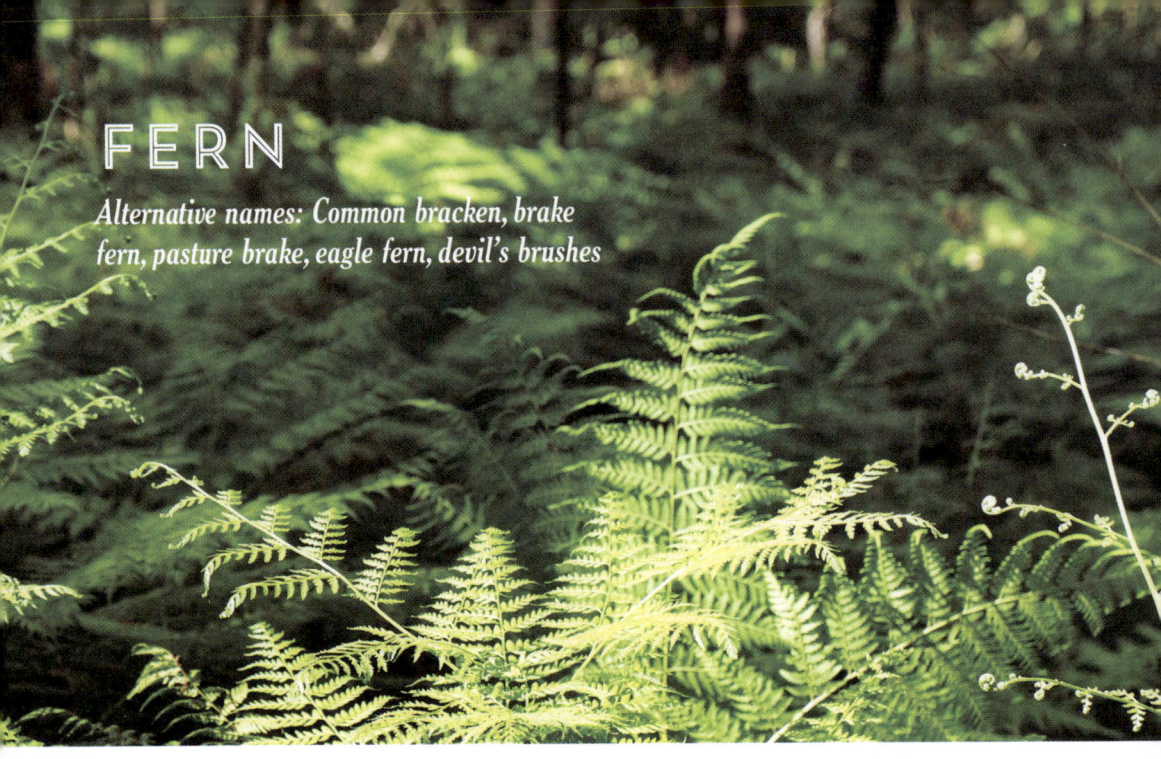

HOW TO IDENTIFY: Fern is believed to be the most widespread plant in the world and can be found everywhere apart from Antarctica. Bracken leaves are large, triangular, much-divided and can be seen slowly unfurling in the spring. Bracken grows anywhere between 1–2 m (3–6 ft) tall, forming dense clumps on the forest floor. Unlike many species of fern, bracken dies back in the winter, leaving brown, withered fronds.

HISTORY: Ferns have been a common sight in woodlands for millions of years so it makes sense that early Brits made good use of this abundant plant. It was used as bedding and fodder for cattle, as fertilizer and as a thatching material for stables and dwellings. Remnants of bracken have been discovered in Iron Age excavations and were believed to be discarded animal bedding.

In the twentieth century, country folk and farmers constructed underground "root clamps" filled with layers of bracken, to preserve potatoes and carrots over winter. Fishmongers would also proudly display their wares laid out on a bed of fresh bracken, and growers of soft fruit packed bracken around their precious produce to protect it from damage as it was transported to market.

Fast-forward to the twenty-first century and bracken is being harvested again, this time mixed with sheep's wool and comfrey to make a nutritious peat-free compost.

FOLKLORE: In Scotland, bracken was said to be a representation of the devil's footprints and thought to reveal a portal to the underworld or the kingdom of the fae. One English folk tale tells of a young girl who accidently sat on some ferns. A faery man appeared before her and made her promise to look after his son in faery land for a year and a day. She swore on her promise by kissing the fern. Whether she returned after a year and a day the folk tale doesn't tell us!

Bracken doesn't bear any flower or fruit, which led to speculation that the seeds might be invisible and that if you found some and carried them, you would become invisible too. This power was clearly common knowledge as Shakespeare references it in *Henry IV*: "We have the receipt of fern seed – we walk invisible."

FOLK MEDICINE: Burning bracken was used as a remedy against aches and pests. Traditionally, people walked through smoking bracken to alleviate the symptoms of sciatica and other aches in the legs. Culpeper wrote that the smoke from the burning of bracken could *"driveth away serpents, gnats, and other noisome creatures"*.

And it wasn't only the leaves that were valued. Culpeper continues, *"The roots boiled in mead [...] killeth both the broad and long worms in the body."*

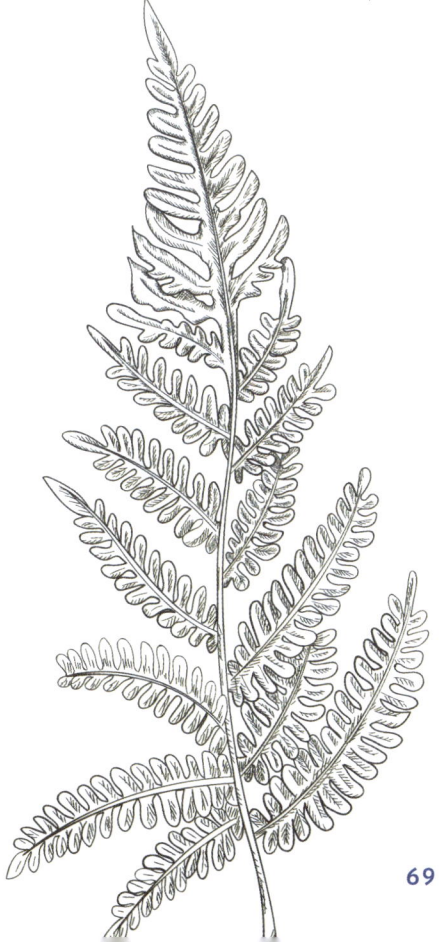

FEVERFEW

Alternative names: Featherfew, bachelor's buttons, flirtwort, midsummer daisy, nosebleed, featherfoil

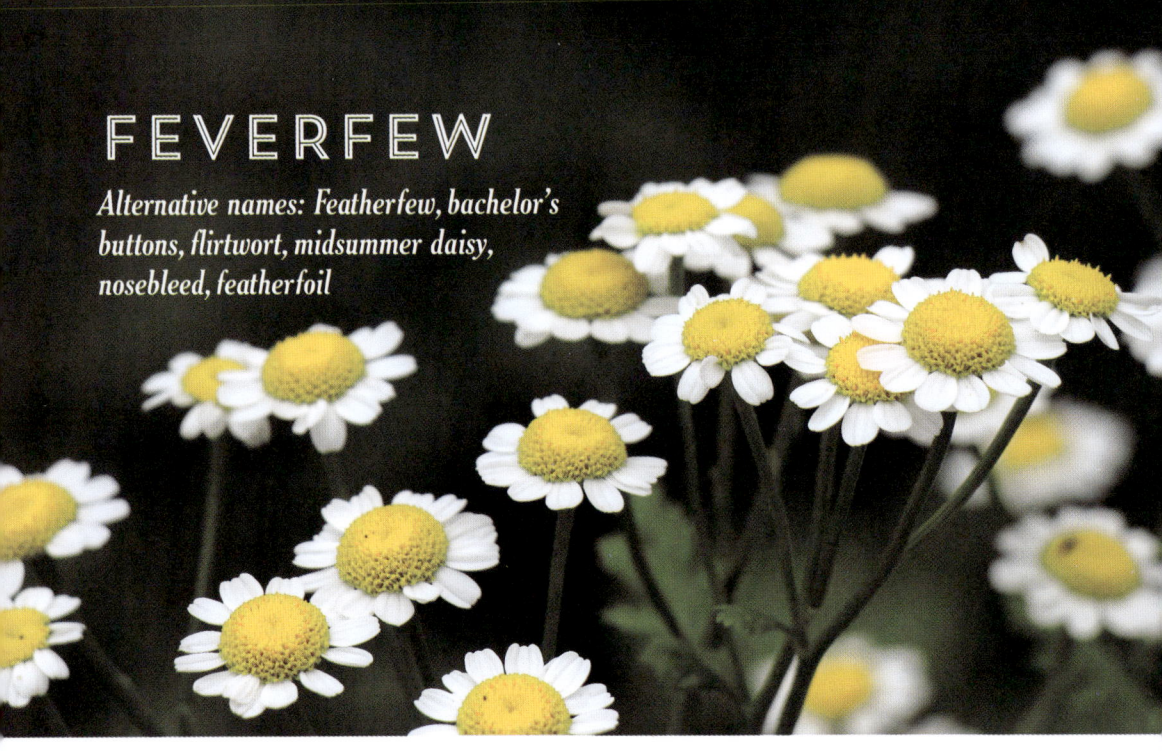

HOW TO IDENTIFY: Feverfew is a bushy perennial plant with a profusion of yellow-centred daisy-like flowers that bloom from July to September. The leaves are yellowish-green and feather-like with a pungent smell and bitter taste. Feverfew likes to grow in confined spaces such as cracks in pavements and walls.

HISTORY: Feverfew was originally introduced from southeastern Europe in the Middle Ages, possibly for medicinal use in monastery gardens, and is now widely naturalized throughout the UK and Ireland.

FOLKLORE: The causes of many diseases weren't fully understood in medieval Europe, and certain ailments suffered by cattle, horses or humans would be attributed to supernatural forces. A person suffering from what we now know to be rheumatism, arthritis, or muscle cramps could well have believed that they had been "elf-shot". During the sixteenth century, many references were made to sharp pains inflicted by elves or witches who fired sharp arrowheads causing wounding and even death.

Horses and cattle were particularly vulnerable to being elf-shot and would fall over, be unable to stand, and suffer breathing difficulties and stomach issues. Sometimes an "elf arrow" or "fairy arrow" would be found near to the afflicted animal. Sudden paralysis in humans and animals was known as "elf-stroke" (now referred to as a stroke or brain haemorrhage) and ultimately led to death.

Feverfew and plantain were prized as a remedy for dreaded elf arrows due to their arrow-shaped leaves. This was due to the medieval belief in the "law of similarity" – where things that resembled each other were thought to be related in some way.

Feverfew was also believed to have protective qualities. Planted around doorways, its strong odour was believed to safeguard against the plague.

FOLK MEDICINE: In Culpeper's *Herbal*, he describes feverfew as being particularly beneficial to new mothers as *"a general strengthener of their wombs, and to remedy such infirmities as a careless midwife has there caused [...] make use of the herb boiled in white wine, and drink the decoction, it cleanses the womb, expels the afterbirth, and does a woman all the good she can desire of an herb".*

Modern herbalists still prescribe feverfew for the treatment of migraine headaches. Culpeper recommends that it *"is very effectual for all pains in the head coming of a cold cause, the herb being bruised and applied to the crown of the head: as also for the vertigo; that is a running or swimming of the head".*

In addition, Grieve advises that, *"A decoction with sugar or honey is said to be good for coughs, wheezing and difficult breathing. The herb, bruised and heated, or fried with a little wine and oil, has been employed as a warm external application for wind and colic."*

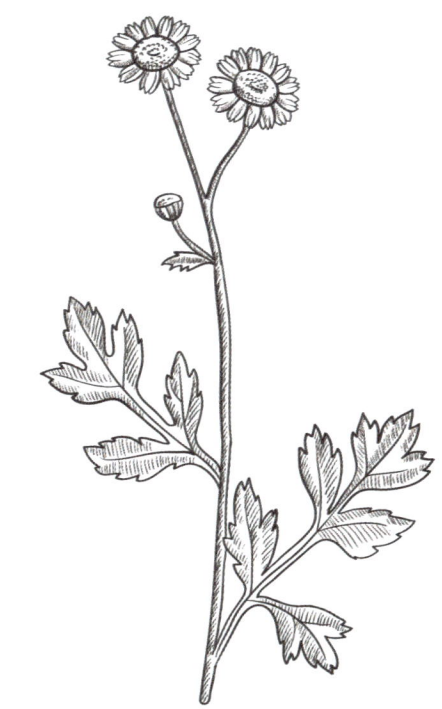

FLEABANE

Alternative names: Harvest flower, pig daisy, mare's fat, Job's tears, middle fleabane, tick weed

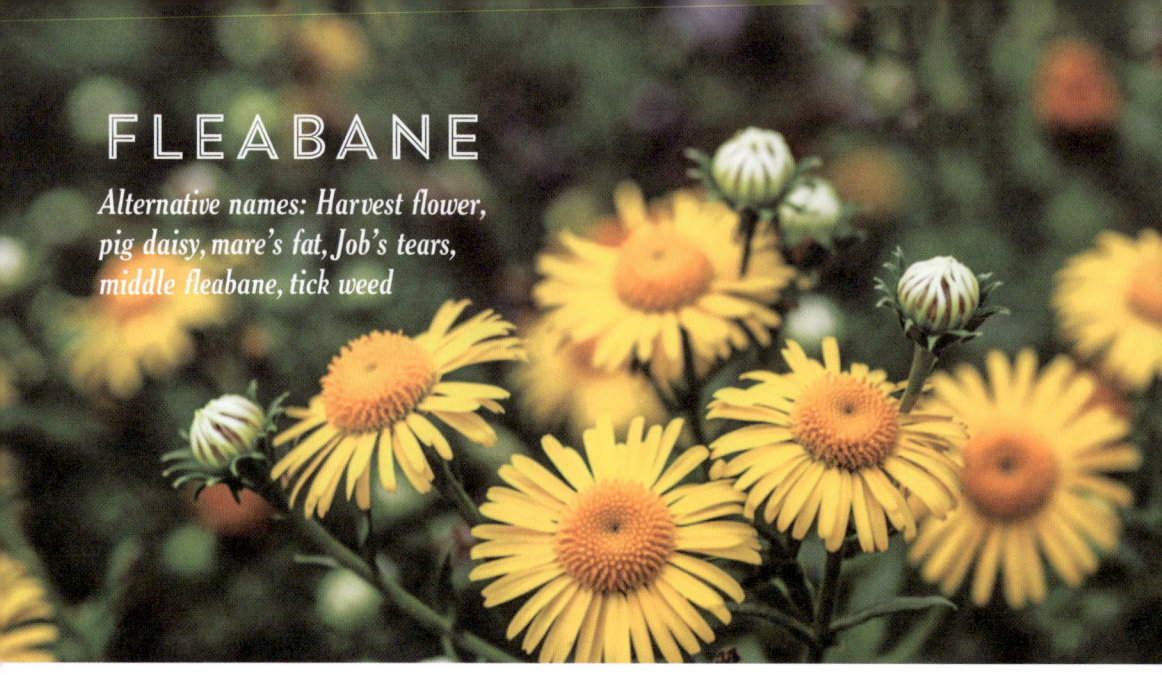

HOW TO IDENTIFY: With its golden-yellow, daisy-like flowering heads that bloom in late summer through to early autumn, fleabane is most likely to be seen in damp, open meadows and the edges of ditches. The oval, crinkly leaves grow all the way up the hairy stem and, once dried, smell a little like carbolic soap and chrysanthemum, which is why fleas consider them a bane!

HISTORY: Records show that powdered fleabane was mixed with charcoal and sprinkled onto floors to deter insects. Natron salt (traditionally used in embalming) mixed with water and fleabane was an effective flea repellent, while dried bunches of the leaves were burned as a fumigant or hung up in windows and doorways to deter fleas and insects. Culpeper even stated that *"the very smell of the herb is said to destroy fleas"*.

The floors of medieval dwellings were carpeted with mats woven from straw, rushes or reeds which were only changed or cleaned once or twice a year. As you would expect, they soon became dirty and smelly. Fleabane was one of several "strewing herbs", chosen for their insect-repelling properties and sweet smell, that were "strewn" onto floors where people slept. Other strewing herbs included pennyroyal to repel ticks, lavender for its sweet scent, and rose petals.

FOLKLORE: In her 1922 book *Old English Herbals*, Eleanour Sinclair Rohde quotes a ritual used in ancient Babylonia:

> *"Fleabane on the lintel of the door*
> *I have hung,*
> *St. John's wort, caper and wheatears,*
> *With a halter as a roving ass,*
> *thy body I restrain.*
> *O evil spirit, get thee hence!*
> *Depart, o evil demon."*

The combination of the four herbs was regarded as very protective and was hung over doorways and windows to prevent evil spirits and negative energy from entering the home.

In the bed chamber, a few fleabane seeds sprinkled in the bed linen was a sure way to ensure the faithfulness and chastity of your loved one.

And in Italian folklore, fleabane was associated with the Madonna and was believed to have the power to heal and protect against disease.

FOLK MEDICINE: When it came to fleabane, Culpeper recommended that the juice of the whole plant should be used as a cure for itching and:

> *"The mucilage of the seed made with plantain water, whereunto the yoke of an egg or two, and a little populeon are put, is a most safe and sure remedy to ease the sharpness, pricking and pains of the haemorrhoids or piles, if it be laid on cloth, and bound thereto."* (Populeon was an ointment made from poplar.)

Fleabane was bound to the forehead to calm a person who was getting a little over-excited and was also a well-known treatment for dysentery. One seventeenth-century account from General Keit of the Russian army recounts that during expeditions against Persia, his soldiers were successfully cured of dysentery by treating them with fleabane.

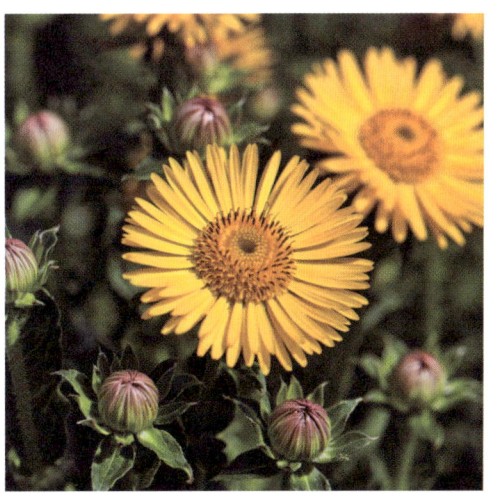

FORGET-ME-NOT

Alternative names: Blue mouse-ear, scorpion grass, bird's eye, love me

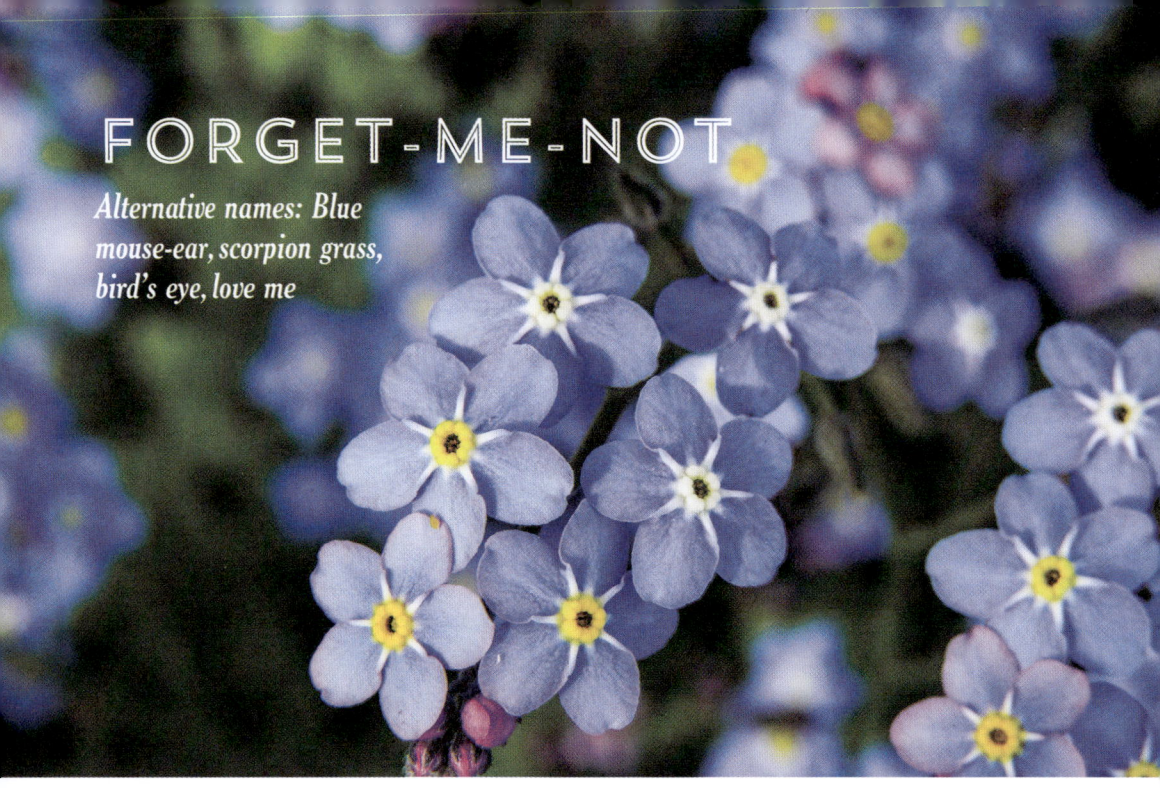

HOW TO IDENTIFY: Look closely in hedgerows and ancient woodlands, for these diminutive azure flowers are easily missed, only growing to 50 cm (20 in.) tall. Clusters of delicate, blue, five-petalled flowers on top of hairy stems with narrow, oval "mouse-ear" leaves begin to appear in April through to June.

HISTORY: Henry V adopted the forget-me-not as his emblem before his exile in 1398, in the hope that it would guarantee that he would never be forgotten.

Throughout history the forget-me-not has been laden with meaning. In the Victorian language of flowers, they signified faithful and enduring love. During World War One, they were used as a symbol to remember fallen soldiers. More recently, the Alzheimer's Society adopted the forget-me-not as their emblem to represent memory loss.

In 1930s Germany, Freemasons faced persecution by the Nazi party. This led to them adopting a forget-me-not badge or lapel pin as a discreet symbol to enable them to recognize each other in a way that would not reveal their identities to those outside the fraternity. It continues to be a Masonic symbol of remembrance, resistance and resilience.

FOLKLORE: There are several legends as to how this delicate flower got its name. One tells that as God was naming all the flowers, he overlooked the tiny plant. The little blue plant called out "Forget-me-not!" Since all the names had been taken, the words spoken by the flower were used instead.

Alternatively, in medieval times, a knight was walking along a river bank with his love. He stopped to pick a posy of the blue flowers for her but, unfortunately, the riverbank was muddy and so he slipped and fell into the river. As he was swept away to his death, he threw the flowers to his love, calling "Forget me not!"

In the West Country, the wearing of forget-me-nots was believed to offer protection against witches, especially during the month of May.

In a rather peculiar claim, juice from the plant is said to make a steel blade so sharp that it could cut through stone.

FOLK MEDICINE: Known in the seventeenth century as "scorpion grass", the forget-me-not was described by Culpeper as having *"a bitterish styptic taste, and is accounted to be drying and binding, and a good vulnerary [wound-healing] herb and helpful for all sorts of fluxes [...] commended for ulcers in the mouth".*

As the folk name suggests, it was believed to be a cure for scorpion stings and snake bites. Made into a concentrated liquid, it was also used to treat sore eyes.

Its properties don't end there. Grieve tells us that, *"the plant has a strong affinity for the respiratory organs, especially the left lower lung [...] it is sometimes made into a syrup and given for pulmonary affections."*

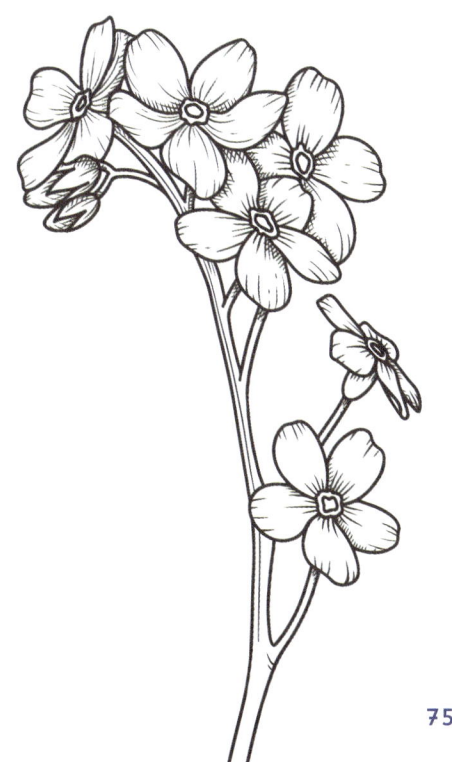

FOXGLOVE

Alternative names: Faery fingers, dead men's bells, folk's gloves, witches' bells

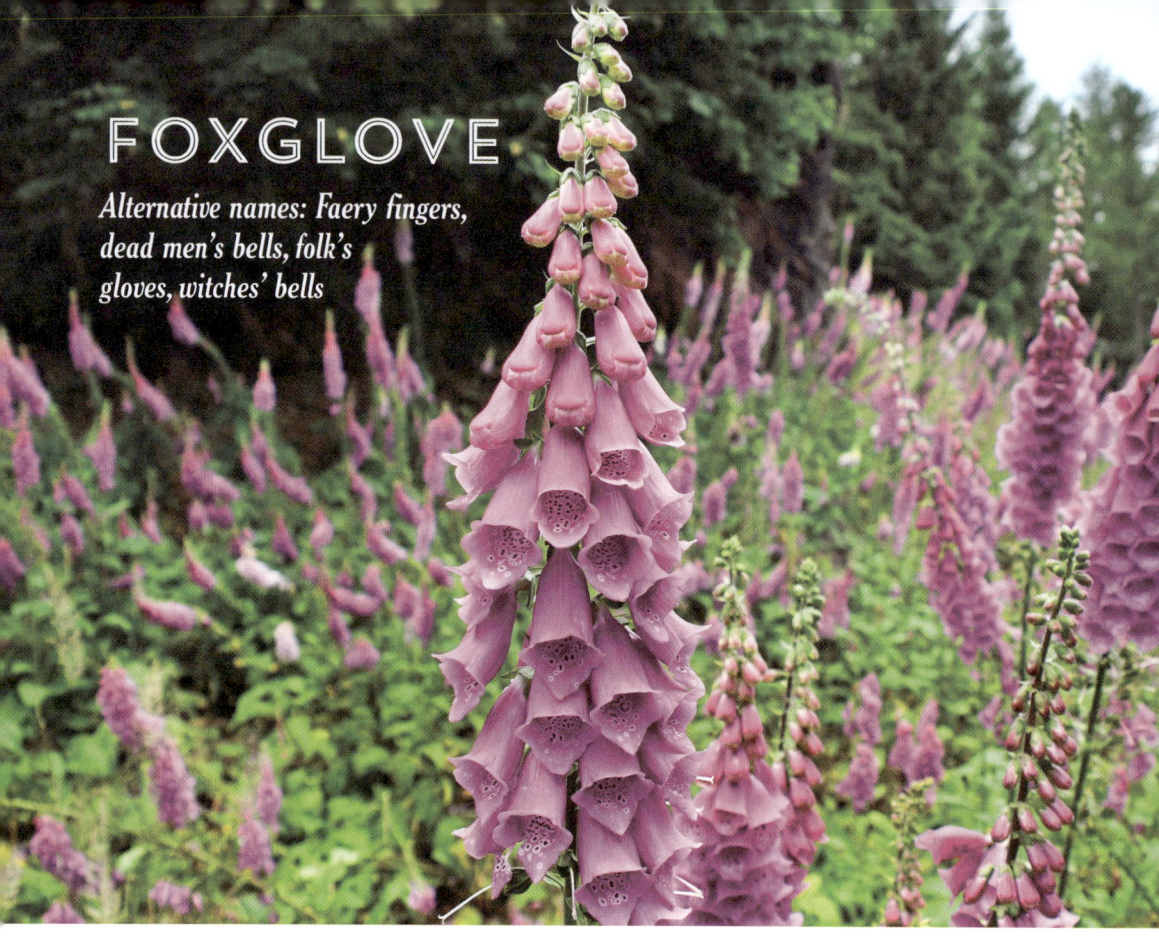

HOW TO IDENTIFY: The foxglove is easily identifiable once in flower but beware – all parts of this plant are potentially poisonous to humans and some animals. Always wear gloves when handling foxgloves and **never** ingest any of the plant.

Foxgloves prefer shady woodland verges, and of course, cottage gardens. They have large, flat leaves at the base followed by majestic tall spikes of bell-shaped purple flowers in early summer that open from the bottom of the spike upwards.

HISTORY: In the eighteenth century, a young country doctor, William Withering, grew frustrated as he watched potential patients visit the local wise woman instead of coming to him. He tried to discredit her by spreading rumours that she was a witch, but her patients were loyal. Withering saw a man who he knew to have heart problems pay a visit to the wise woman. He then observed her gathering foxglove leaves in her garden with which to successfully treat the man. Withering never did make a success of his rural practice, but he went on to write *An Account of the Foxglove and Some of its Medicinal Uses* which led to further research and the development of the heart drug, digoxin.

FOLKLORE: As with bluebells, the distinctive bell shape of the flowers has always been associated with faery folklore. One medieval ritual that is definitely not recommended was designed to deal with badly-behaved, surly children or "changelings" – innocent human children that had been swapped for an unruly faery child. Three drops of foxglove juice were placed on the child's tongue and three drops in each ear, then they were made to sit on a shovel which was swung three times out of an open doorway saying:

"If you're a faery, away with you!"

In Scotland, foxglove leaves were put into babies' cradles to protect them from evil. The connection between foxgloves and children seems to be a common theme; naughty children who knew that faeries hid inside the flowers would strike the flower bell hoping to hear "faery thunder" as the annoyed creature made her escape.

Planting foxgloves in your garden will encourage faeries to live there and hopefully keep evil away. If this doesn't work, black dye made from the leaves can be painted on your cottage floor in the shape of a cross for protection.

Foxes are believed to wear the little bell-shaped flowers on their paws, enabling them to sneak into the chicken coop at night without being heard – hence the name!

FOLK MEDICINE: Foxglove was used as a cure for a number of ailments, from bad knees to eczema in animals. A handwritten note, now held in a Scottish museum and believed to date from the early nineteenth century, gives an insight into one of the remedies:

"For a man in great pain from an internal growth or swelling, a pulp was made from squashed foxglove roots, then applied inside flannel, after the pulp had been heated, as a poultice to the swelling. The man received immediate relief, and continued to do so until the cure was completed."

FUMITORY

Alternative names: Birds on the bush, earth smoke, God's fingers and thumbs, lady's locket, mother-of-thousands, wax dolls

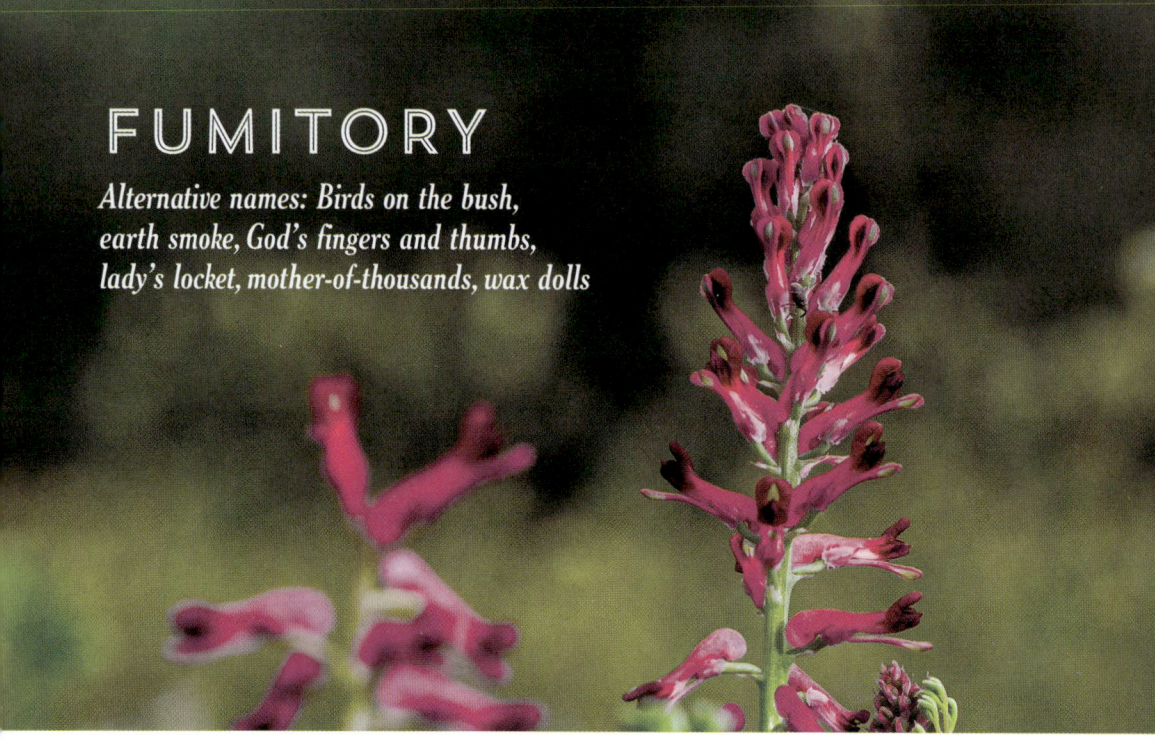

HOW TO IDENTIFY: Preferring well-drained soil, fumitory likes disturbed land and waste ground. It can easily spread in arable fields, where it is quite capable of strangling the whole crop. Upright spikes of pink flowers are tipped with deep red and can be seen from April to October. Common fumitory is a member of the poppy family and has similarly small grey-green, much-divided leaves which are delicate and fern-like.

HISTORY: Common fumitory is vitally important for the survival of turtle doves, a breed that has suffered a 95 per cent decline since the 1990s. Turtle dove chicks are fed "crop milk" by their parents; studies have shown that a major component of this food is fumitory fruits which ripen just as the chicks are born in May.

The first mention of *"fumeterre"* was in Geoffrey Chaucer's *The Nun's Priest's Tale*, written in 1386, where parts of the plant were used as a laxative.

FOLKLORE: Fumitory translates as "smoke of the earth". Some say that this is because the leaves are so delicate that they resemble smoke, while others suggest that this plant was produced not from seed, but from vapours rising from the ground.

Fumitory was burned during exorcisms in the belief that it could help to banish evil spirits from the body. It was also planted around houses to protect and purify.

Rubbing fumitory in your shoes protected you as you set off on a journey and the plant was said to bring you riches, both monetary and spiritual.

Bathing the face with an infusion of fumitory was thought to make you more beautiful and remove spots and freckles. Poet John Clare wrote:

> *"And fumitory too, a name*
> *Which superstition holds to fame,*
> *Whose red and purple mottled flowers*
> *Are dropped by maids in weeding hours,*
> *To boil in water, milk. And whey,*
> *For washes on a holiday,*
> *To make their beauty fair and sleek,*
> *And scare the tan from summer's cheek."*

FOLK MEDICINE: Fumitory appears to have been a very valuable herb much used in many historical remedies and has been used to treat rheumatism, scurvy, fevers, colic and even the plague.

In his book *The British Herbal* (1770), John Edwards writes, "*It is good for obstructions in the viscera [intestines] and jaundice. The juice of fumitory and dock mixed with vinegar, cures scabs, pimples, wheals, or pushes [hives]."*

Grieve recommends it highly: *"A decoction makes a curative lotion for milk-crust [cradle cap] on the scalp of an infant [...] The Japanese make a tonic from it. Cows and sheep eat it and are said to derive great benefit from it. [...] French and German physicians still prefer it to most other medicines as a purifier of the blood; while sometimes the dried leaves are smoked in the manner of tobacco, for disorders of the head."*

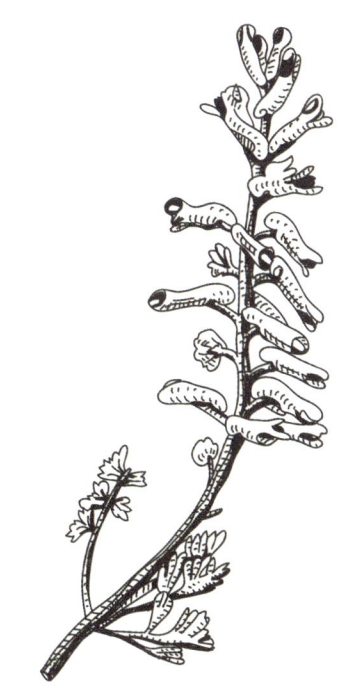

GREEN ALKANET

Alternative names: Dyer's bugloss, Spanish bugloss, blue-eyed Mary, pheasant's eye, water forget-me-not

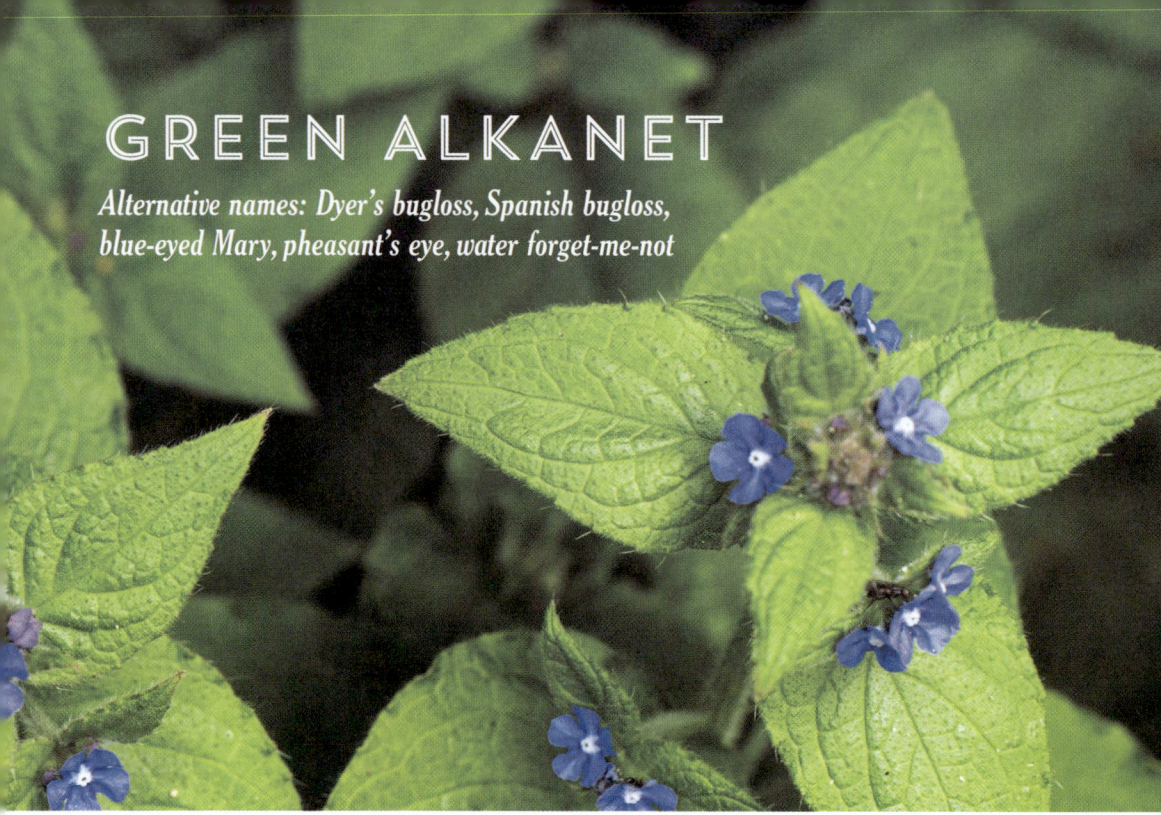

HOW TO IDENTIFY: Green alkanet spreads very readily and could easily be confused with borage or comfrey, as they originate from the same family. The leaves are long, oval and bristly, and sometimes have little white dots on them. The stem grows tall and hairy and can cause skin irritation if handled without gloves. By April, green alkanet is beginning to produce bright blue five-petalled flowers with a white centre, which can be seen well into late summer in damp, shady places.

HISTORY: Green alkanet was introduced into the UK in the 1700s and was first recorded in the wild in 1724. The bark on the roots of green alkanet has long been used to produce a red dye for fabrics, paper and wool. The Romans were known to use this red dye in sweets and cosmetics, and for rather more underhand practices – such as adulterating red wine to make it look more expensive.

More recently it has been discovered that rubbing furniture with oil that has been infused with alkanet root will produce a fine red stain, resulting in a good imitation of mahogany or rosewood.

FOLKLORE: Known for its protective properties, travellers and traders in medieval Europe often carried green alkanet in the belief that it would protect them from poisoned food and drink, since it was thought to have the power to neutralize and detect poison.

Amulets and charms containing the herb provided extra protection from evil spirits that wished you harm. Alkanet allegedly protected against snake bites and helped to control the fear of snakes. It could also aid divination, attract love, deepen existing relationships and, added to a face wash, enhance the complexion.

In modern use, alkanet root burned as an incense is said to give you protection from those who try to trick you out of money, and is believed to give you the edge as far as work or academic success is concerned.

FOLK MEDICINE: Gerard recommends green alkanet if you have been unlucky enough to fall from a height:

"Do boil with the root of alkanet and wine, sweet butter, such as hath in it no salt at all, until such time as it becometh red, which they call red butter, and give it not only to those that have fallen from some high place, but also report it to be good to drive forth measles and smallpox, if it be drunk at the beginning with hot beer."

Later in the seventeenth century, Culpeper talks of green alkanet in great length:

"If you make a vinegar of it, as you make vinegar of roses, it helps the morphew [blemishes usually caused by scurvy] and leprosy [...] It helps the yellow jaundice, spleen and gravel in the kidneys [...] If anyone hath newly eaten it doth spit into the mouth of a serpent, the serpent instantly dies [...] It helps bruises and falls, and is a gallant remedy to drive out the smallpox and measles."

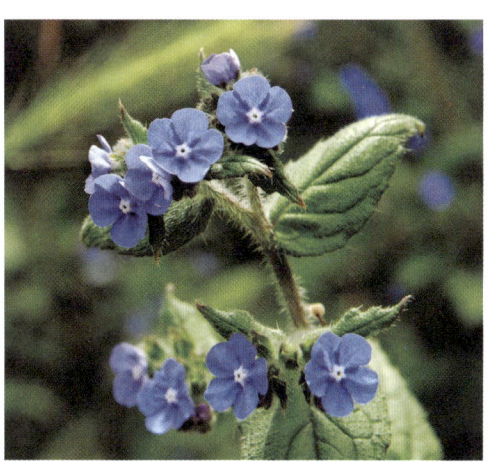

HEATHER

Alternative names: Ling, dog heather, hadder, mountain mist, Scots heather

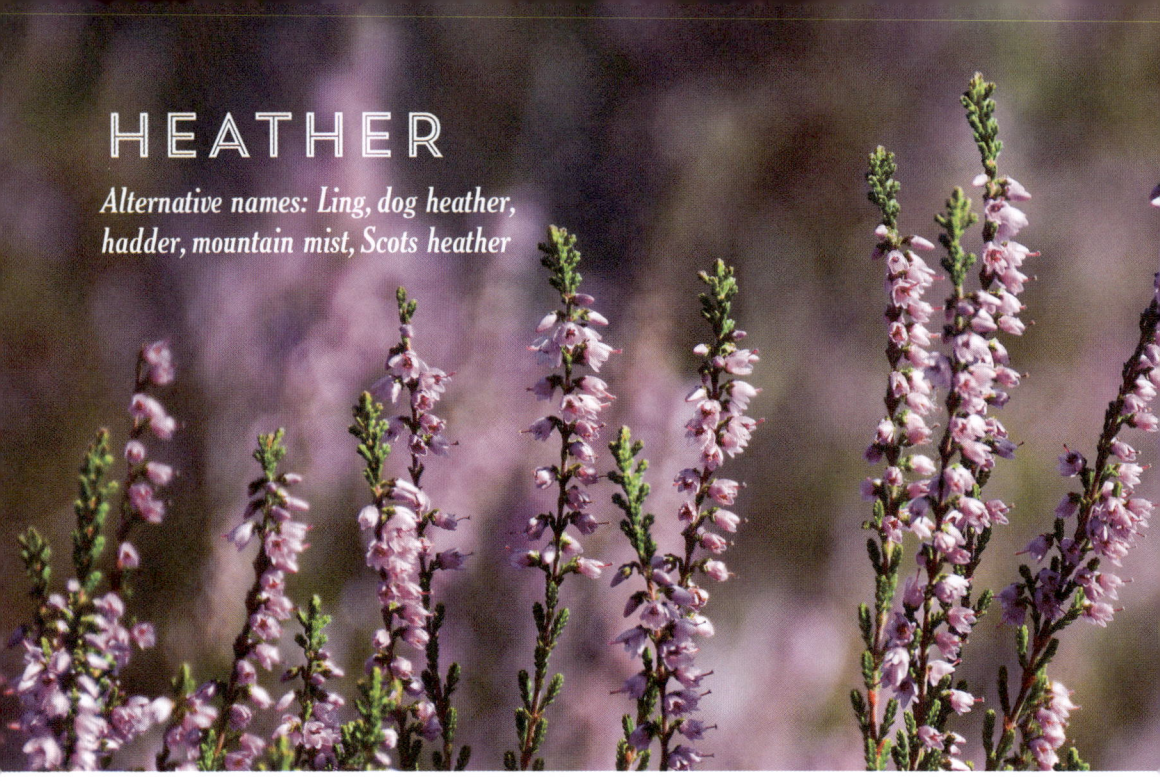

HOW TO IDENTIFY: Heather grows close to the ground on coarse, woody stems, creating a carpet of tiny purple, pink, red or white bell-shaped flowers. Heathers prefer to grow in acidic soil on wild heathlands and open woodlands, and can be seen in flower from August to October.

HISTORY: Native to Scotland, Ireland and western Europe, the name heather is believed to derive from the Scots word *haeddre*, used to describe heathland or "heather place".

Covering an impressive five million acres of Scottish moorland, it's no wonder that the Scots found many practical uses for this prolific flower. Especially useful on remote Scottish islands, heather has had a vital role in the building of dwellings, being used to thatch roofs, build walls and make pegs, mats, baskets, brooms and ropes.

Dried Scottish heather made a fragrant filling for mattresses and promised a comfortable night's sleep. Also, in textiles, different varieties of heather were used in the dyeing of wool and cloth, and could produce many different colours from yellow to green and purple, which of course feature in traditional Scottish tartan.

For culinary purposes, heather honey is much-prized for its delicate floral taste and in the making of mead and traditional ale.

FOLKLORE: Sprays of white heather have been added to bridal bouquets for centuries as it was considered to be the luckiest of all the heather colours. In 1884, on a visit to the Highlands, Queen Victoria commented on the actions of one of her Scottish servants:

> *"he espied a piece of white heather, and jumped off to pick it. No Highlander would pass by it without picking it, for it was considered to bring good luck."*

Many superstitions surround this humble little plant. White heather only grows on the final resting place of faeries or where blood has been spilled. Chiefs of the Clan McDonald are said to have attached heather to their spears before battle, and all soldiers would wear a sprig to ensure victory. Clan Ranald attributed their victory in 1544 at the oddly named Battle of the Shirts (apparently the day was so hot that both sides discarded their chainmail and fought in shirts) to the wearing of white heather.

Up until the eighteenth century, when it was outlawed in favour of hops, heather was used as a traditional ingredient to ferment ale. Despite being illegal, heather continued to be used in brewing in the home and has now been commercially revived under the name of Fraoch.

FOLK MEDICINE: Heather is a powerhouse of medicinal properties, being antiseptic, anti-inflammatory, disinfectant and diuretic. Heather has also been used as a gargle for tonsillitis, a cure for blindness and poisoning, and as a treatment for arthritis and rheumatism.

In the Scottish Highlands, an infusion of heather was recommended for insomnia, as well as being taken as a tonic by tuberculosis patients.

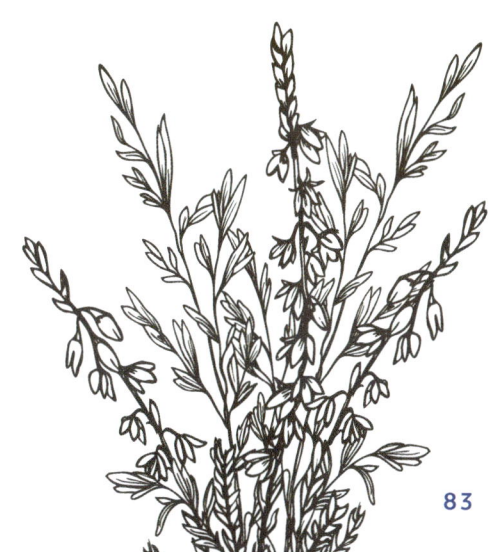

HEDGE WOUNDWORT

Alternative names: Red archangel, hedge stachys, clown's woundwort, wild nettle grass, hock heal, hercules, whitespot

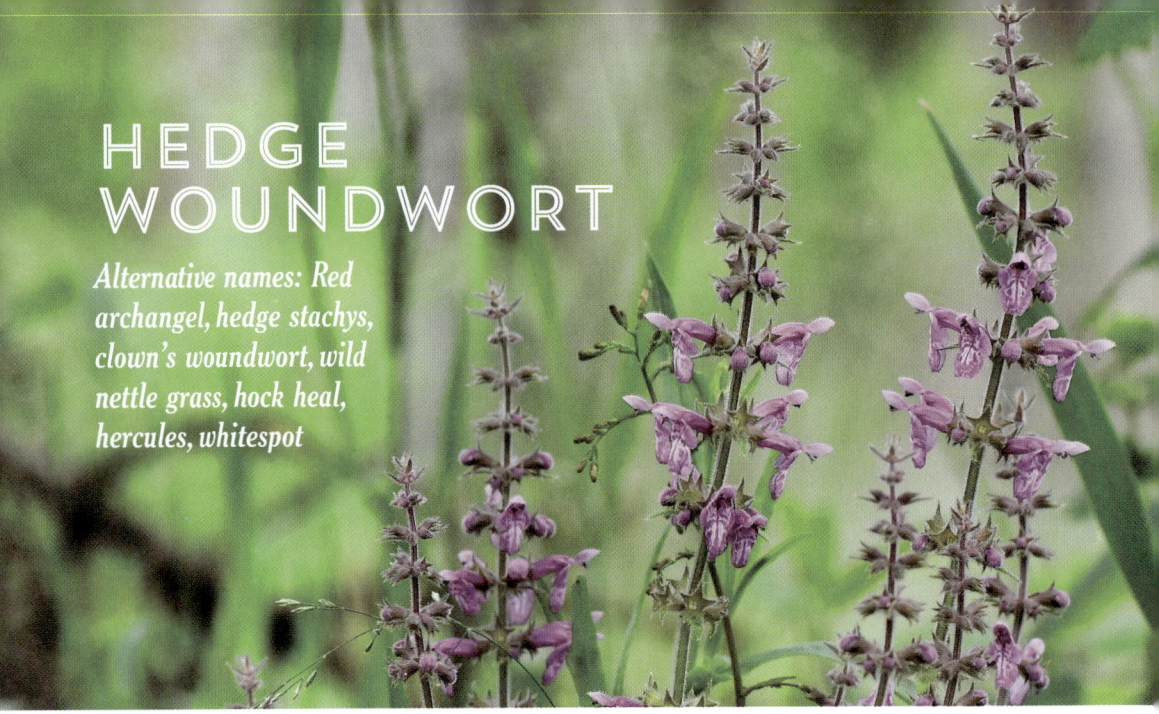

HOW TO IDENTIFY: The purple-magenta hooded flowers of hedge woundwort are a common sight, flowering in woodlands, and along hedgerows and roadside verges from June to October. Similar in appearance to nettles but without the sting, hedge woundwort can grow to around 1 m (3 ft) tall on square-shaped stalks. These heart-shaped leaves give off a strong smell to entice insects to pollinate the flowers, particularly favoured by the bronze shield bug.

HISTORY: As its name implies, hedge woundwort has been an invaluable plant in times of conflict for its fabulous antiseptic properties and plentiful availability all over medieval battlefields.

In the Middle Ages, hedge woundwort was used as a substitute for lint when dressing wounds and cuts, and proved to be very effective in the management of pain, inflammation and swelling.

FOLKLORE: Some cultures believed that hedge woundwort had magical properties and that planting the herb near the home could protect the occupants from evil spirits.

Allowing hedge woundwort to grow freely in your garden would not only attract numerous amounts of bees to protect you from bad luck, but would also allow abundance to enter your home.

Don't be tempted to weed out your hedge woundwort or it could result in bad luck and injury heading your way. In folk magic, hedge woundwort was traditionally carried by travellers who believed that it would keep them safe from injury and attack on their journey.

FOLK MEDICINE: Gerard had his own experience of the amazing healing powers of woundwort. He once witnessed a man in Kent cut his leg very badly with a scythe while harvesting peas:

"Wherein he made a wound to the bones and withal very large and wide, and also with great effusion of blood [...] The poor man crept unto this herb, which he bruised with his hands, and tied a great quantity of it unto the wound with a piece of his shirt, which presently staunched the bleeding, and ceased the pain, insomuch that the poor man presently went to his day's work again, without resting one day."

Gerard continues:

"I saw the wound, and offered to heal the same for charity; which he refused, saying I could not heal it so well as himself; a clownish answer I confess, without any thanks for my goodwill; whereupon I have named it clown's woundwort."

Culpeper says of woundwort: "A syrup made from the juice of it, is inferior to none for inward wounds, ruptures of veins, bloody flux, vessels broken, spitting, ruining, or vomiting blood."

Four hundred years later, Grieve tells us that a yellow dye can be extracted from the plant and that it is *"used to make the heart merry, to make a good colour in the face, and to make the vital spirits more fresh and lively."*

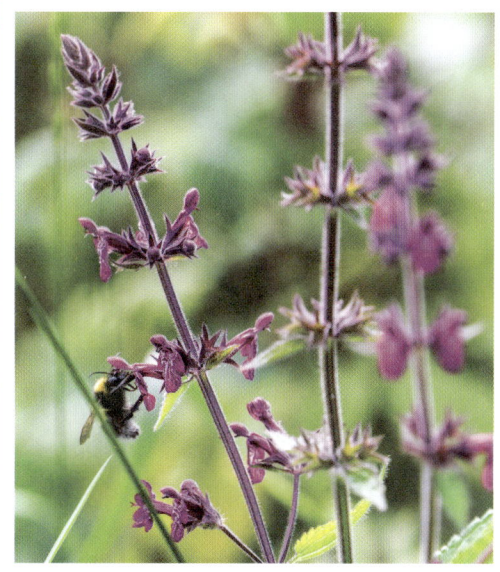

HEMP AGRIMONY

Alternative names: Holy rope, jack-o-lantern, raspberries and cream, water agrimony, water hemp

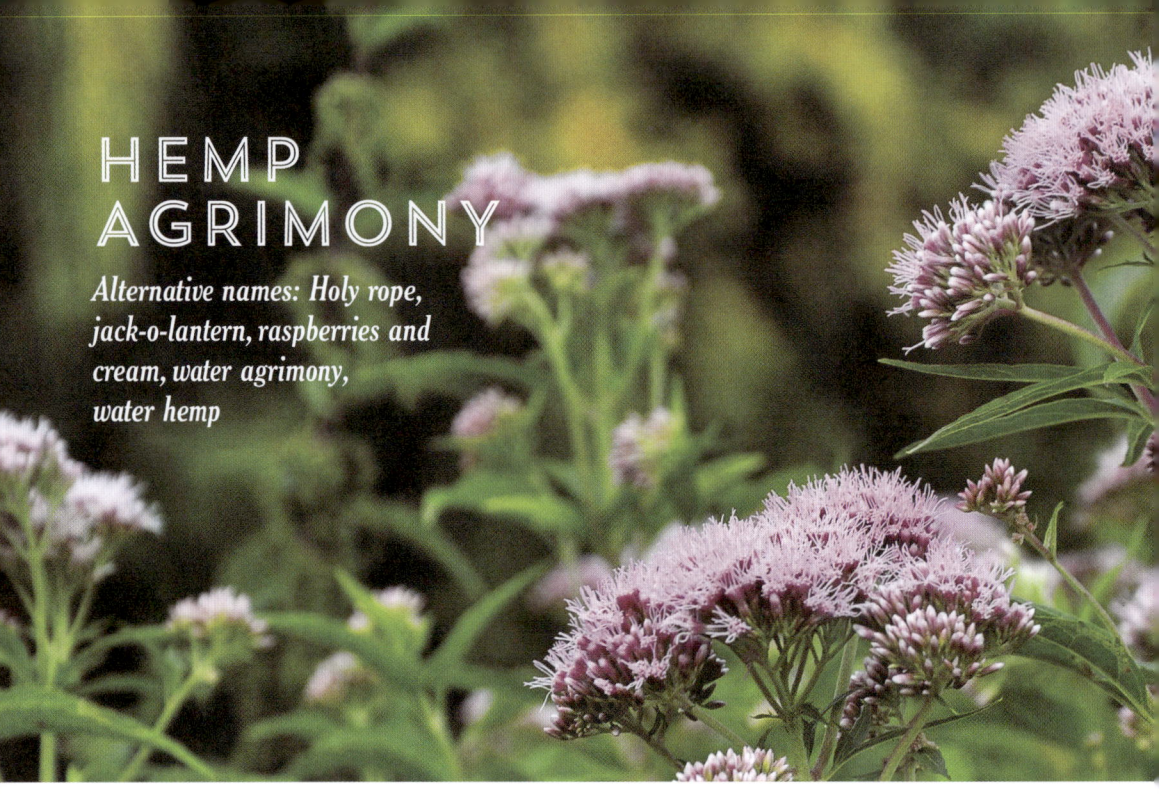

HOW TO IDENTIFY: Hemp agrimony is a perennial plant that likes to have its roots in damp soil. Look for it along riverbanks, in wet woodlands and marshland. Between July and September, numerous tiny pink tubular flowers can be seen massed together to form a large, flat-topped, frothy head atop a tall, red stalk. Leaves resemble the cannabis plant, although the two species are not related.

HISTORY: The first written record of hemp agrimony was in 1548 by naturalist William Turner, the "father of English botany", who named it "water hemp" because *"It groweth about watersydes and hath leaves like hemp."*

In medieval times, hemp agrimony was laid onto bread in the belief that it would prevent it from becoming mouldy, while Culpeper recommended that hemp agrimony was burned in order to create smoke that would drive away wasps.

Hemp agrimony is a wildlife haven attracting a multitude of pollinators to its nectar-rich flowers – especially the larger varieties of butterfly such as the red admiral, peacock and tortoiseshell. Wasps, bees and hoverflies can be seen covering the flowerheads in the height of summer, making hemp agrimony a brilliant plant for your wildlife-friendly garden.

FOLKLORE: The Celts thought that hemp agrimony was blessed by the faery folk and could shield their sacred and hallowed woodlands from unwelcome visitors.

Hemp agrimony planted in the garden was believed to revitalize tired soil and ensure a bountiful harvest. These enriching qualities extended to relationships, too. A sprig of hemp agrimony worn by lovers would ensure fidelity, as well as promoting a deep and loving relationship. It was also believed to bring good luck and protection from evil spirits.

In a more sombre connection, hemp agrimony was known in the Middle Ages as "holy rope", from a belief that the ropes that bound Christ on his way to the crucifixion were made from fibres of the plant.

FOLK MEDICINE: According to the words of Culpeper, hemp agrimony was able to *"Help with the cachexia [unexpected weight loss] or evil disposition of the body; also, the dropsy [fluid retention] and yellow jaundice. It opens obstructions of the liver, mollifies the hardness of the spleen [...] it provokes urine, it kills worms, and cleanseth the body of sharp humours."*

Juice made from the leaves was believed to be an excellent insect repellent when rubbed into the skin.

And Grieve listed other uses for hemp agrimony: *"Though now little used medicinally, herbalists recognise its cathartic, diuretic and anti-scorbutic [scurvy curing] properties, and consider it a good remedy for purifying the blood, either used by itself, or in combination with other herbs."*

In Nepal the herb is known as *banmara* or *kalijhar* and is still used to stop bleeding, treat ulcers and relieve fevers. Fresh leaves and stems are crushed and the juice applied to the wound in the form of a poultice to reduce and even stop the bleeding.

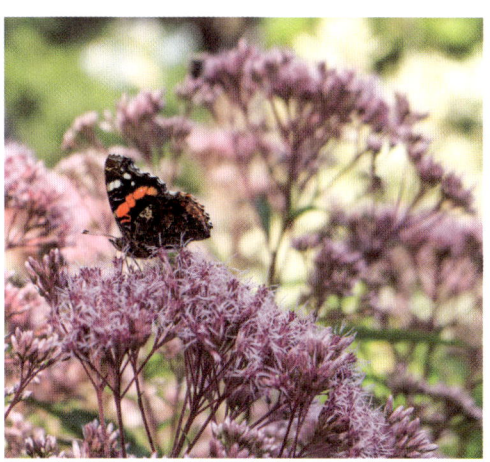

HERB BENNET

Alternative names: Avens, wood avens, blessed herb, clove root, hare foot, star of the earth, yellow strawberry

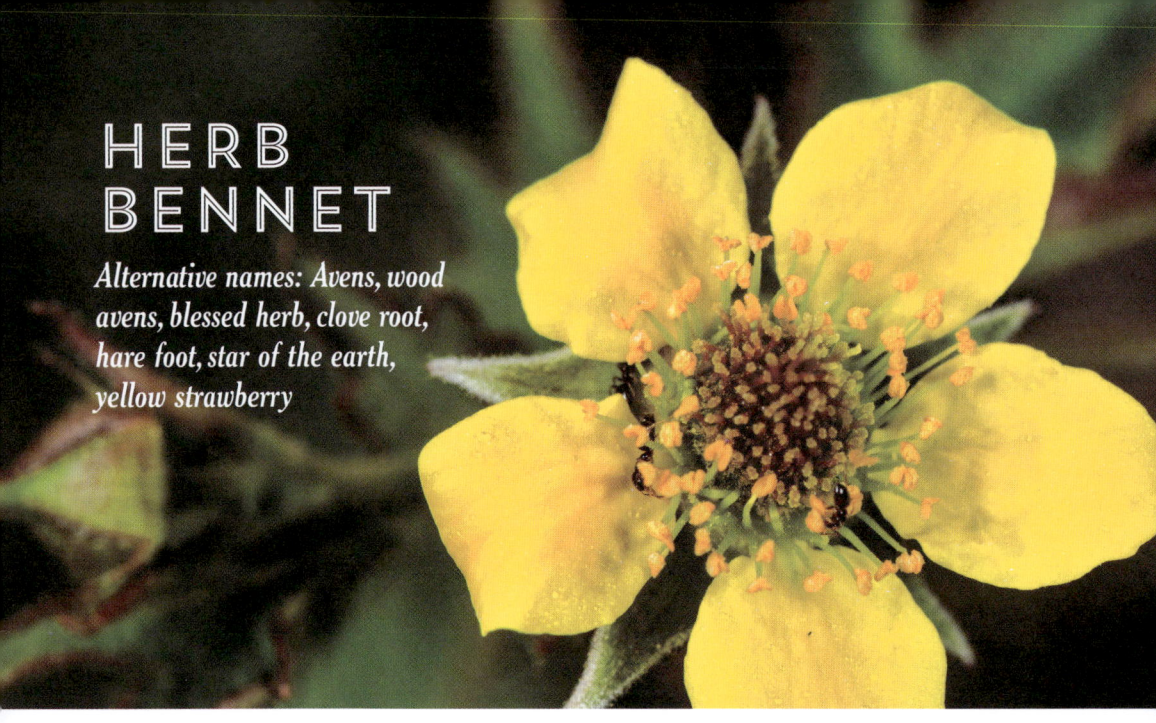

HOW TO IDENTIFY: Found in woodlands, grassland and farmland, herb bennet has leaves similar to strawberry plants. Yellow five-petalled flowers appear on the end of long stalks from May to September, followed by red-hooked seed heads that easily latch onto animal fur for efficient seed distribution.

HISTORY: The Latin name for herb bennet is *Geum urbanum*, meaning "to yield a pleasant aroma" (*Geum*) and "of towns" (*urbanum*).

Sometimes herb bennet is referred to as the "blessed herb", due to religious associations: it has a trefoiled leaf and five yellow petals, which are said to represent the Holy Trinity and the five wounds of Christ. For this reason, representations of the plant were often depicted in architectural sculptures that appeared on columns and wall patterns in churches.

The root has a delicious smell and flavour of cloves when freshly dug up and has been used as a seasoning in cooking for centuries, well before the spice cloves made it to British shores.

Augsburg ale brewed in southern Germany places a small bag of herb bennet in each wooden cask to impart a subtle clove-like flavour to the drink, as well as preventing it from turning sour.

FOLKLORE: With its reputation of being a "blessed herb", no wonder herb bennet was regarded as an incredibly powerful tool of protection.

The 1491 Latin natural history encyclopedia, *Ortus Sanitatis*, which translates as "the garden of health", states:

> *"Where the root is in the house, Satan can do nothing and flies from it, wherefore it is blessed before all other herbs, and if a man carries the root about him no venomous beast can harm him."*

Hanging herb bennet above your door was believed to prevent the devil from entering your home. The roots were used as a protective amulet carried against evil spirits, snakes and rabid dogs as well as being used in purification rites and exorcisms.

FOLK MEDICINE: Culpeper had many uses for herb bennet:

> *"The root in the spring time steeped in wine, give it a delicate savour and taste, and being drank fasting every morning, comforteth the heart, and is a good preservative against the plague, or any other poison."*

Grieve is very specific in telling us when the root should be dug up: *"25th of March was fixed for procuring the root. At this time the root was said to be most fragrant."* She cautions us that the root *"must be dried with great care [...] and powdered as required"*.

Grieve lists a vast number of ailments that herb bennet was used to treat, including sore throat, diarrhoea, fevers, catarrh and headaches, while an infusion was used as a wash to remove spots and freckles.

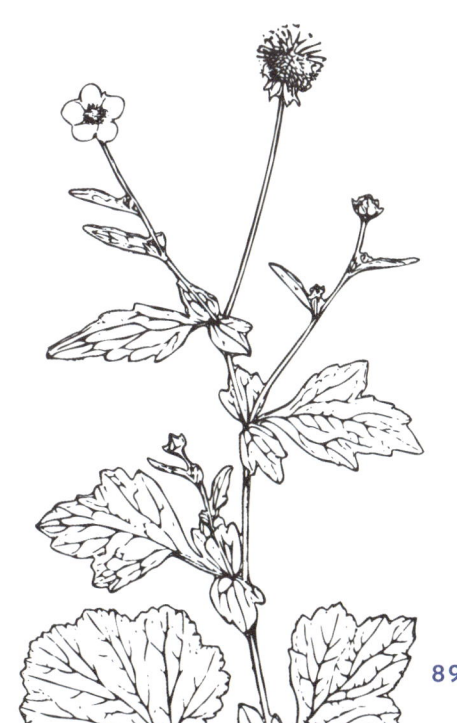

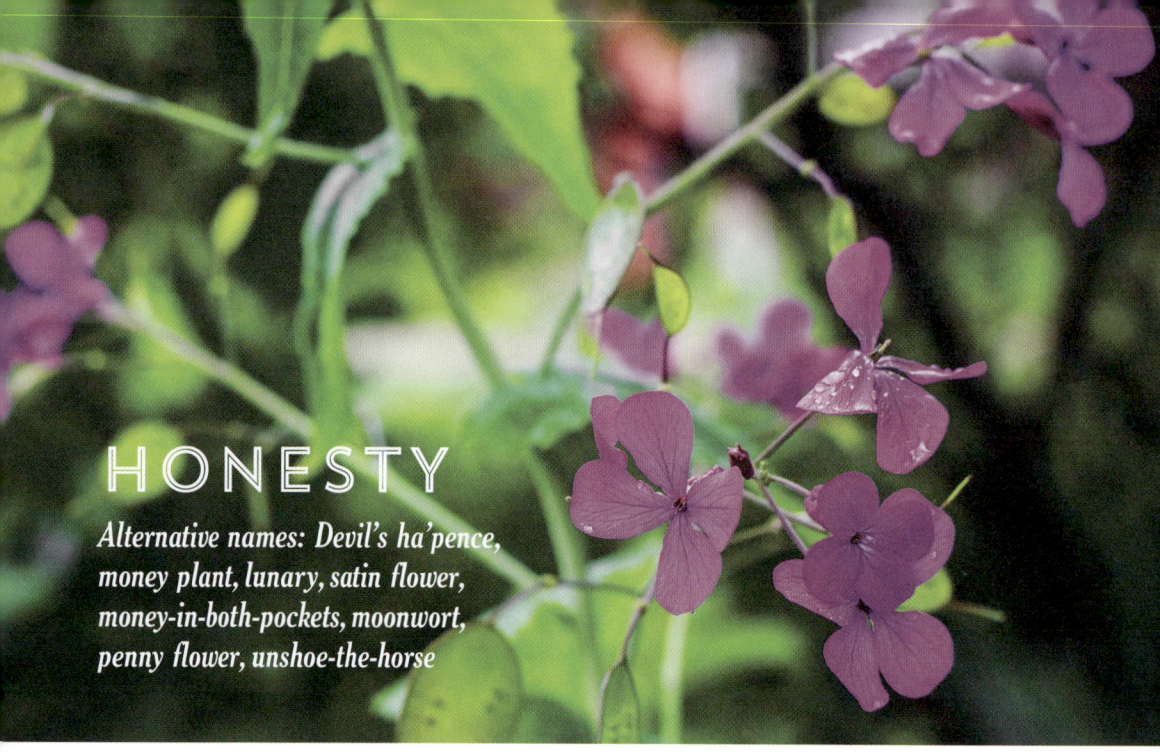

HONESTY

Alternative names: Devil's ha'pence, money plant, lunary, satin flower, money-in-both-pockets, moonwort, penny flower, unshoe-the-horse

HOW TO IDENTIFY: Probably the most recognizable feature of honesty is its seedpods which are oval and translucent, rather reminiscent of the full moon. Magenta four-petalled flowers growing on slender stems burst into life from April to June along riverbanks, waste ground and hedgerows.

HISTORY: The name "honesty" is believed to be a reference to the fact that the seedpods are completely transparent.

Originally introduced into the UK as a garden plant in the sixteenth century from southern Europe, honesty soon escaped the garden gate and became widely naturalized. In 1597, Gerard recorded in his *Herbal* that it could be found *"wilde in the woods about Pinner and Harrow on the Hill, twelve miles from London".*

Honesty is still a cottage-garden favourite. With its sweet scent and blousy dark pink flowers, it is a useful plant to attract butterflies, moths and other beneficial insects.

FOLKLORE: Not surprising considering their resemblance to coins, honesty seed heads are used in money spells: place them in your purse or pocket at the time of the new moon to attract prosperity. As well as being useful to keep away monsters, evil spirits and demons, honesty can break chains, and it can help you to enter the faery realm and magically create gold.

As well as giving his medical opinion, Culpeper shares a little folklore:

> *"Moonwort is an herb which (they say) will open locks and unshoe horses as tread upon it. This some laugh to scorn [...] but country people, call it unshoe the horse. I have heard commanders say that on White Down in Devonshire, near Tiverton, there were found thirty horse shoes, pulled off from the feet of the Earl of Essex's horses, many of them being newly shod, and no reason known."*

In Christianity, honesty is known as "the plant of thirty silver coins" or "Judas' plant", and as a consequence many will not have it in their gardens.

The image of witches flying on broomsticks is one of many popular misconceptions; witches "flew" but perhaps not in the way you expect. The earliest surviving recipe for "flying ointment" was recorded in 1440 by the Bavarian doctor Johannes Hartlieb. Flying ointment was a salve consisting of a variety of plants including honesty, foxglove, hellebore and mugwort, along with some hallucinogenic herbs. Recipes varied from area to area. Witches applied the ointment liberally to their skin, seemingly to get an intense flying experience – what would now be called a "high".

FOLK MEDICINE: Culpeper writes the following of honesty, or "moonwort": *"The moon owns this herb. It stays bleeding, vomiting, and other fluxes. It helps all blows and bruises, and to consolidate all fractures and dislocations. It is good for ruptures..."*

Despite Culpeper's endorsements, honesty hasn't been used widely in folk medicine except for the treatment of skin conditions and as a digestive stimulant.

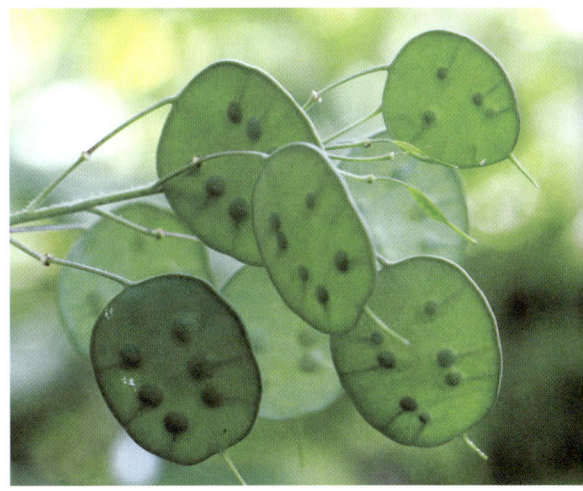

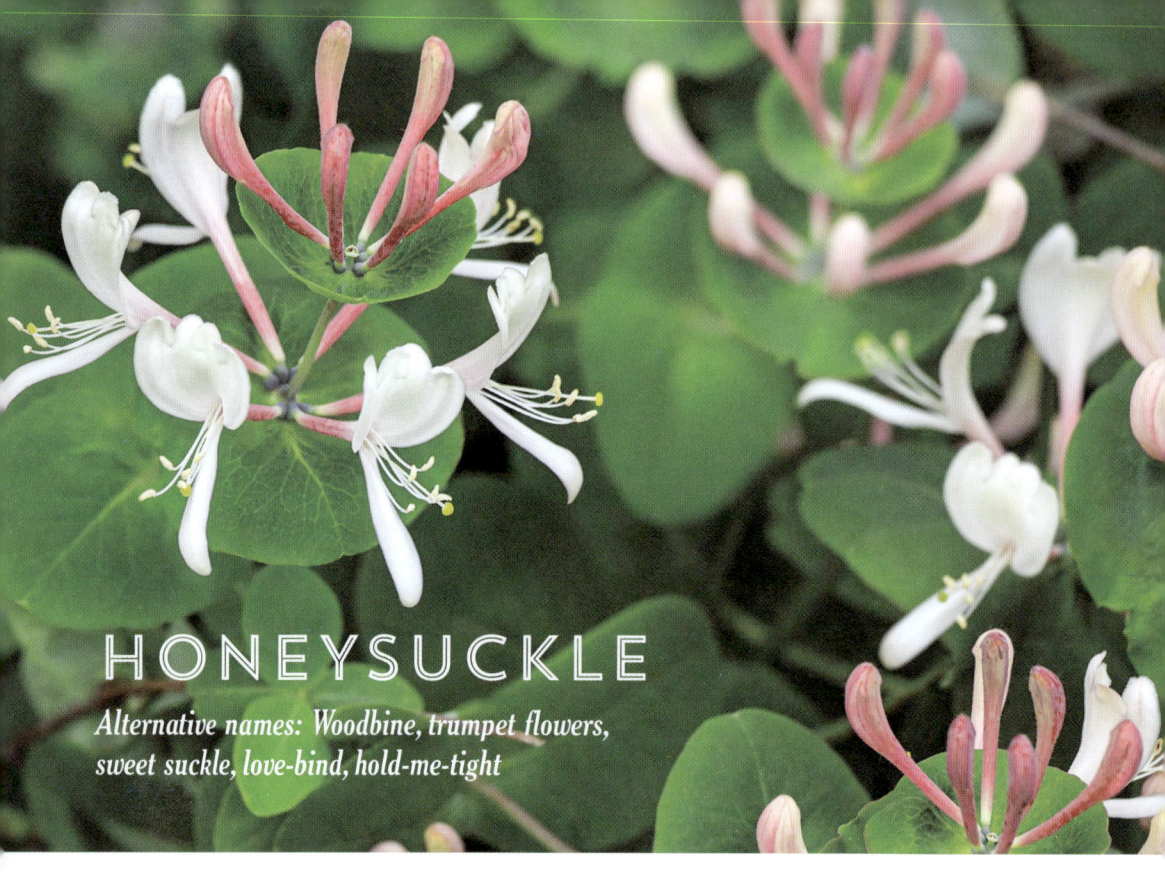

HONEYSUCKLE

Alternative names: Woodbine, trumpet flowers, sweet suckle, love-bind, hold-me-tight

HOW TO IDENTIFY: Slightly smaller than the cultivated variety, wild honeysuckle twirls its way up and around hedgerows and trees creating a heady, sweet scent that is carried on the breeze. Distinctive yellowy-white, trumpet-shaped flowers appear in summer, attracting pollinators at dusk when their scent is at its most fragrant. Clusters of red berries ripen in the autumn to be gratefully devoured by warblers, thrushes and bullfinches.

HISTORY: Countless children over the years have enjoyed sucking the sweet honey-tasting nectar from the base of the trumpet-shaped flowers, hence the name "honeysuckle".

When honeysuckle grows, it winds itself tightly around the host tree, sometimes causing spiralling grooves. Hazel sticks that were misshapen in this way were known as "honeysuckle sticks" and were used as walking sticks, with the added bonus that they were thought to attract luck – especially with the ladies.

FOLKLORE: Honeysuckle is the perfect plant to grow around your doorways. It will bring you wealth and protect your family from illness and black magic, as well as being attractive with a gorgeous fragrance.

Opinion seems to vary from region to region as to whether it was a good idea to bring honeysuckle into the house. In Wales it was considered unlucky, but in Somerset its intertwining stems were believed to encourage a strong marriage and even promote erotic dreams if placed in the bedroom.

Gently crushing fresh honeysuckle flowers on your forehead was said to heighten your psychic powers, while entwining young shoots into a ring and placing them over a candle, preferably a green one, would attract money into the home.

Dreaming of honeysuckle was a bad omen as it indicated that there would be arguments between partners; however a gift of a posy of honeysuckle would ensure fidelity.

FOLK MEDICINE: The leaves are rich in salicylic acid, a component of aspirin, which makes them a useful and effective treatment for headaches, flu, colds and general aches and pains.

The twelfth-century Welsh herbalists, the Physicians of Myddfai, documented their remedy for toothache:

> *"Take the inner bark of the ivy, and the leaves of the honeysuckle, bruising them well together in a mortar, expressing them through a linen cloth into both nostrils, the patient lying on his back, and it will relieve him."*

An infusion of honeysuckle flowers was regularly used in the treatment of asthma and other lung complaints. Culpeper held honeysuckle in very high regard as he knew *"no better cure for asthma"*.

Between the sixteenth and nineteenth centuries, those suffering from migraines, coughs and asthma were encouraged to sit over a bowl of the flowers infusing in hot water, with a cloth over their heads and to breathe in the smell.

Warts were also treated with honeysuckle. A poultice containing the dried flowers was applied to the skin growths – far nicer than some medieval cures for warts involving the use of slugs.

HONEYSUCKLE AND WILD ROSE LIP BALM

This delicious lip balm captures the spirit of two of our most delightful hedgerow flowers, honeysuckle and wild rose.

Honeysuckle flowers are anti-inflammatory, anti-viral and antimicrobial so may help to speed up the healing of cold sores. Rich in antioxidants and vitamin C, rose petals can help to soothe and nourish the lips, leaving them soft and hydrated.

Gather your flowers and petals on a dry day, away from the pollution of busy roads, and try to ensure that they haven't been sprayed with any chemicals.

Remember, anything that you put onto your skin may be absorbed into your bloodstream.

Makes approx. 60 ml

INGREDIENTS

50 ml honeysuckle-and-rose-petal-infused carrier oil (see pages 20–21)

7 g shea butter or mango butter

7 g unbleached beeswax (or 3 g candelilla wax for a plant-based version)

5 drops rose essential oil (optional)

For cold sores, add 5 drops lemon balm essential oil

EQUIPMENT NEEDED

Heatproof bowl

Saucepan

Small jars or tins with lids

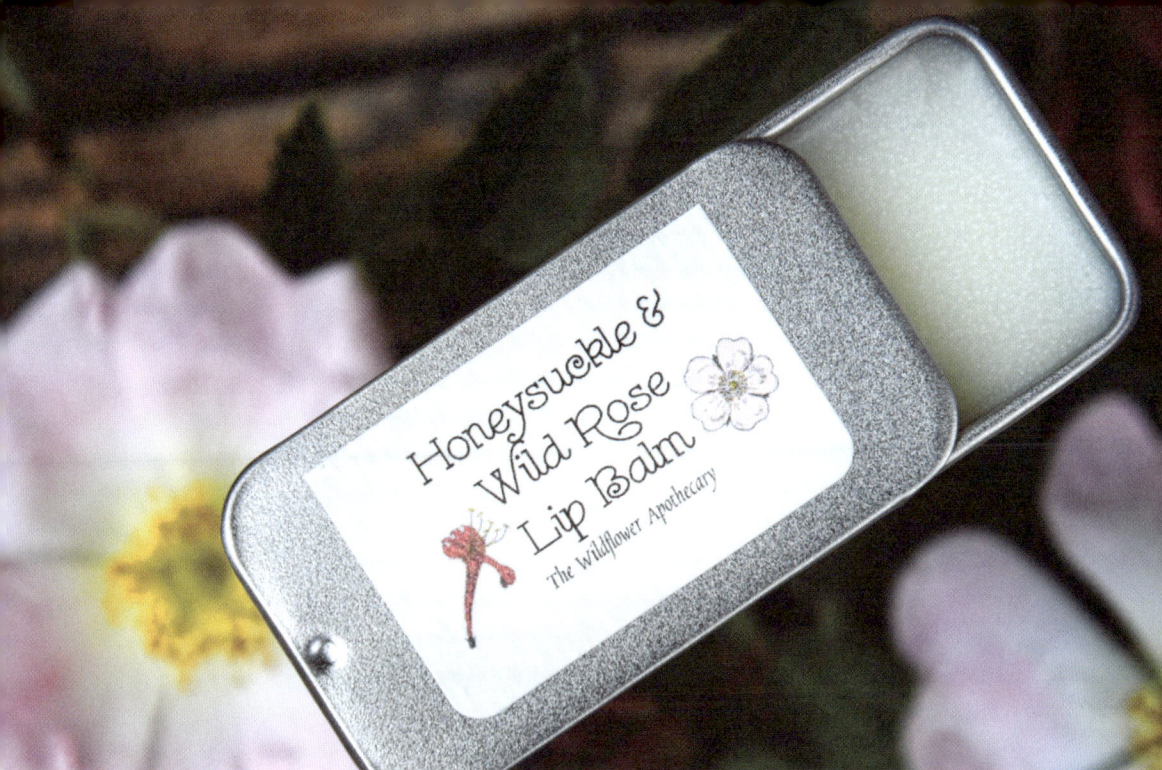

METHOD

Place a heatproof bowl over a pan of boiling water. Put all your ingredients except for the essential oils into the bowl.

Stir gently until everything melts together.

Carefully remove from heat and allow to cool for a couple of minutes.

Stir in your essential oils if using.

Pour the cooled lip balm into jars or small lip balm tins.

Allow to cool completely before popping on the lids.

The lip balm will keep for 6–12 months.

Not recommended if taking anti-coagulant medications. Always do a patch test.

LADY'S BEDSTRAW

Alternative names: Lady's golden bedstraw, creeping Jenny, cheese rennet, maiden's hair, robin-run-the-hedge

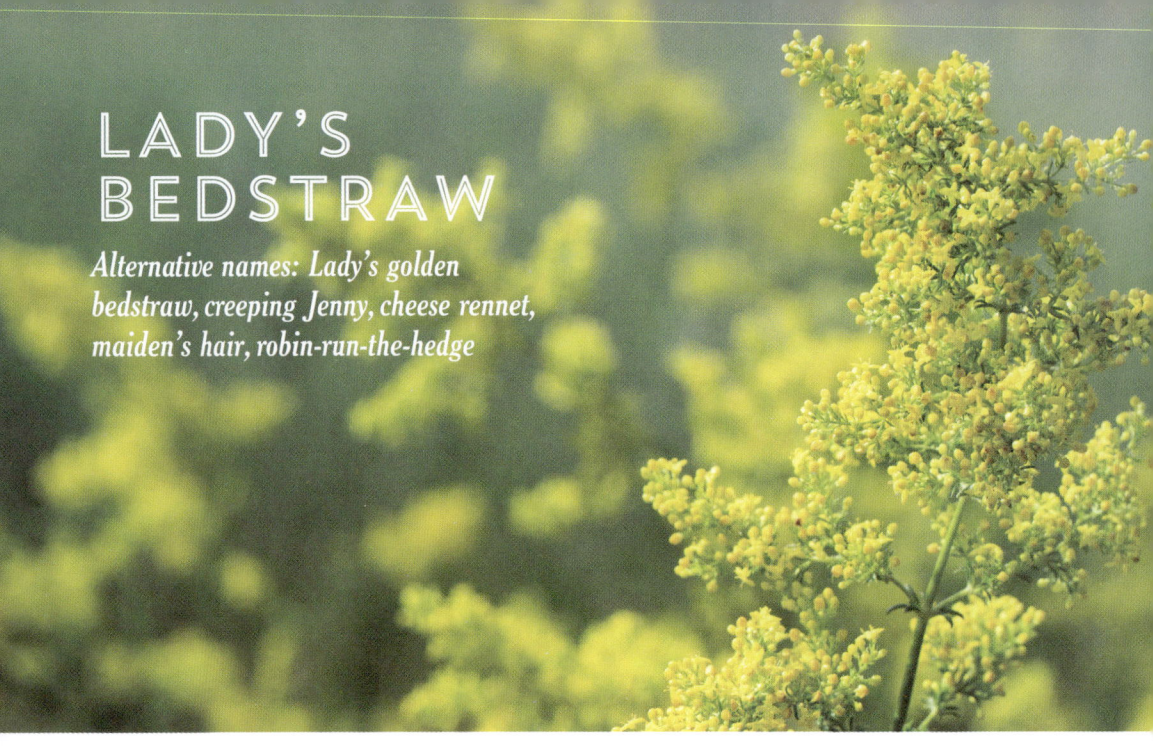

HOW TO IDENTIFY: Flowering from June to September, lady's bedstraw is most likely to be found on chalk downlands, meadows, sand dunes and in hedgerows, growing only to about 30-cm (12-in.) tall with whorls of shiny leaves growing up its angular stem. Small, frothy, densely packed yellow flowers erupt which some say smell of honey, others of new-mown hay.

HISTORY: The pleasant scent of lady's bedstraw has been much-utilized over the centuries. Once dried, it was placed among medieval clothing to repel moths and make the garments smell sweet. Lady's bedstraw was the perfect choice for the stuffing of mattresses and pillows, since it was soft and springy, smelled divine, had insect-repellent properties and was believed to bring sweet dreams and protection from nightmares.

Historically lady's bedstraw has been used in cheesemaking. The flowers have the ability to curdle milk without the use of animal rennet, giving double Gloucester cheese its distinctive yellow colour for many centuries.

Ladies in the court of Henry VIII gave their hair a yellow tint by packing the flowers under their caps. Red, orange and yellow dye can be obtained from the plant, which was once used to dye wool for the Harris Tweed industry.

FOLKLORE: The plant's use in bedding was believed to be particularly beneficial for ladies giving birth, ensuring a safe and easy childbirth. One German custom suggests that the plant got its name because the baby Jesus was placed in a crib filled with lady's bedstraw and bracken. Bracken refused to acknowledge the baby Jesus and as a result her flowers were taken away. Bedstraw blossomed to welcome the baby and its plain white flowers were turned to gold.

In Romania, it is believed that on 9 March every year the lady's bedstraw faery is born. She is fully grown by 24 June and is celebrated in the festival of sânziană to thank her for granting abundance to crops and for the healing powers of her flowers.

FOLK MEDICINE: Gerard recorded in 1636 that lady's bedstraw *"is used in ointments against burnings, and it stancheth blood: it is put into cerote [wax] or cere-cloth of roses [cloth soaked in wax;] it is set a sunning in a glass, with olive oil, until it be white: it is good to anoint the wearied traveller: the root thereof drunk in wine stirreth up bodily lust; and the flowers smelled unto work the same effect".*

In 1653, Culpeper refers to its usefulness to *"stay inward bleedings, and to heal inward wounds; the herb or flower bruised, and put up into the nostrils, stayeth their bleeding likewise".* He states that an ointment made from infusing lady's bedstraw can *"helpeth the dry scab, and the itch in children; and the herb with the white flower is also very good for the sinews, arteries and joints, to comfort and strengthen them after travel, cold and pains".*

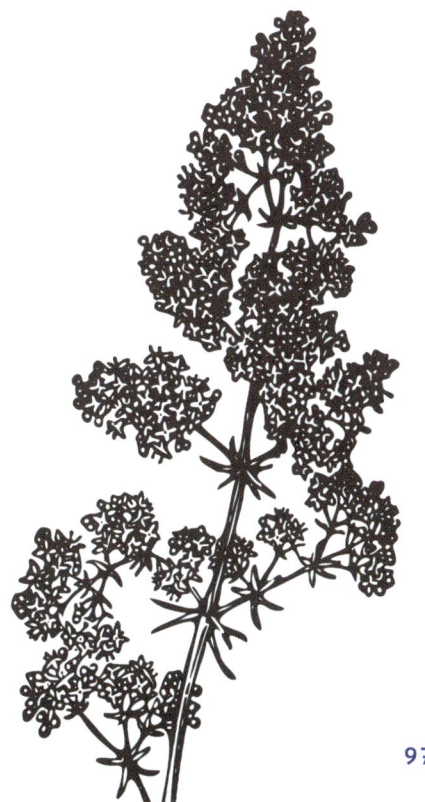

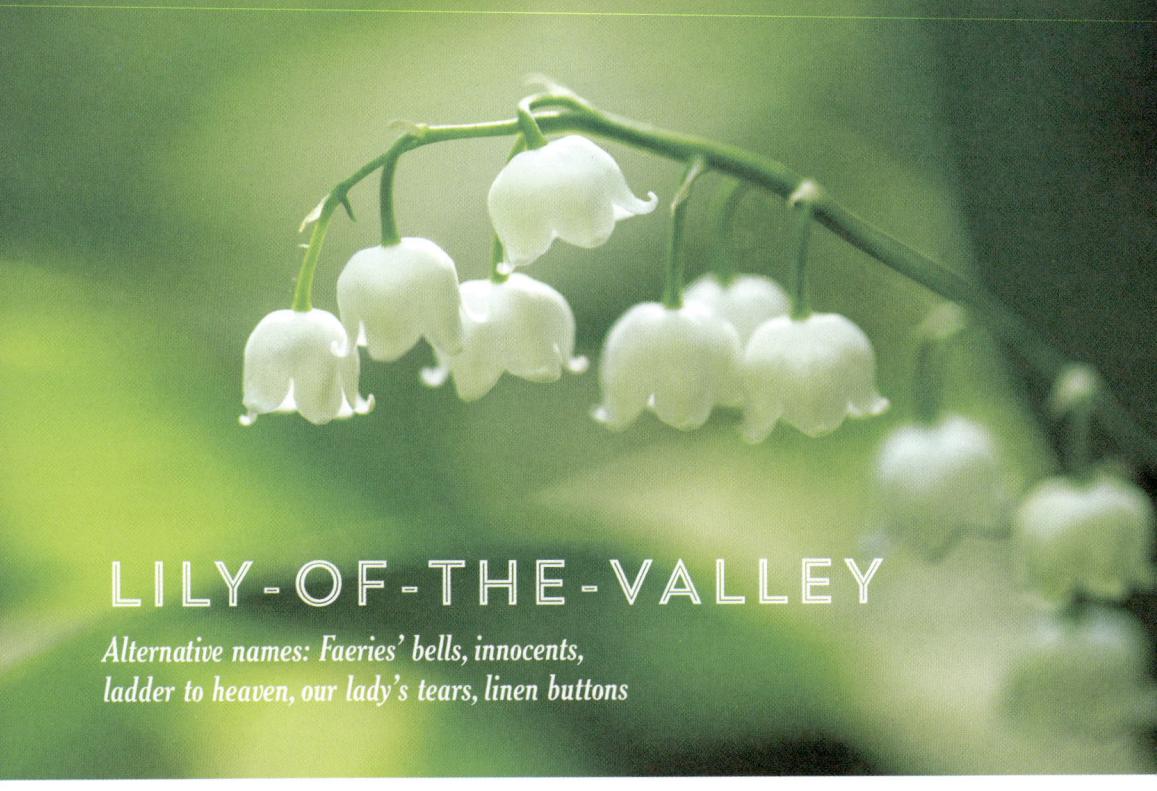

LILY-OF-THE-VALLEY

Alternative names: Faeries' bells, innocents, ladder to heaven, our lady's tears, linen buttons

HOW TO IDENTIFY: Most likely to be found on woodland floors, lily-of-the-valley is a diminutive plant with an incredibly powerful scent. Delicate white bell-shaped flowers dangle from bowed stems, which emerge from pairs of large, glossy, spear-like leaves from May to June.

HISTORY: Ancient woodlands are areas that have not been disturbed since 1600 CE in England, Wales and Northern Ireland or 1750 CE in Scotland. These woodlands host an incredibly diverse ecosystem, making them important habitats for many of our threatened species.

Ancient woodland indicators include lily-of-the-valley, bluebell, dog's mercury, red campion and wild garlic, plus lichen, ferns and spindle. If you see any or a combination of these, chances are you are fortunate enough to have discovered an ancient woodland.

These precious habitats cover only 2.5 per cent of the UK compared to 16 per cent in the seventeenth century. Sadly they are under constant threat from development, pollution and encroachment of invasive species.

FOLKLORE: In Christian symbolism, the lily-of-the-valley is revered as a symbol of purity, humility and redemption. Christian lore tells that the Virgin Mary's tears at the cross blossomed into these flowers, earning them the name "our lady's tears".

To protect the home from evil spirits and ghosts, British folklore tells us to plant lily-of-the-valley in gardens, although another piece of lore tells us that a gardener who plants a bed of lily-of-the-valley will suffer an untimely death.

In Ireland, a charming folklore tells us of the creation of lily-of-the-valley:

> *"Five fairy sisters were sent out to gather dew for the fairy queen in tiny white cups. The naughty faeries hung their cups on a blade of grass and danced and played unaware that the sun was coming up. No faerie should be caught outside after sunrise, in fright they ran to get their cups only to find that the handles had stuck fast to the blade of grass and could not be freed! Luckily for them their kindly godmother appeared who, wanting to protect the little girls from the queen's anger, tied a big green leaf to either side of the cups to hide them."*

FOLK MEDICINE: In the Middle Ages, lily-of-the-valley was believed to improve your cognitive ability. The little flower was acclaimed for its ability to enhance mental acuteness and rejuvenate memory. Herbalists prescribed it in concoctions aimed at clarifying thoughts and sharpening perception.

Culpeper agrees with the medieval herbalists, stating: *"It strengthens the brain, recruits a weak memory, and makes it strong again"*, and that *"the distilled water dropped into the eyes, helps inflammation there; as also the infirmity which they call a pin and web [cataracts]."*

He quotes his predecessor Gerard: *"that flowers being close stopped up in a glass, put into an ant hill, and taken away again a month after, ye shall find a liquor in the glass, which, being outwardly applied, helps the gout".*

All parts of lily-of-the-valley are toxic.

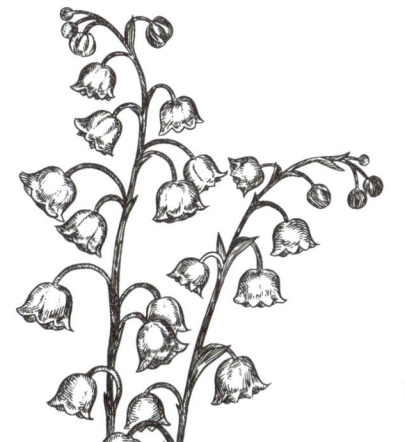

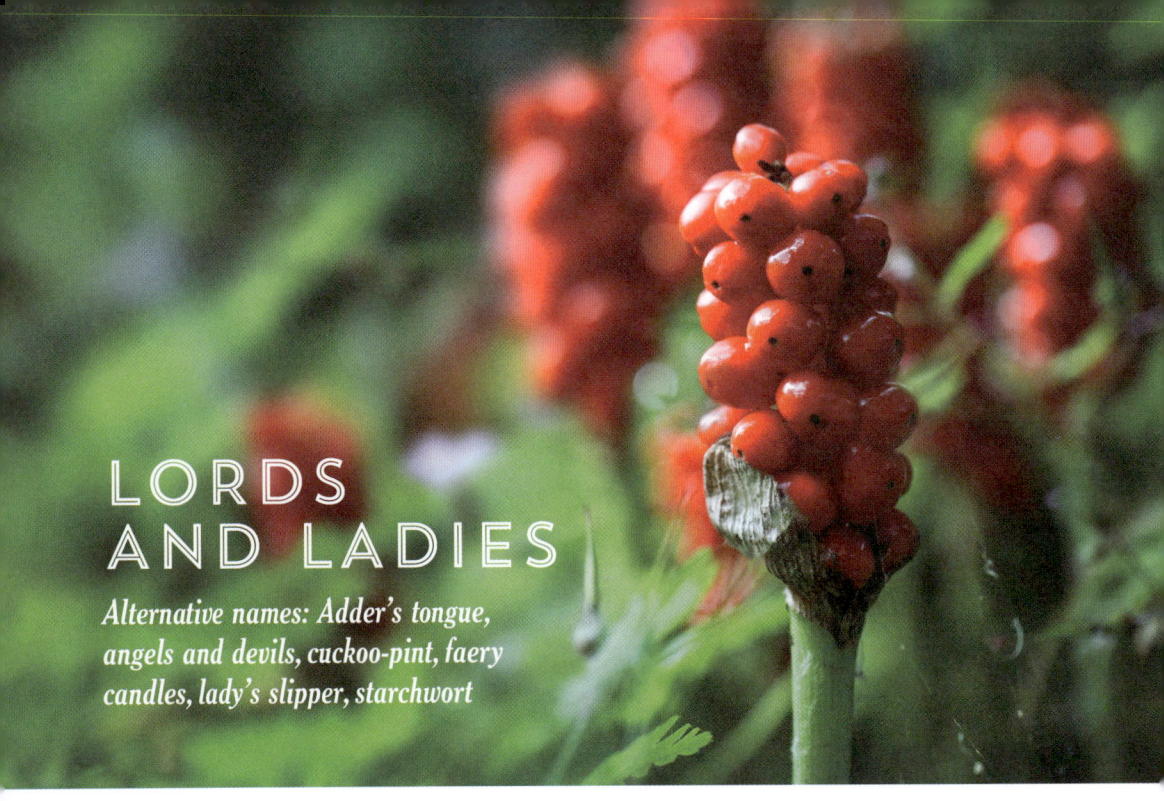

LORDS AND LADIES

Alternative names: Adder's tongue, angels and devils, cuckoo-pint, faery candles, lady's slipper, starchwort

HOW TO IDENTIFY: Large, shiny, arrowhead-shaped leaves appear in early spring, sometimes dotted with black splodges. In April and May, a pale green pointed sheath surrounds a spike of tiny yellow flowers, then in autumn the spike turns into a stalk of bright red berries. Lords and ladies are a lover of shady spots and can be spotted along hedgerows and in woodlands.

HISTORY: The elaborate ruffs worn around the necks by the upper classes in the sixteenth century needed to be stiffened in order to keep their shape. Known as "starchwort" to country folk, lords and ladies provided the answer. Gerard commented:

"The most pure and white starch is made of the roots of Cuckoo-Pint [lords and ladies]; but most hurtful to the hands of the laundress that hath the handling of it for it choppeth, blistereth, and maketh the hands rough and rugged, and withal smarting."

Starch could also be obtained from bluebells and wheat, but lords and ladies were considered to be far superior despite the detrimental effect on the poor laundry workers. It was in constant use until ruffs went out of fashion and the use of lords and ladies was pretty much forgotten.

FOLKLORE: The mythology of lords and ladies is studded with tales of mystery, snakes, sexual activity and death. The Victorians, being extremely prudish, viewed it with deep suspicion – although in the language of flowers it had a very clear meaning: "My heart is aflame with passion!"

Lords and ladies seems to have had quite a reputation as a powerful aphrodisiac, due to parts of the plant resembling sexual organs. In some rural areas it was even believed that a maid could become pregnant just by touching or looking at the plant.

In order to catch the attention of the prettiest girl at a dance, a man should take a small piece of the flowering spike in his shoe while reciting:

*"I place you in my shoe,
Let all the young girls be drawn to you."*

When it's ready for pollination, the spike emits a smell and a warm glow. In Ireland this led to the plant being known as "faery lamps", when in fact the fluorescence is a clever way for the plant to attract insects.

FOLK MEDICINE: Despite its caustic nature, Culpeper still used lords and ladies in his remedies:

"The green leaves bruised, and laid upon any boil or plague-sore, do very wonderfully help to draw forth the poison."

He wasn't even particularly cautious about its use for cataracts:

"The water wherein the root hath been boiled, dropped into the eyes, cleanseth them from any film or skin, or cloud or mist, which begin to hinder the sight."

In the eighteenth century, the juice was distilled and applied to the face as an anti-ageing treatment, while the root was used to help cure asthma, ruptures, scurvy and wind.

All parts of lords and ladies are poisonous and can irritate the skin.

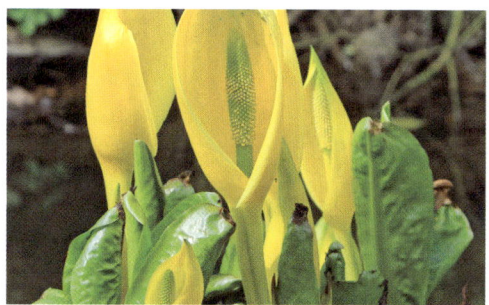

LUNGWORT

Alternative names: Soldiers and sailors, Joseph and Mary, spotted Mary, Mary-spilt-the-milk, spotted dog, Jerusalem cowslip, Mary's tears

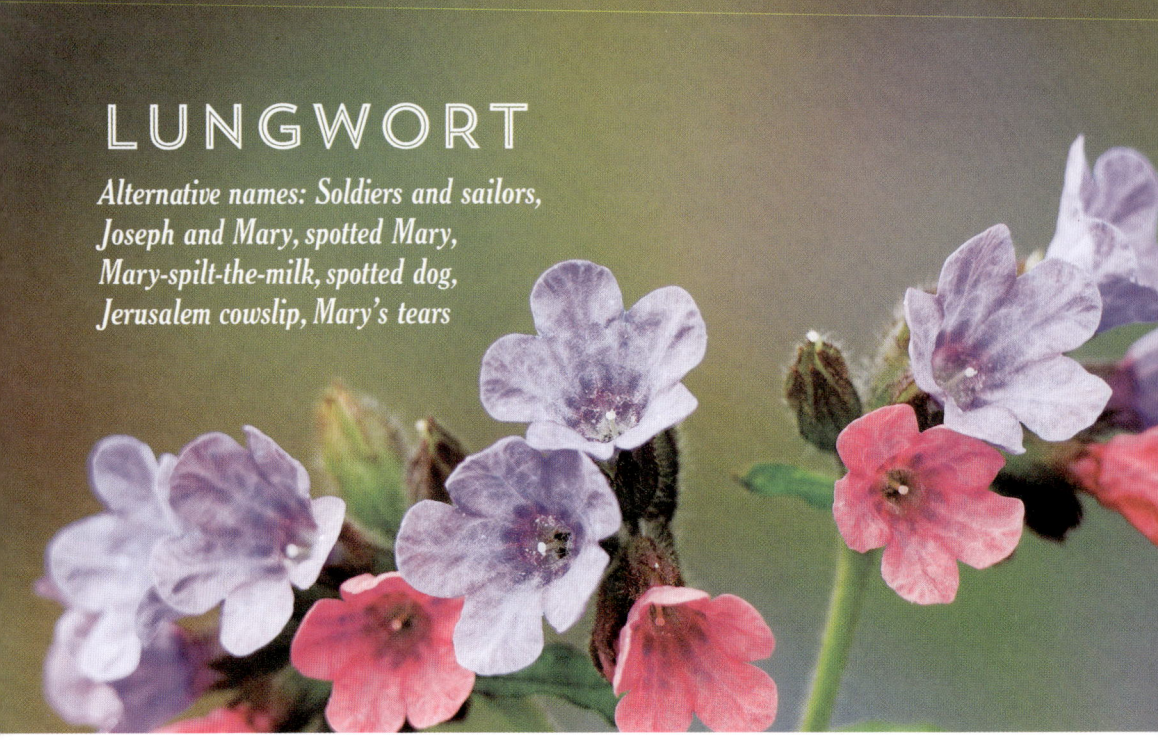

HOW TO IDENTIFY: The most distinctive feature of lungwort is its oval leaves covered in white spots, said to resemble lungs, hence the name. Lungwort prefers to grow in clumps in damp, shady woodlands. Clusters of funnel-shaped pink flowers appear in March, changing gradually to blue in June.

HISTORY: Lungwort is one of the original wildflowers of the European woodlands and for centuries has been one of many herbal ingredients in the alcoholic drink vermouth.

The leaves of the plant contain a purple pigment which has been used for dyeing wool and other textiles. The colour can be altered from purple to grey, depending on the pH of the mordant used.

FOLKLORE: In Christian folklore lungwort was also known as "Mary's tears" as the white spots on the leaves supposedly came about as Mary wept at the crucifixion of Jesus. The flowers' colours of blue and pink represented her eyes – she had wept so much that her eyes had become sore.

In Russian folklore, the changing colours of the lungwort flower were said to embody the different stages of life: young pink blooms to represent youth and young, blue flowers for healing during adult life. The older blue flowers were said to have lost their strength and were ready to be absorbed back into the soil.

Lungwort is associated with youth, beauty, good luck and happiness, and is said to have the power to restore physical and spiritual welfare.

FOLK MEDICINE: Lungwort was named according to the "doctrine of signatures", which believes that God put every plant onto the earth for the benefit of man and created it to resemble the part of the body that it could heal. Lungwort has a long history of being used to treat many ailments of humans and animals, particularly those of the lungs.

In the eleventh century, German abbess Hildegard von Bingen wrote of lungwort: *"If sheep eat Lungwort often, they will become healthy and fat [...] But if, as we have said, one who has a swollen lung frequently drinks Lungwort cooked in wine, his lung will return to health, since the lung has the nature of a sheep."*

Gerard tells us that *"The leaves are used among pot-herbs. The roots are also thought to be good against the infirmities and ulcers of the lungs."*

Culpeper expands on the uses of lungwort: *"It is of great use to physicians to help the diseases of the lungs, and for coughs, wheezings, and shortness of breath, which it cures in both man and beast [...] It is an excellent remedy boiled in beer for broken-winded horses."*

He goes on to detail other uses: *"It is very profitable to put into lotions that are taken to stay the moist humours that flow to ulcers, and hinder their healing, as also to wash all other ulcers in the privy parts of a man or woman."*

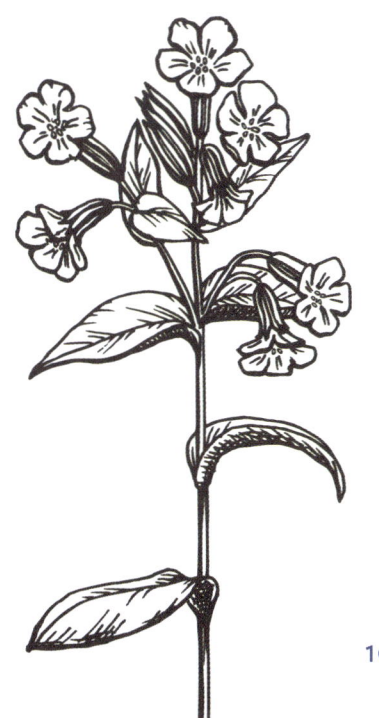

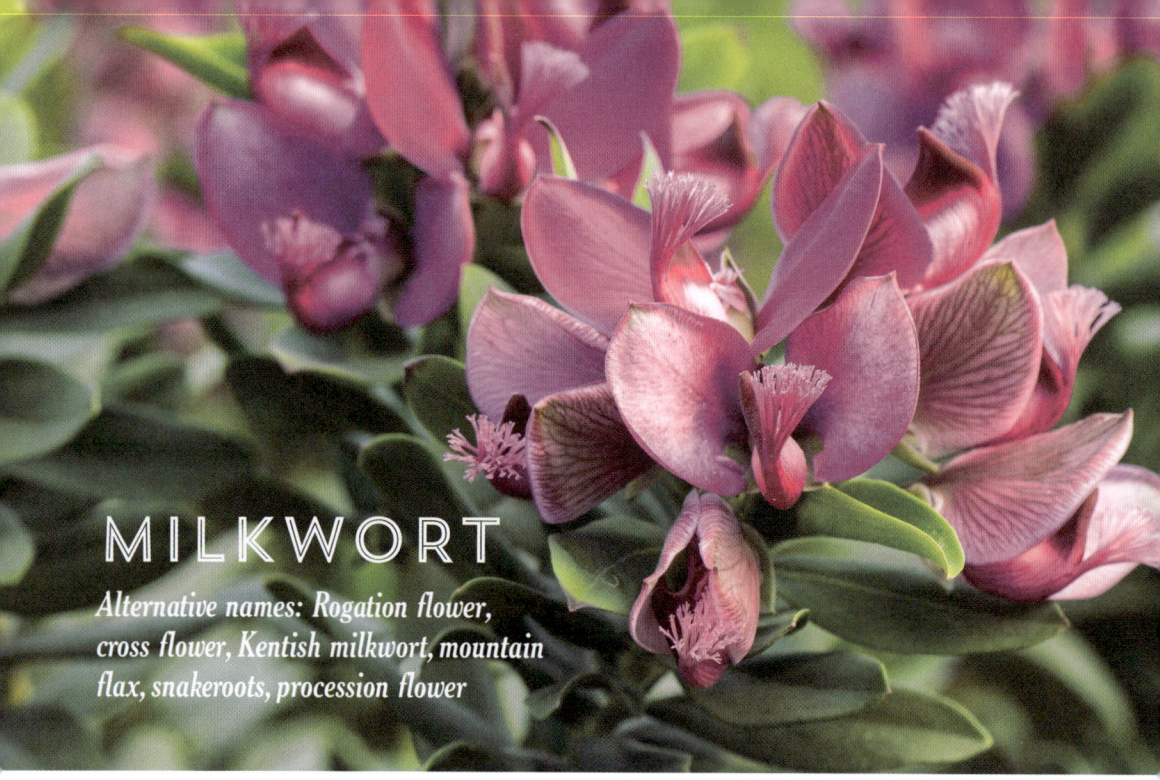

MILKWORT

Alternative names: Rogation flower, cross flower, Kentish milkwort, mountain flax, snakeroots, procession flower

HOW TO IDENTIFY: This dainty blue flower thrives in chalk grassland, sand dunes and moorland. The blooms can also be seen in pink or white from May to September. With narrow pointed leaves similar to thyme, milkwort is low-growing with clusters of flowers on top of the stems.

HISTORY: Part of the Catholic Church's Easter calendar, Rogation days are the Monday, Tuesday and Wednesday leading up to the feast of Ascension, which is the fortieth day after Easter Sunday. On these days the priest would lead the congregation around the local fields to bless the crops and livestock, pray for a good harvest and confirm the parish boundaries. Village children would join the procession, carrying a pole decorated with a profusion of flowers, including milkwort.

This practice was recorded as early as 550 CE and carried on despite protests that it was too superstitious, seeming to continue the pagan rituals it had replaced. Some modifications were introduced during the reign of Elizabeth I to disassociate the custom from its Catholic roots. It became known as "beating the bounds", which still happens in some rural parishes to this day.

FOLKLORE: Milkwort has long been used in rituals and spells to ward off evil spirits, false friends, liars and "snakes in the grass", as well as actual snakes. Powdered milkwort dusted into shoes could shield you from any spells laid in the dirt to trap you.

In Nordic mythology, milkwort was associated with the goddess Frigg, who was said to have used the plant to increase her power and influence.

And in medieval times, dairymaids worried that their milk could be bewitched, rendering it useless as it could not then be made into cheese or butter. A "magic hoop" was fashioned out of flowers, including milkwort, and the dairy bowl placed inside it to protect it from witches. Milkwort was put into milk that was believed to have been bewitched to reverse the spell.

FOLK MEDICINE: As the name and perhaps the udder-shaped flowers suggest, milkwort was believed to have the ability to increase milk production in new mothers and animals. A mother who was struggling to breastfeed her baby should boil up milkwort and drink the resultant bitter-tasting beverage, as this was sure to increase her milk flow.

Gerard makes little mention of the maternal benefits of milkwort, but recommends it to cure angry and ill tempers: *"An handful hereof steeped all night in wine, and drunk in the morning, will purge choler [bad temper] effectually by stool without any danger."*

Traditionally, milkwort has been made into infusions for the treatment of coughs and bronchitis. It was also boiled in milk and used as a lotion to help heal the scars of smallpox.

On Guernsey, milkwort is known as *herbe de paralysie* and was used in the treatment of strokes and paralysis.

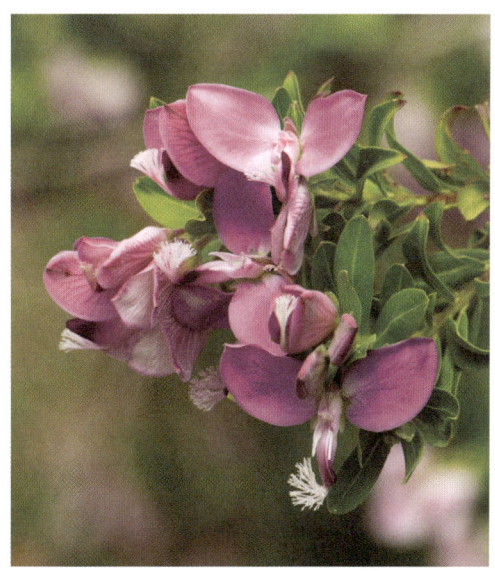

MUGWORT

Alternative names: Maiden's wort, naughty man, crone wort, witch herb, sailor's tobacco

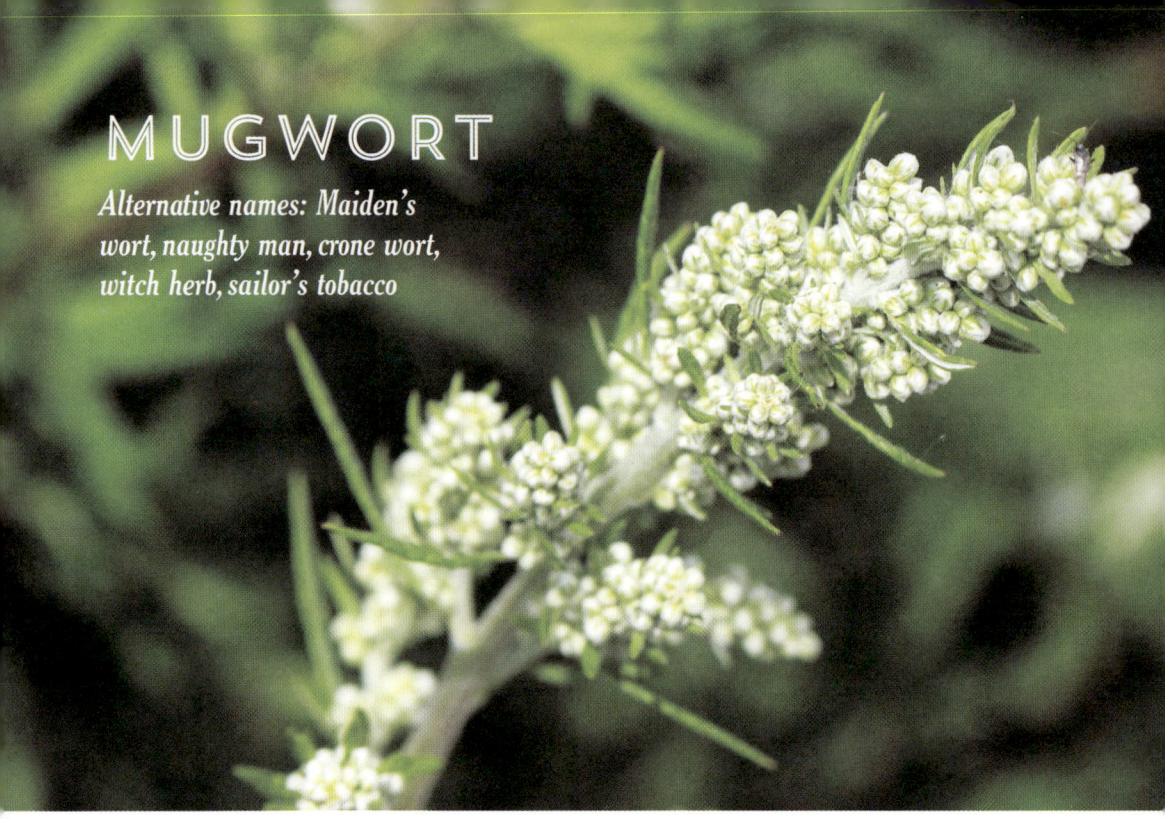

HOW TO IDENTIFY: This hardy plant grows on wasteland and verges and can grow up to 2 m (6 ft) tall. The leaves are delicate and finely lobed, dark green on the uppermost side, and covered in dense silvery hairs on the underside. Mugwort is in bloom from June to September, with tiny clusters of whitish-green flowers and a distinct fragrance of sage.

HISTORY: One of the nine sacred herbs of the Anglo-Saxons, mugwort was dried and burned during rituals and ceremonies to protect and cleanse, as well as to enhance spiritual awakening.

Medieval ale called "gruit" was brewed using mugwort, myrtle and yarrow, and was to be served in large "mugs"; it is thought this is how the plant got its name. However, other theories suggest that the name comes from the plant's ability to deter midges and moths, or "muggia".

In twelfth-century Wales, the Physicians of Myddfai knew the usefulness of mugwort as an insecticide: *"to destroy flies, let the mugwort be put in a place where they are frequent and they will die."*

FOLKLORE: Mugwort has a long association with protection. St John the Baptist is believed to have worn a girdle of mugwort around his waist to protect himself from the Devil when he went into the wilderness. Later, in medieval times, it was thought that if you dug up a mugwort plant on Midsummer's Eve you would find a "coal". Carrying this with you protected you from witchcraft, lightning, plague, infected swellings and burning.

Bunches of mugwort were hung above medieval doorways to protect against evil entering the home. As recently as the nineteenth century, German people wore headdresses of mugwort and vervain while looking at a bonfire through bunches of larkspur to keep their eyes healthy for another year. As they left the fireside, they threw their headdresses into the fire, saying, *"May all my ill luck depart and be burnt up with these."*

Mugwort was used to predict the future, with an infusion used to clean crystal balls and scrying mirrors. Burning incense made from mugwort and sandalwood was used to aid concentration for the psychic.

FOLK MEDICINE: Known as *mater herbarum* or "mother of herbs", mugwort was traditionally used in childbirth, for fertility and virginity. It was widely used for "women's problems": for balancing the menstrual cycle and helping with cases of difficult childbirth. Culpeper considered it *"an herb of Venus"*, writing: *"Its tops, leaves and flowers are full of virtue, they are aromatic, and most safe and excellent for female disorders."*

It was also used to relieve aching feet. Roman soldiers wrapped mugwort around their feet to prevent weariness while marching. And in 1656, William Coles wrote: *"And if a footman take mugwort and put it into his shoes in the morning, he may goe forty miles before noon and not be weary."*

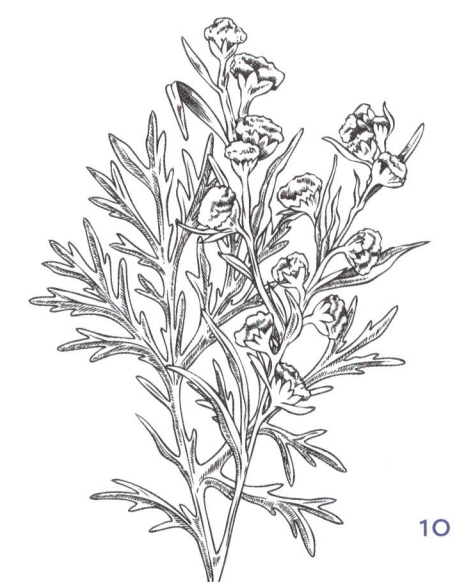

NAVELWORT

Alternative names: Pennywort, marsh pennywort, penny-pies, kidneywort, ladies navell

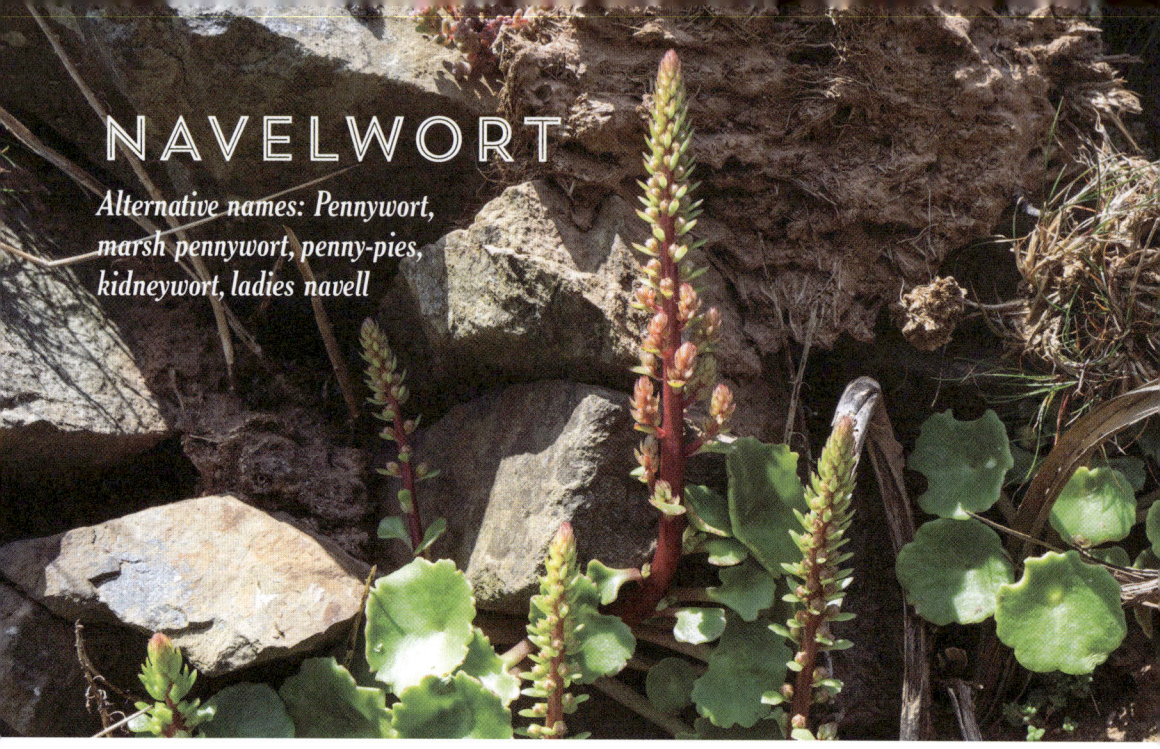

HOW TO IDENTIFY: If a plant ever resembled its name, then navelwort is definitely it. Navelwort leaves are fleshy and circular with a dimple in the centre, quite clearly resembling tummy buttons. Living in the cracks of walls or stony outcrops, navelwort throws up tall, flowering spikes covered in pink or white bell-shaped flowers, similar to foxgloves, from June to August.

HISTORY: Gerard recorded a few places that he had seen pennywort, as he called it, noting the plant *"groweth plentifully in Northampton upon every stone wall about the town, at Bristol, Bath, Wells [...] it groweth upon Westminster Abbey, over the door that leadeth from Chaucer's tomb to the old palace".*

Botanist Richard Anthony Salisbury (1761–1829) was responsible for giving navelwort its Latin name *Umbilicus rupestris*. *Umbilicus* as, unusually, the leaf stems emerge from the centre of the leaf, similar to an umbilical cord, and *rupestris*, meaning to live on rocks. Salisbury was a controversial figure, shunned by his botanist contemporaries for his methods of classifying plants. Robert Brown said of Salisbury: *"I scarcely know what to think of* him except that he stands between a rogue and a fool." Salisbury's work was later re-examined by The International Code of Nomenclature and he was declared *"an accomplished and painstaking botanist".*

Children used to prick a hole through the middle point of the green, succulent leaves and put posies of small flowers through the opening. The circular leaves were also used as imitation coins for games.

FOLKLORE: Traditional folkloric uses for navelwort are very thin on the ground; however there exists one of unknown origin for predicting the weather:

> *"Select two of the largest navelwort leaves that you can find, spit on them generously and stick the two together. Throw them up into the air, if they come apart then dry weather is expected, if they stick together then rain is on the way."*

FOLK MEDICINE: In Ancient Rome the plant was nicknamed "Venus's navel" after the goddess of love and fertility. Looking at the photo, it's easy to see what they used it for!

In Irish folk medicine it was a cure for corns, chilblains, jaundice, worms and kidney stones, and the sap was dripped onto bee stings to ease the pain. In Cornwall the skin was removed from the underside of the leaf which was then applied to corns, chilblains and warts, and it was a handy plaster to help draw out splinters and thorns.

Gerard describes navelwort as *"a singular remedy against all inflammations and hot tumors, as erysipelas [skin infections], Saint Anthony's fire [a disease caused by eating contaminated rye] and such like, and is good for kibed [cracked] heels [...] one or more of the leaves laid upon the heel".*

Culpeper observes: *"Being used as a bath, or made into an ointment, it cools the painful piles or haemorrhoidal veins".*

Grieve tells us rather disparagingly that *"It is applied by the peasantry in Wales as a remedy in some diseases. The leaves, bruised, to a pulp and applied as a poultice [...] are recommended as an application for slight burns or scalds."*

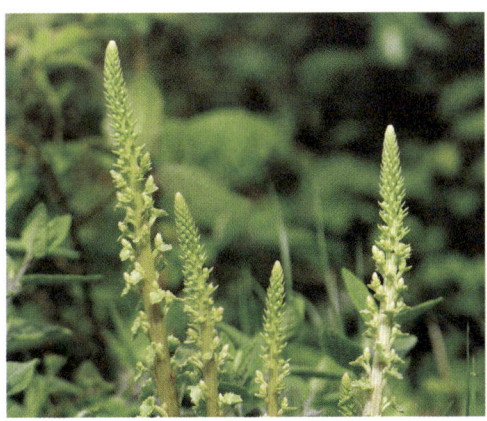

NETTLE

Alternative names: Stinging nettle, devil's plaything, burn nettle, hoky-poky, naughty man's plaything

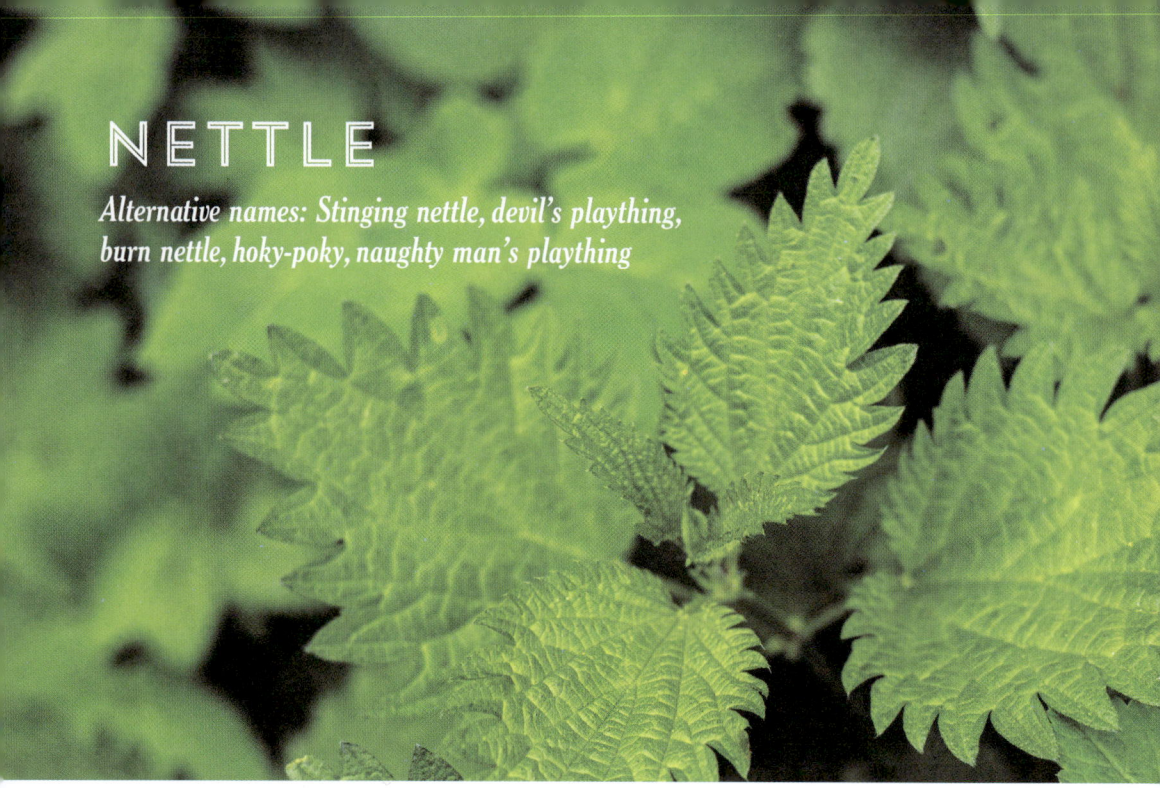

HOW TO IDENTIFY: Growing everywhere that there may be vulnerable bare arms and legs, nettles are often felt before they are seen! Dark green, hairy, heart-shaped stinging leaves are set opposite each other in pairs along a tall, straight stem. The flowers form at the base of the leaves and are greenish-white with yellow anthers.

HISTORY: The nettle stem contains long, strong fibres that have been spun into thread since the Bronze Age for weaving into cloth and making cord.

During World War One, when cotton was scarce, nettle fibre was cultivated on a huge scale to be woven into uniforms for German and Austrian soldiers. Green dye made from the nettles helped to make camouflage uniforms for the British Army during World War Two, and there were even plans to construct aircraft wings from nettle fibres.

Wartime shortages led to many people using nettles in their cooking, as they were a good source of iron and vitamin C. However, according to folklore, nettles are best eaten young and certainly before May

Day as after this they will become tough, because the devil is gathering them to make his shirts.

FOLKLORE: Nettles were used to thrash the devil out of poor souls believed to be possessed. Sprinkling chopped nettle around the house would offer protection from evil; nettles in the dairy stopped witches curdling the milk; and to keep the family safe from danger, some nettle would be thrown into the fire.

Folklore surrounding this stinging plant extends beyond the spirit world. Holding a nettle during a thunderstorm, if you could tolerate the stings, would prevent you from getting struck by lightning, while carrying yarrow with nettles would help you become fearless – useful during a thunderstorm!

Finally, if you desired luscious locks, you could try combing nettle juice through your hair and massaging it onto your scalp. Nettle was believed to stimulate hair growth, and this remedy would make your hair soft and glossy and prevent it from falling out.

FOLK MEDICINE: It was believed that a fever could be cured by picking a nettle by its roots while reciting the name of the sick person and the names of their parents. An old remedy for arthritis and rheumatism involved whipping the affected joints with fresh nettles – this reportedly gave some pain relief, despite the nasty nettle rash!

Gerard was clearly a fan of nettles:

"It is good for them that cannot breathe unless they hold their necks upright, and for those that have the pleurisy, and for such as be sick of the inflammation of the lungs if it be taken in a lohoch or licking medicine, and also against the troublesome cough that children have, called the chincough [whooping cough]."

In the seventeenth century, earache was soothed by dripping freshly squeezed nettle juice into the ears. Mix nettle juice with egg white and rub onto temples to cure insomnia or use it to ease burns and rashes.

When foraging for nettles for a folk remedy, it must be gathered in complete silence at midnight for the best results.

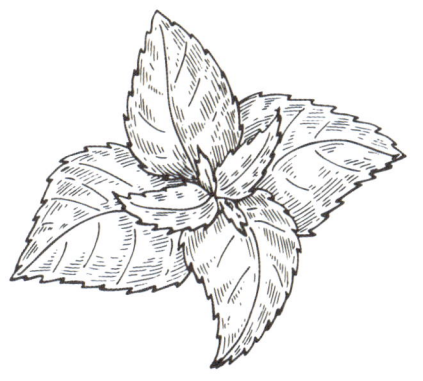

NETTLE LOTION BAR FOR STIFF JOINTS

Dried nettle leaves and seeds are known to have potent anti-inflammatory properties making it incredibly useful to relieve the pain and stiffness of sore joints and muscles. Adding a few drops of ginger essential oil will gently help to warm the joints and improve circulation, and lavender or camomile work well too.

Rubbing your skin with lotion bars delivers beneficial oils and you benefit from a soothing massage at the same time. There are some beautiful silicone moulds available online, but paper or silicone cupcake cases or any flexible container can also be used to set your lotion bar.

Makes two 60-ml bars

INGREDIENTS

45 g unrefined beeswax

35 g organic shea butter

35 ml nettle-infused carrier oil (see pages 20–21)

20 drops ginger essential oil

EQUIPMENT NEEDED

Heatproof bowl

Saucepan

Silicone moulds

METHOD

Place a heatproof bowl over a pan of boiling water. Melt the beeswax, shea butter and nettle oil in the bowl.

Once melted, take the mixture off the heat and stir in the essential oil. Try not to create bubbles.

Pour into silicone moulds and allow to cool completely for about an hour before popping them out

The lotion bar will melt gently when rubbed over your skin and will keep for about a year.

Always do a patch test before using.

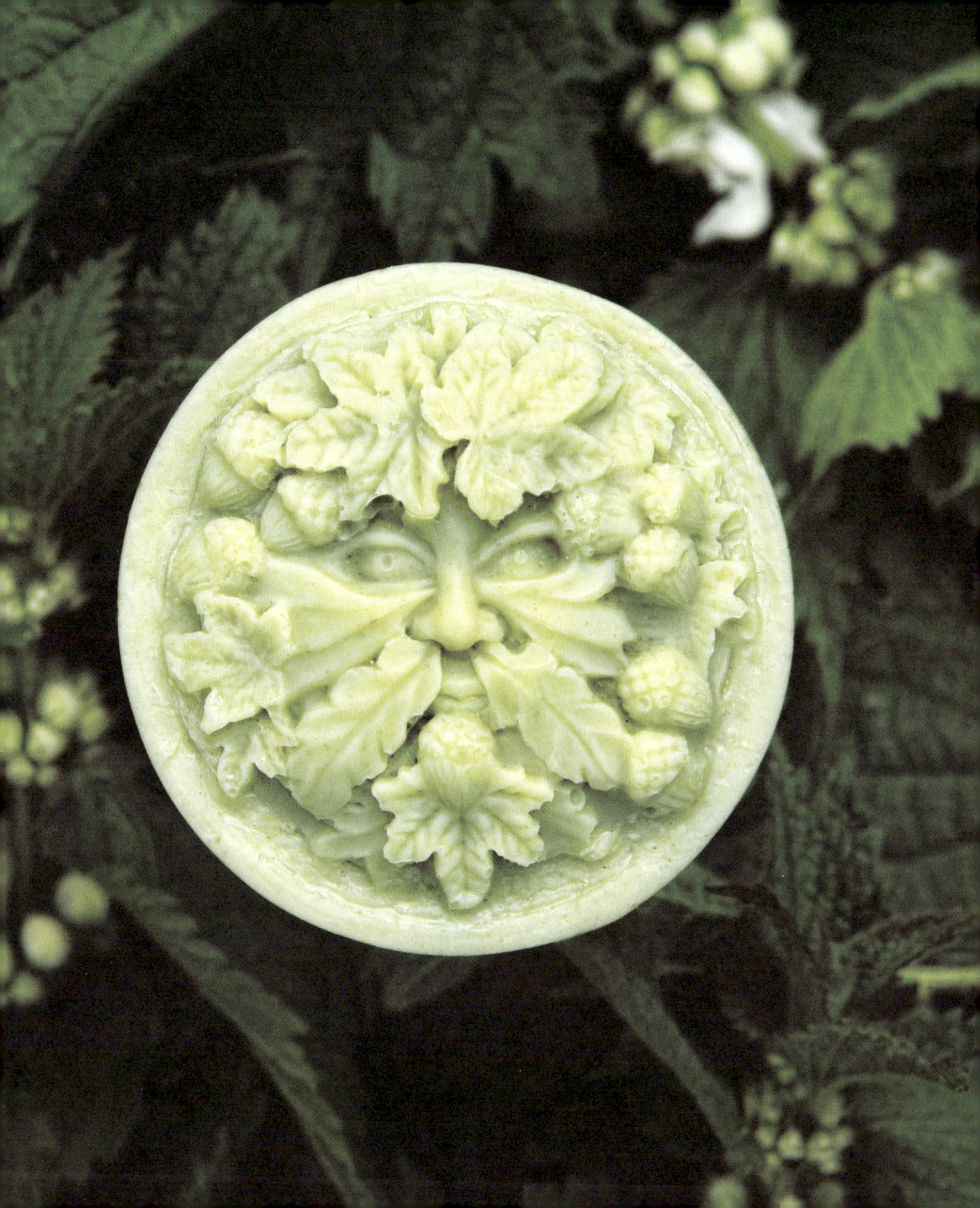

OXEYE DAISY

Alternative names: Marguerite, field daisy, gypsy daisy, moon penny, midsummer daisy, poverty weed

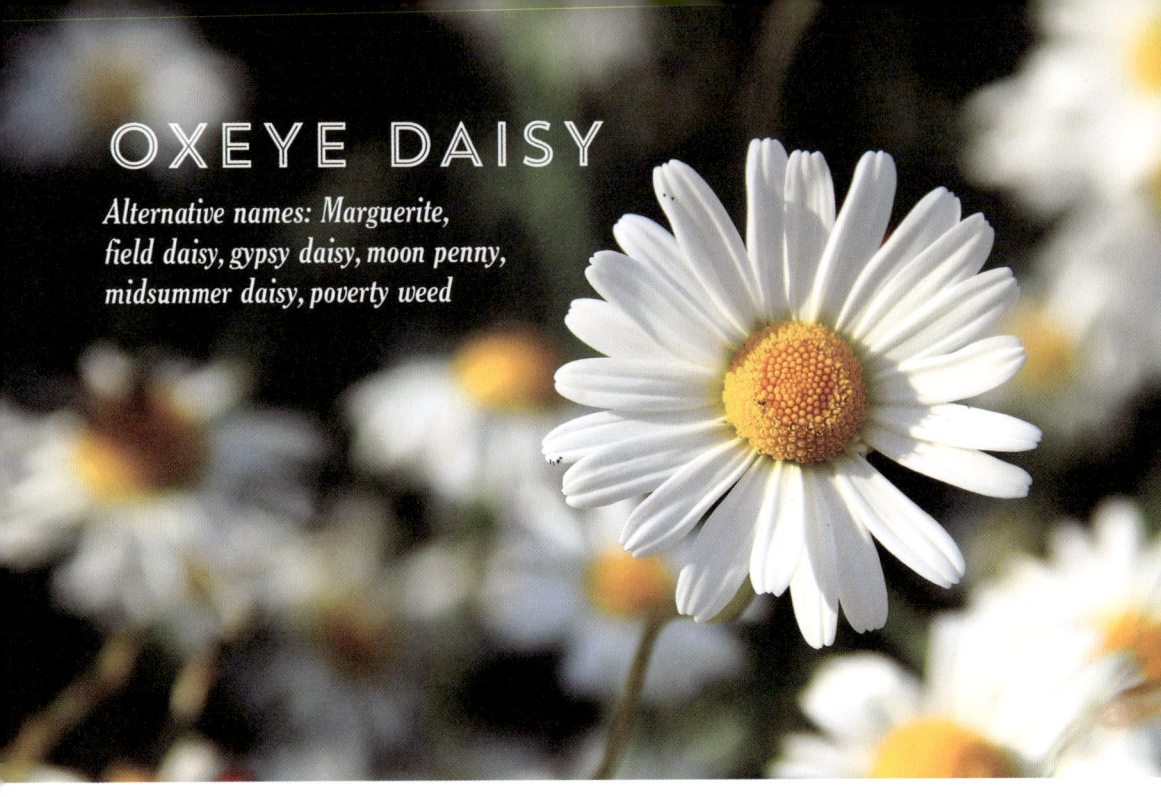

HOW TO IDENTIFY: Native to the UK, oxeye daisies are a very familiar sight in hay meadows, on waste ground and along roadsides and verges from June to September. The oxeye daisy is very easy to identify by its tall, thin stems topped with large daisy-like flowers, and its spoon-shaped leaves at the base, becoming thin and jagged further up.

HISTORY: In Christianity the oxeye daisy was known as "maudlin wort", and was associated with Mary Magdalen.

We are all familiar with the childhood game of "he/she loves me, he/she loves me not", played all summer long in fields and parks by girls and boys desperate to know if their love would be reciprocated. Originating in France, the game *effeuiller la marguerite* was traditionally played using an oxeye daisy. The petals would be removed alternately, with the hope that the final petal would fulfil the player's desire that "they love me".

English farmers who had too much oxeye growing among their crops were looked upon as indolent, and in the sixteenth century King Henry VIII introduced severe punishments for these lazy practices. In Scotland, oxeyes or "gools" as they were known were considered to be a substantial pest, as they were invasive and could taint the milk of dairy cattle. "Gool riders" patrolled the parish and farmers risked being fined one wether (castrated) male sheep or 3 shillings and 4 pence if they didn't keep their fields free from oxeye daisies.

FOLKLORE: Early Brits dedicated the oxeye daisy to Artemis, goddess of women, believing that the plant was particularly helpful for "women's health problems". However, it was also held that unmarried women should never take oxeye into the house if they wished to see a wedding day. If it was your beloved's fidelity that was troubling you, on the other hand, unfaithful lovers could be brought back to you by sleeping with an oxeye under your pillow.

Due to their bright white appearance, oxeyes represented childhood and innocence. In a divine example of this connection, star-like oxeyes growing by a stable helped the three wise men to find the baby Jesus. However, in sadder lore linking oxeye with babies, the Celts believed that the flowers were the spirits of infants who had died at birth.

In more earthly matters, oxeyes were suspended on the rafters of medieval barns and hayricks for protection from fire. It was believed the flower had the power to keep farm buildings safe from this very real risk – flames could swiftly engulf entire farmsteads and lead to devastating food shortages for livestock and people.

FOLK MEDICINE: Culpeper referred to oxeye as *"a wound herb of great respect, often used in those drinks and salves that are for wounds, either inward or outward [...] very fitting to be kept both in oils, ointments, plasters and syrups".*

He recommended that leaves should be bruised and used to reduce swellings, and an infusion of the flowers in asses' milk would ease consumption (tuberculosis).

Oxeye was also used to treat coughs and bronchitis. In 1812, Sir John Hill wrote that the *"great daisy"* is *"balsamic [curative, restorative] and strengthening for the lungs."*

In the Scottish Highlands, oxeye juice was dropped into sore eyes, pressed onto wounds, mixed with honey as a remedy for coughs, and infused into beer to cure jaundice.

OXEYE DAISY CHEST RUB

Historically, oxeye daisy flowers have been recommended to ease bronchitis and help relieve coughs. My all-natural oxeye chest rub utilizes some of nature's best medicines in the form of essential oils: eucalyptus, a natural expectorant and antimicrobial; peppermint oil, for its antibacterial and anti-inflammatory properties; rosemary, which clears a groggy head; and lavender, which helps the body relax and get the rest needed when recovering from a cough.

This recipe can easily be made plant-based by replacing the beeswax with candelilla wax – don't forget to halve the amount, though.

Makes approx. 110 ml

INGREDIENTS

100 ml oxeye daisy-infused oil (see pages 20–21)

10 g unrefined beeswax (or 5 g candelilla wax)

10 drops eucalyptus essential oil

6 drops peppermint essential oil

4 drops lavender essential oil

4 drops rosemary essential oil

EQUIPMENT NEEDED

Heatproof bowl

Saucepan

Small tins or jars

METHOD

Place a heatproof bowl over a pan of boiling water. Add the oxeye-infused oil and beeswax to the bowl.

Once the beeswax has melted, remove from heat.

Allow to cool for 5 minutes.

Stir in the essential oils, combining well.

Pour into clean jars or tins.

Allow to cool completely before popping on lids.

Rub onto chest and neck as needed.

Use within a year.

Do not use on broken skin. Always do a patch test before using; do not use if you are allergic to daisies. Not recommended for pregnant women or children under three years.

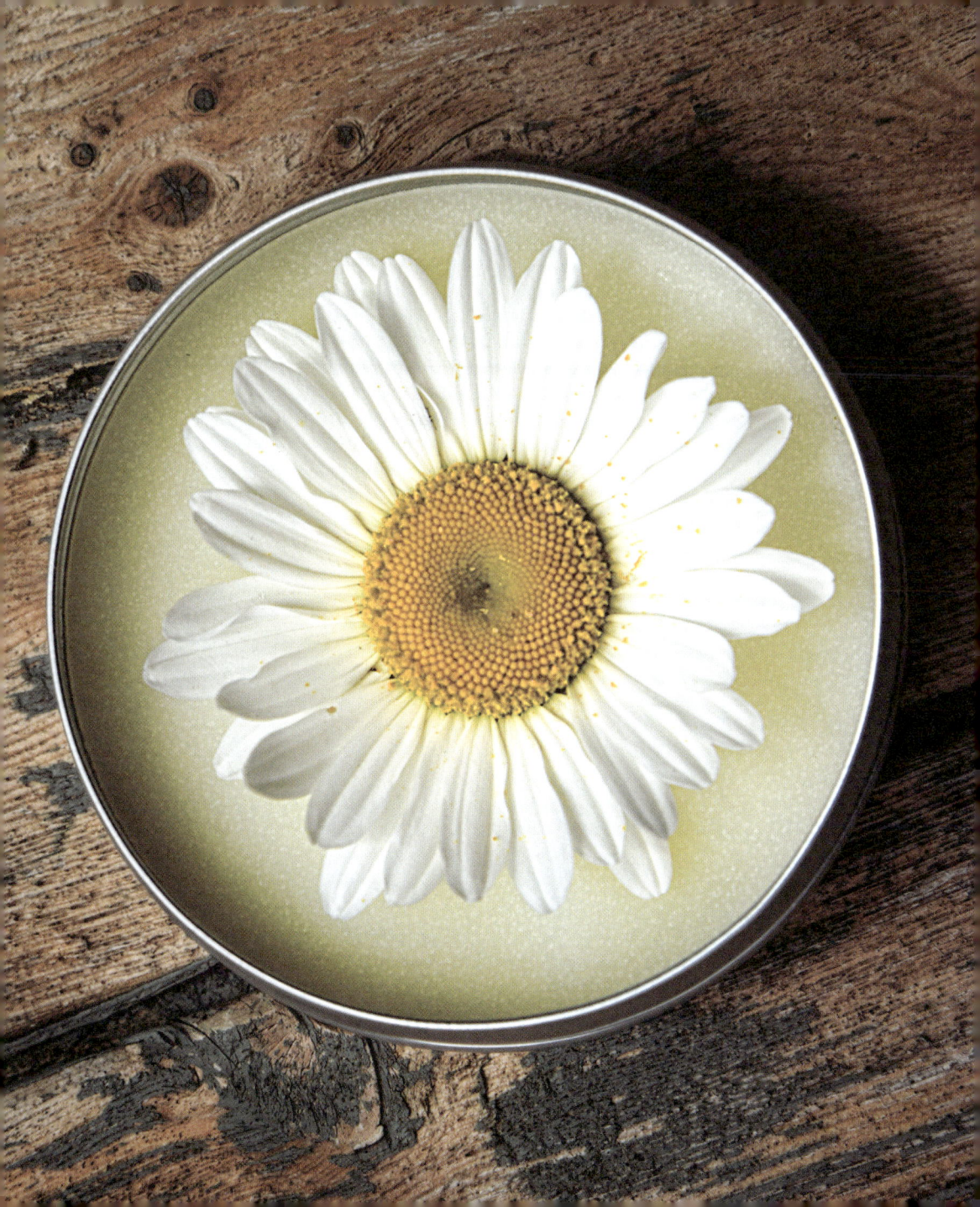

PINEAPPLE WEED

Alternative names: Disc mayweed, pineapple camomile, pavement weed, wild camomile

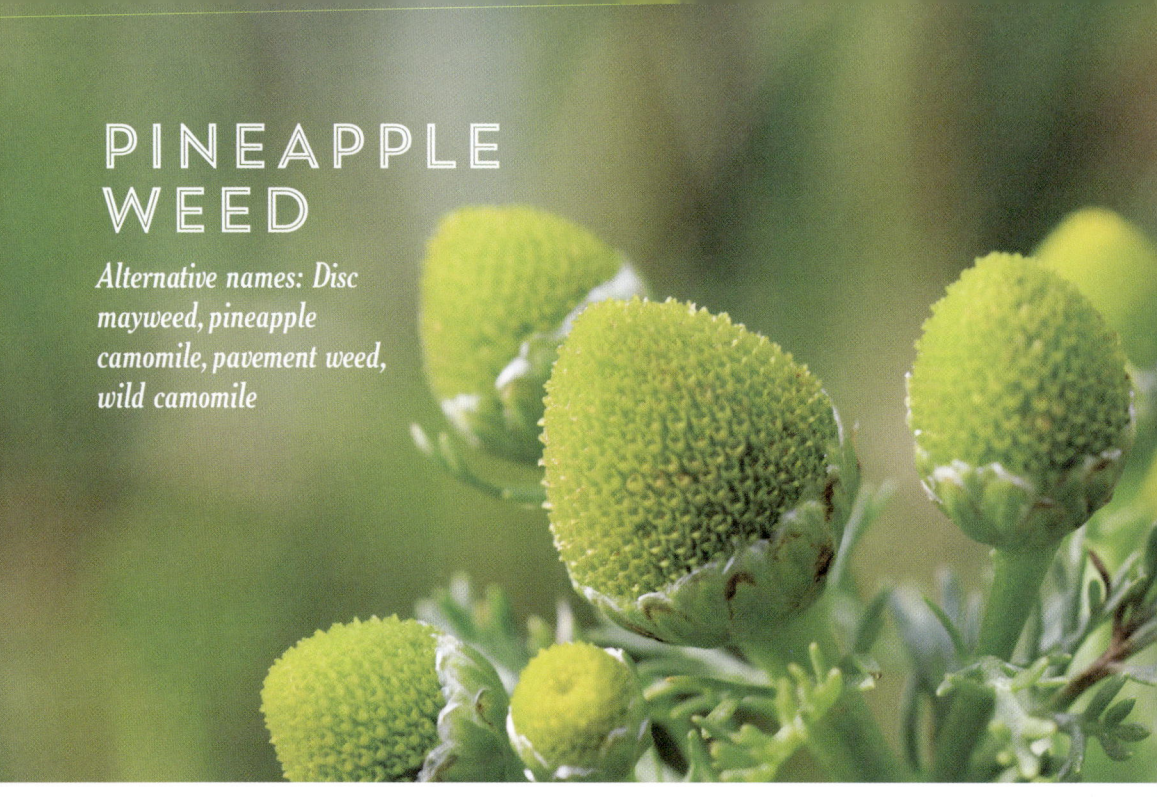

HOW TO IDENTIFY: Pineapple weed certainly lives up to its name – gently crush the feathery leaves and they will instantly release a delicious, fruity pineapple scent. The small flowers (5–9 mm/0.2–0.3 in.), which appear from May to November, look very similar to tiny pineapples too. You'll find pineapple weed growing in cracks in pavements, on wasteland, gravel paths and field edges from June to September.

When foraging for pineapple weed, try to pick flowers that are almost completely yellow, since these have the most flavour, are the freshest and smell most deliciously of pineapple.

HISTORY: Pineapple weed is a native of Asia and North America; it was accidentally introduced into the wild when it escaped from Kew Gardens in the London borough of Richmond in 1871. It became one of the fastest-spreading invasive species of the twentieth century, crowding out many native plants in its wake. Its rapid spread is believed to have been exacerbated by the introduction of cars and buses, the seeds being easily carried on muddy tyres from rural roads and washed off by rain.

This tough little plant seems to not only survive regular trampling, cracks in the concrete and heavily compacted soils – it positively thrives in them. English botanist John Hutchinson wrote that *"the more it is trodden on, the better it seems to thrive".*

FOLKLORE: Every year on the summer solstice, the Cheyenne people of Montana, Oklahoma, and North and South Dakota perform a ritual sun dance to renew, bless and cleanse the earth and the tribe. The whole tribe as well as family and friends gather together to chant, sing, dance and make personal sacrifices for their community.

Pineapple weed, known as *Ononevoneshke-moxeshene* or "prairie dog mint", is chewed during the ritual and blown onto the dancers to cool them down.

When burned with human hair, pineapple weed is believed to prevent a loved one from leaving. Adding horse hair keeps your steed close to you as well.

The flowers are prized for their fragrant scent and are dried and worn as necklaces, or placed in babies' cribs to repel insects.

FOLK MEDICINE: Mainly used by Indigenous American tribes throughout the United States in the form of a tea, pineapple weed is said to help relax the nervous system, ease gas in the stomach, relieve indigestion, help with diarrhoea and combat intestinal worms. Women drink the tea for its pain-relieving properties after childbirth, and it also helps with delivery of the afterbirth and eases menstrual cramps.

A wash made from pineapple weed can soothe itches and sores, and the leaves rubbed on insect bites will give instant relief. Be careful though as this may cause an allergic reaction, especially if you suffer from hay fever. Pineapple weed is a perfect substitute for its cousin camomile and is still used to treat insomnia and ease anxiety.

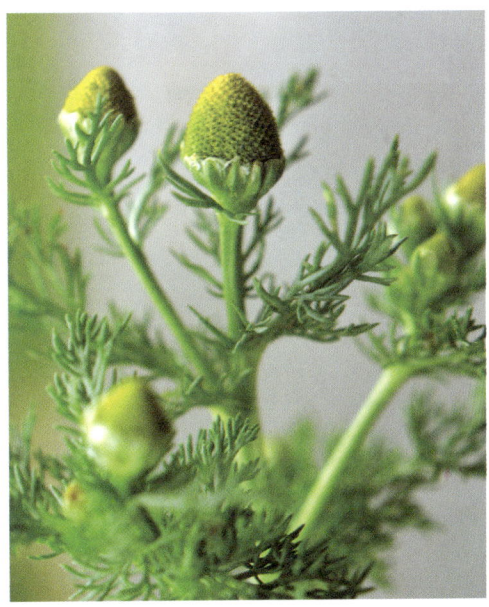

PINEAPPLE WEED POSSET

A posset in the fifteenth century was a hot drink of curdled milk, alcohol and lemon which was often spiced and served to invalids or as a remedy for colds and flu. Some were thickened with eggs while others used oatmeal or grated biscuits which would soak up the liquid and float on the top.

Thankfully, the recipe evolved over the years and in the nineteenth century became the silky-smooth creamy dessert that we now recognize.

Possets were widely used as an aphrodisiac and were believed to have anti-ageing properties preserving beauty – which was often regarded as witchcraft. Because of this, they were often viewed a little suspiciously as a "cure-all".

As always, forage away from busy roads, dog-walking areas and places that may have been sprayed by pesticides.

Serves six

INGREDIENTS

Good handful of pineapple weed flower heads

600 ml double cream (or plant-based alternative)

50 g caster sugar

Juice and finely grated zest of 1 organic lemon

Pineapple weed flowers to decorate

EQUIPMENT NEEDED

Pestle and mortar/rolling pin

Saucepan

Whisk

Six ramekins/small pots

METHOD

Thoroughly crush the pineapple weed flower heads using a pestle and mortar or the end of a rolling pin.

Pour the cream into a large pan, adding the pineapple weed and caster sugar.

Gently bring the cream to the boil, stirring to dissolve the sugar.

Boil for 3 minutes, then remove from the heat and allow the cream to cool completely.

Once cooled, strain out the pineapple weed.

Add the lemon juice and zest to the cream and whisk until it thickens to the desired texture.

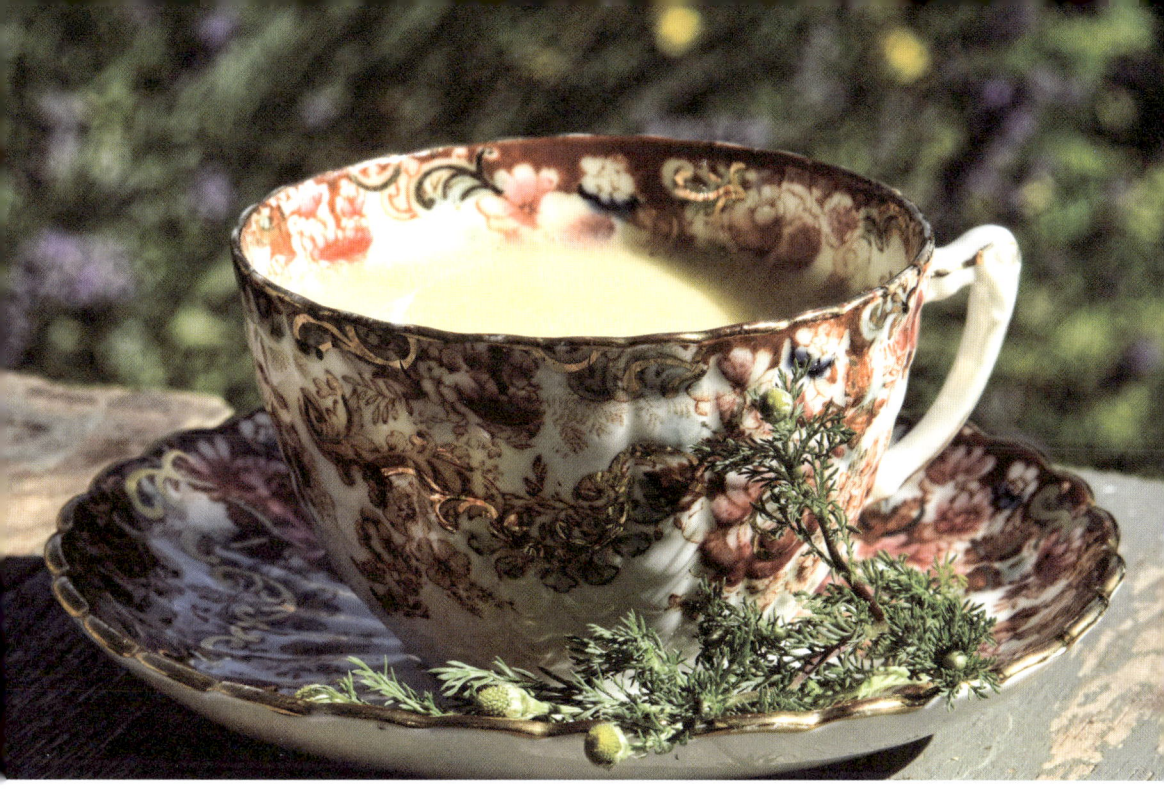

Pour into small pots (I like to use vintage china teacups) and chill for about 3 hours to set the posset.

Decorate with pineapple weed flowers.

ALTERNATIVE USES FOR PINEAPPLE WEED FLOWER HEADS

Pineapple weed tea: Pop some fresh pineapple weed flower heads into a teapot. Pour over boiling water and steep for 5 minutes. Sweeten with honey or sugar.

Pineapple weed syrup: Cover a couple of handfuls of flower heads with water, simmer for 5 minutes, allow to cool and strain. Add 100 g sugar to every 100 ml liquid. Pop back onto the heat until the sugar has dissolved and the liquid has thickened slightly. Dilute for drinks, pour over pancakes or use in salad dressings.

Not recommended if you are allergic to the daisy family.

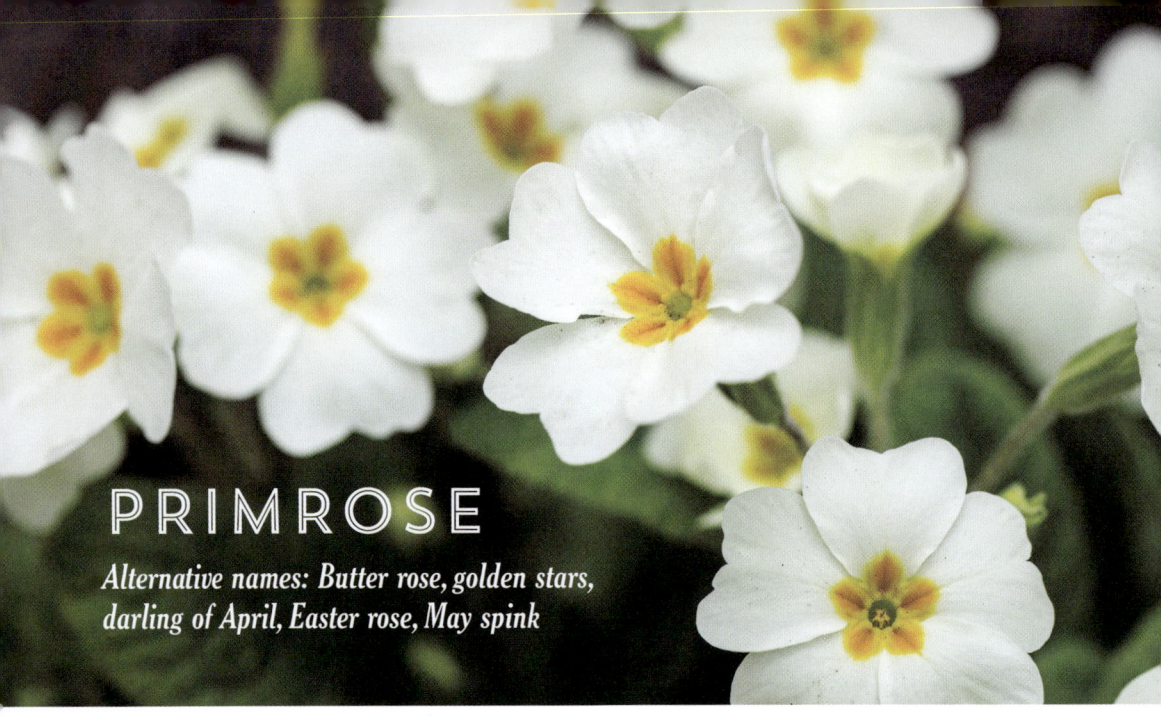

PRIMROSE

Alternative names: Butter rose, golden stars, darling of April, Easter rose, May spink

HOW TO IDENTIFY: This pretty woodland perennial heralds the start of spring. It grows in neat clumps of pale lemon flowers dotted with a deeper yellow or orange centre. The single flowers have five notched petals on upright furry stalks. The crinkly-wrinkly short-stemmed leaves have hairy undersides that form a rosette at the base of the plant.

HISTORY: Primroses were so popular in Victorian times that country people would gather them into posies and send them to London to sell to city dwellers. Unfortunately they often dug up the plant too, which could be one of the reasons why we just don't see as many primroses in the wild nowadays.

FOLKLORE: Some folk tales credit primroses with the supernatural ability to enable people to see faeries, either by eating their petals or by placing a bunch on a faery rock or faery mound. In Ireland, the flowers were scattered by the cow byre to stop faeries from stealing the milk.

In many counties it was considered unlucky to bring primrose flowers into the house and a primrose flowering in winter was taken as an omen of death.

Bunches of primroses were hung in cowsheds during the Celtic festival of Beltane to protect the cattle. Primroses were used to decorate churches, and they were also placed on doorsteps to prevent malignant forces and bad faeries from entering.

On the contrary, some folklore said that bringing primroses into the house could be a good thing. The primrose has long been associated with the hatching of eggs, both goose and hen. If a bunch of primroses was gathered, the corresponding number of eggs would hatch. A broody hen's clutch would traditionally number thirteen so you should gather a minimum of thirteen primroses.

Parents would sew primroses into their children's pillows to ensure eternal love and loyalty. When worn, primroses were believed to cure madness and to attract love.

If you'd like to try some primrose lore, placing a primrose under your pillow is reputed to cure your insomnia. For spots and blemishes simply rub primrose sap onto your face, while to dream of primroses means that you will find happiness in a new friendship.

FOLK MEDICINE: Culpeper found that primroses had numerous benefits:

> *"They remedy all infirmities of the head coming of heat and wind, as vertigo, ephialtes [nightmares], false apparitions, frenzies, falling sickness, palsies, convulsions, cramps, and pain of the nerves."*

Healing salves were traditionally made from primrose flowers. The leaves were infused into boiled water to make a soothing eyewash or gargle for sore throats. Meanwhile, juice from primroses and cowslips was applied to soften wrinkles. Their crinkly leaves resembled wrinkly skin so it was a reasonable assumption that it would work at a time when people believed in the doctrine of signatures.

When boiled with lard, primroses were made into a salve for cuts and minor wounds. Primrose tea is purported to alleviate anxiety, and the roots and plant were made into cough medicine.

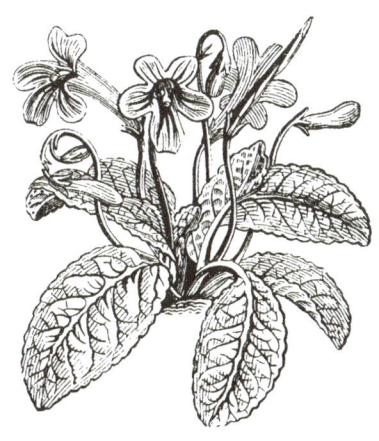

PURPLE LOOSESTRIFE

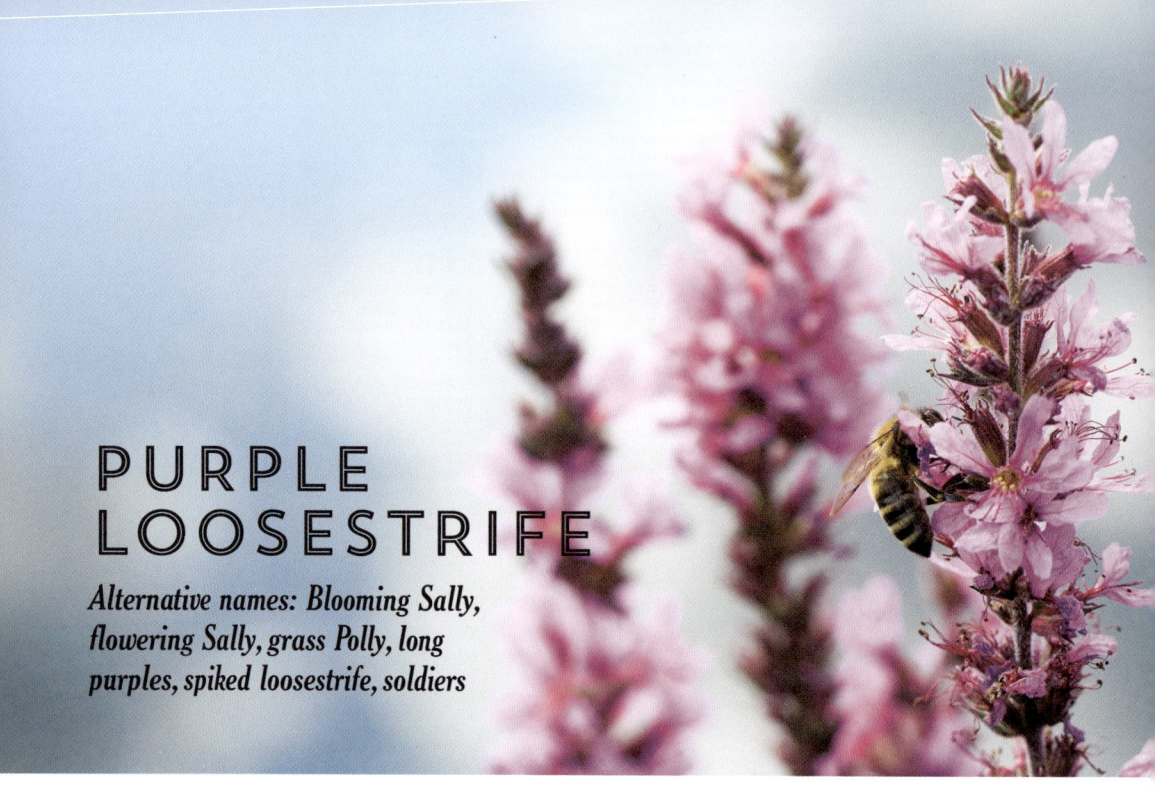

Alternative names: Blooming Sally, flowering Sally, grass Polly, long purples, spiked loosestrife, soldiers

HOW TO IDENTIFY: Purple loosestrife can be found flowering between June and August in wet habitats such as riverbanks, marshes and fens. It is a tall plant growing up to 1.5 m (5 ft), with six-petalled magenta flowers growing in spikes. Long green leaves grow in opposite pairs along the stem.

HISTORY: William Turner was the first to formally record, *"The plant may in englishe be called red loosestrife or purple loosestrife"* in his *New Herball* of 1548.

The leaves were found to have a high tannin content, and in the past were used in the commercial tanning industry to treat leather, as well as for preserving wood or ropes to prevent rotting in water. In addition, the plant was used as a pigment: the flowers make an edible red dye which was at one time used for desserts and sweets, and also hair dye.

Gerard recommended burning purple loosestrife as an early fly killer and snake deterrent: *"This I found in a watery lane leading from the Lord Treasurer his house* called Theobald's, unto the backside of his slaughter-house, and in other places [...] The smoke of the burned herbe driveth away serpents, and killeth flies and gnats in the house." Garlands of the herb were tied around horses and cattle to deter biting insects during the summer months.

And in literature, Gerard's contemporary, Shakespeare, uses the old country name of "long purples" in *Hamlet* when he describes the sad discovery of Ophelia:

> *"There is a willow grows aslant a brook*
> *That shows his hoar leaves*
> *in a glassy stream.*
> *There with the fantastic*
> *garlands did she come.*
> *Of crowflowers, nettles, daisies*
> *and long purples."*

FOLKLORE: As the name suggests, historically the herb has been used to help "loose strife", to heal arguments, bring people back together and disperse negative energy.

Purple loosestrife was believed to be able to soothe difficult horses and oxen, especially when they were tethered together to plough fields, as confirmed by Gerard: *"a special virtue that it hath in appeasing the strife and unruliness which falleth out among oxen at the plough, if it be put about their yokes".*

In the Victorian language of flowers, purple loosestrife is associated with royalty, wisdom and deep contemplation, while in certain circumstances it can represent unchecked growth or disruption due to its vigorous growing habit.

In European folklore, purple loosestrife was believed to be able to give protection from evil spirits as well as bringing harmony and security to the household, and to grant psychic powers.

FOLK MEDICINE: Purple loosestrife has a long history of being used for nosebleeds and to stanch bleeding anywhere in the body. According to Gerard:

> *"It is excellent good for green wounds, and stancheth the blood: being also put into the nostrils, it stoppeth the bleeding at the nose [...] This herb is good for all manner of bleeding at the mouth, nose, or wounds, and all fluxes of the belly, and the bloody-flux, given either to drink or taken by clysters [enema]."*

Culpeper concurs, referencing its use to control heavy menstruation: *"it stays also the abundance of women's courses; it is a singular good wound-herb [...] it quickly close together the lips of the wound, if the herb be bruised, and the juice only applied".*

RAGWORT

Alternative names: Cankerweed, faeries' horses, St James' Wort, stinking Billy, yellow daisy, cradle-dock, bolyawn

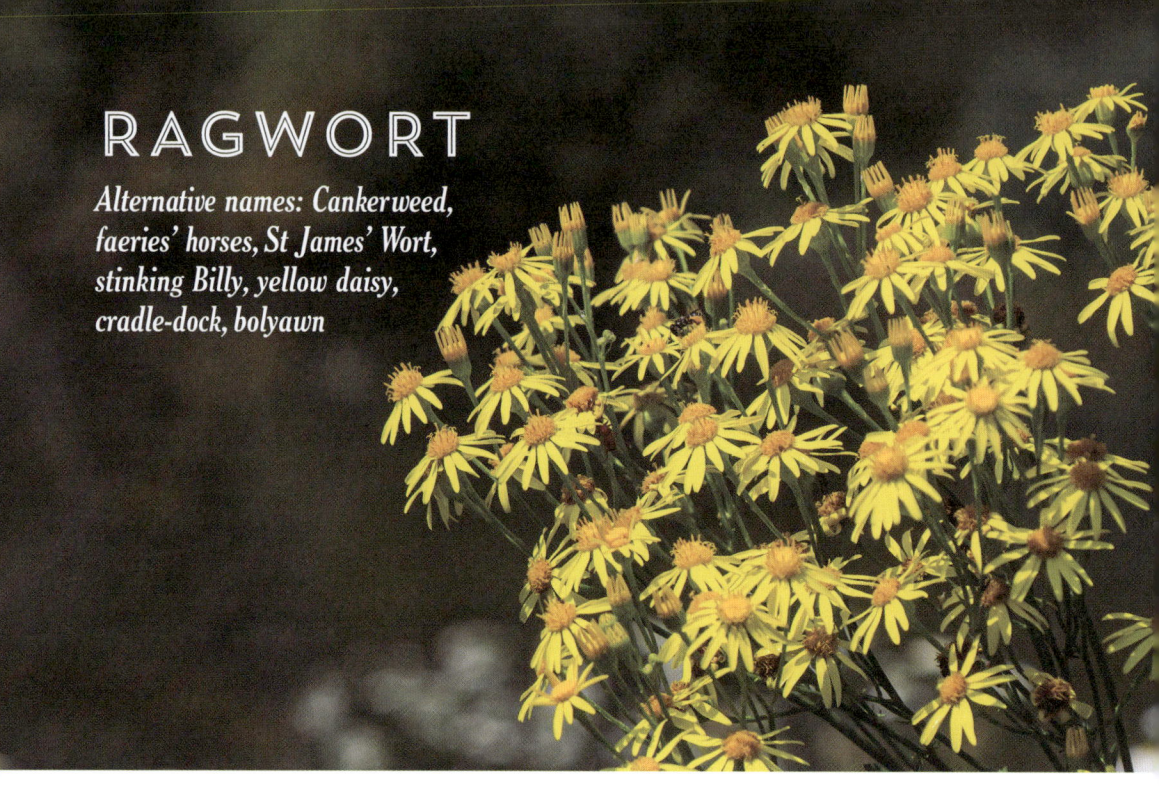

HOW TO IDENTIFY: The bright yellow daisy-like flowers are much-loved by bees and moths, but much-disliked in paddocks and pastures as the plant can be harmful to horses and cattle if eaten. Flowering stems appear from late June onwards, with flat-topped clusters of yellow flowers sitting atop tall stems with "tattered" leaves that can grow to over 1 m (3 ft) tall.

HISTORY: Ragwort is a native biennial plant that has a very efficient way of using the wind and its parachute-shaped seeds to spread relentlessly. A single plant can produce thousands of seeds, resulting in it becoming classified as an invasive species. Although not popular with gardeners, ragwort provides a food source for a huge variety of insects, particularly the black and red cinnabar moth, whose numbers are declining rapidly.

In 1959 the British Government classified ragwort as one of five "injurious weeds" along with spear thistle, field thistle, curled dock and broad-leaved dock. This means that farmers have a duty to control the growth of these weeds on agricultural land and to prevent them from getting into the animal food chain.

However, with a romantic's eye, poet John Clare saw nothing but beauty in the plant in his 1832 poem "Ragwort":

*"Ragwort, thou humble flower
with tattered leaves
I love to see thee come & litter gold."*

FOLKLORE: One charming folk tale originates from Ireland where ragwort is known as bolyawn:

A lazy lad named Tom was strolling along a country lane in an effort to avoid having to do any work, when he was lucky enough to meet a leprechaun in the hedgerow. Grabbing hold of the little fellow, he rudely demanded good luck or he wouldn't let him go. The leprechaun reluctantly took Tom to a field full of bolyawns, indicated a tall plant in full bloom and told him that if he dug there, he would find a pot of gold. Before Tom released the leprechaun and ran off to find a spade, he tied a handkerchief around the plant so that he would be able to find it again. On his return Tom found that the pesky leprechaun had tied an identical handkerchief to every single bolyawn plant in the field, leaving Tom empty-handed and very cross!

In sixteenth-century England, it was thought that witches could ride the long stems of ragwort at midnight, while in Ireland it was believed that faeries also used ragwort to fly from the Isle of Arran to the Emerald Isle.

FOLK MEDICINE: Historically ragwort was mixed with pig fat to make an ointment to treat pain in the legs, hips and arms, and used too for sciatica, gout and rheumatism. In some parts of the UK, it was carried when visiting a sick friend, for the plant was believed to have the power to prevent the carrier from becoming infected.

Ragwort was used as a gargle due to its antimicrobial and anti-inflammatory properties. Gerard wrote that *"the decoction hereof gargarised [gargled] is much set by as a remedy against swellings and impostumations [abscesses] of the throat, which it wasteth away and thoroughly healeth."*

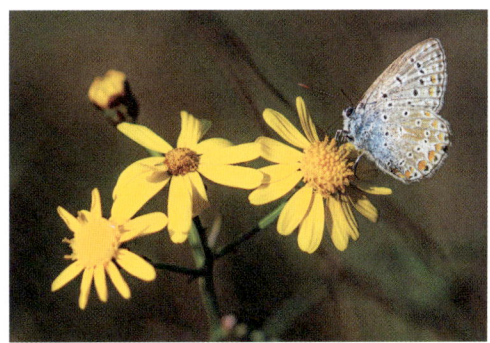

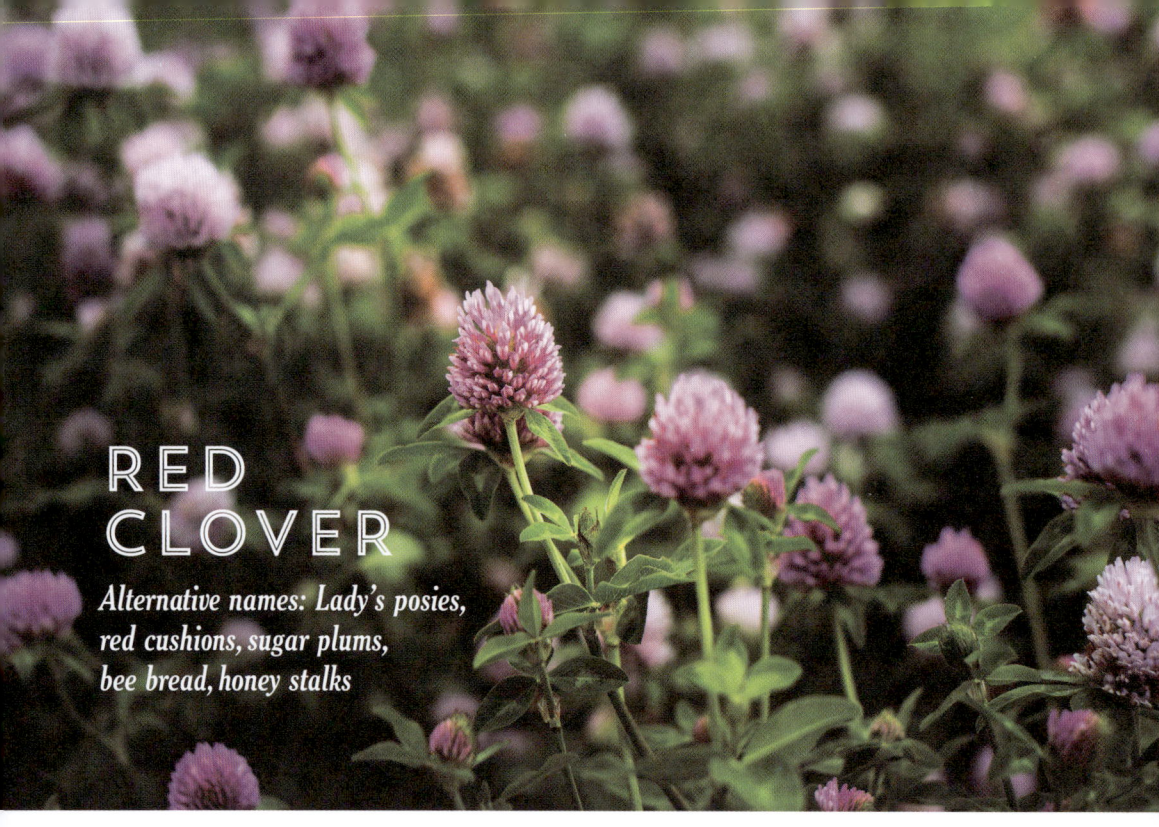

RED CLOVER

Alternative names: Lady's posies, red cushions, sugar plums, bee bread, honey stalks

HOW TO IDENTIFY: This three-leaf clover is commonly found growing in grassy areas and lawns all over Europe. The petite bobble-topped magenta wildflower is a constant irritant to "stripey lawn" gardeners, but a firm favourite with bees, rabbits and cattle.

HISTORY: Introduced from Europe in the seventeenth century as an important pasture crop for cattle, red clover's nitrogen-producing roots make it extremely useful for crop rotation, helping plants to photosynthesize and stimulate healthy growth.

FOLKLORE: Having three leaves, clover has always been associated with the Holy Trinity, giving it the ability to keep away evil spirits. However, it is the four-leafed clover that is considered especially lucky. Medieval children believed that carrying a four-leafed clover would allow them to see faeries, but their chances of finding one were slim – only one in 10,000 clovers have four leaves. Legend has it that Napoleon dodged a fatal bullet (literally) because he bent over to pick a four-leafed clover.

Witches, meanwhile, were believed to become more powerful if they managed to find a five-leafed clover, while maidens hoped to find a two-leafed clover, allowing them to see their future spouse.

In Christian lore, St Patrick used the threefold shape of the clover leaf to preach the Holy Trinity (Father, Son and Holy Spirit), while Eve took some four-leafed clover with her when she was banished from the Garden of Eden as a reminder of her happy time in Paradise.

Its reputation as a plant of luck and prosperity is most prevalent in Celtic countries, and some of its lore predates Christianity. For the Celts, clover was dedicated to the goddesses as a symbol of contentment, and was used as a charm to ward off spells and protect against evil spirits. The flowering clover revealed the footsteps of the goddesses and if you followed them, you would be blessed.

In other beliefs, washing with an infusion of red clover made with the morning dew would make freckles disappear, to bathe surrounded by clover would bring you wealth, and mopping the floor with clover water would chase away unwelcome spirits.

FOLK MEDICINE: Pliny the Elder recommended that red clover be used to treat bladder stones and dropsy (swellings under the skin), and as a diuretic for cleansing the liver and improving the circulation.

Honey infused with red clover flowers was considered to be an effective treatment for coughs, bronchitis, asthma and whooping cough. Gerard, who called it "meadow trefoil", cites other uses for this honey-clover remedy:

> *"The meadow Trefoil (especially that with the black half-moon upon the leaf) stamped with a little honey, takes away the pin and web in the eyes [cataracts], ceaseth the pain and inflammation thereof, if it be strained and dropped therein."*

Red clover is also believed to relieve skin irritation. Bathing in a solution of red clover can give relief from eczema and psoriasis, help soothe itchy scalps and speed up the healing of wounds. The flowers can be rubbed onto insect bites and stings for instant relief from itching.

The plant has returned to popularity in recent years, used by menopausal women to help treat hot flushes and night sweats, and to balance hormones.

RED CLOVER BLOSSOM SYRUP

White and pink clover blossoms contain magnesium and calcium, which have historically been used to cleanse the lymphatic system and help support immune function.

This delicately flavoured syrup is delicious poured over pancakes or ice cream, or diluted with sparkling water or prosecco for a summer cocktail. The taste is very similar to honey, with a floral note. Red clover blossom syrup will keep in the fridge for six to eight weeks, or frozen into ice cubes it should last a year.

Makes two to three small bottles

INGREDIENTS

2 generous handfuls gently washed red clover flowers

250 ml water

150 g granulated sugar

2½ tbsp lemon juice

EQUIPMENT NEEDED

Saucepan

Muslin or tight-meshed sieve

Measuring jug

Scales

Small bottles with lids

METHOD

Place the blossoms and water in a saucepan and bring to the boil. Simmer for 15 minutes. Remove from the heat, cover and allow to cool overnight.

Once cool, strain the liquid through a muslin cloth or tight-meshed sieve. Don't be tempted to press the flowers or your syrup will become cloudy.

Measure your liquid.

For every 100 ml liquid, add 60 g sugar and 1 tbsp lemon juice into a saucepan.

Bring the liquid slowly to the boil, stirring to dissolve the sugar.

Boil for 5 minutes to thicken slightly.

Decant into sterilized bottles.

Red clover is best avoided if you are suffering from breast, uterine or ovarian cancer and during pregnancy.

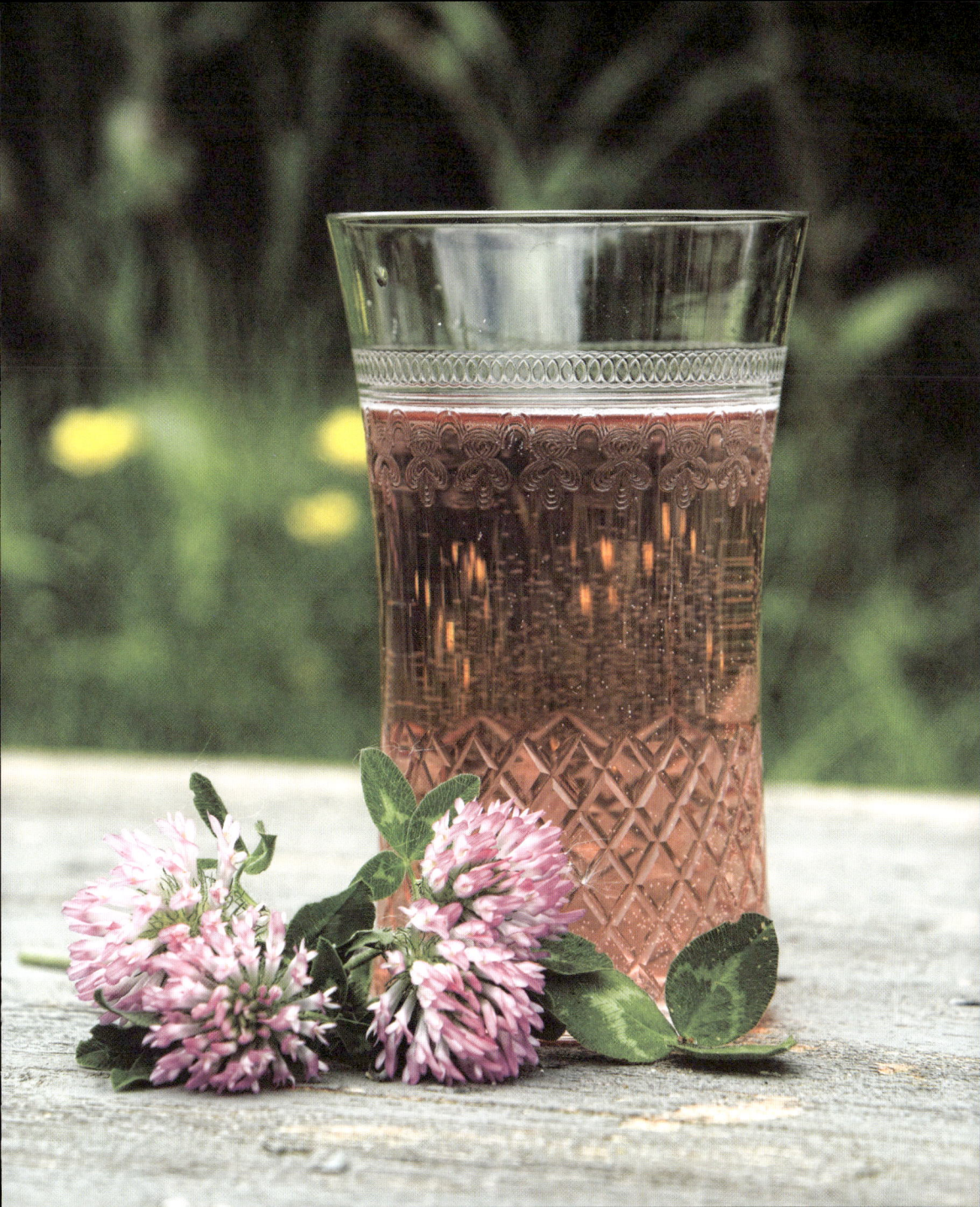

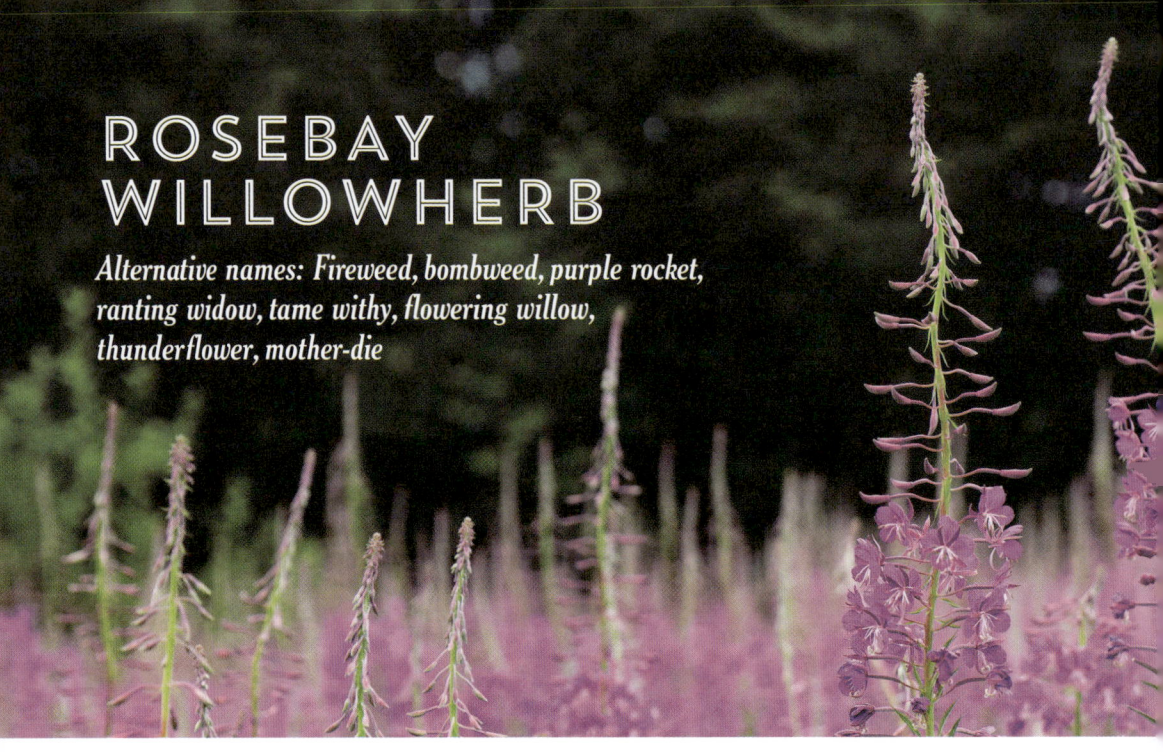

ROSEBAY WILLOWHERB

Alternative names: Fireweed, bombweed, purple rocket, ranting widow, tame withy, flowering willow, thunderflower, mother-die

HOW TO IDENTIFY: Spreading by means of underground rhizomes, rosebay willowherb is quick to colonize grasslands, woodland clearings and waste ground. Tall, deep-pink flower spikes form a cluster at the top of the stalk, blooming from June to September, and the leaves are long, green and pointed. Tiny seeds are covered in soft fluffy down, enabling them to be easily dispersed by the slightest breeze in autumn.

HISTORY: If you lived in Britain in the eighteenth century, rosebay willowherb would have been quite a rare sight and only found in gravelly or damp areas. So how did it become so widespread? The answer seems to lie with the revolutionary expansion of the railway network during the nineteenth century. A large amount of soil was disturbed as the rail network forged ahead relentlessly and rosebay willowherb took full advantage, rapidly going from being scarce to being incredibly abundant – making it one of only a few wildflowers that have actually increased their numbers.

Rosebay loves to grow in dusty, dry and exposed conditions; it even gained the nickname "bombweed" during World War

Two, being one of the first plant species to establish itself in a bomb crater. On 24 July 1944, the New York Herald Tribune reported:

> "London, paradoxically, is the gayest where she has been most blitzed [...] There is the brilliant rose-purple plant that Londoners call rose-bay willow herb [...] It sweeps across the pock marked city and turns what might be scars into flaming beauty. You see it everywhere – great meadows of it in Lambeth, where solid tracts were blitzed; waves of it about St. Paul's. Behind Westminster Abbey bits of it are high up where second-story fireplaces still cling to the hanging walls."

FOLKLORE: In the Macclesfield area of the UK, where the plant was known as "thunderflower", it was believed that rosebay willowherb should never be picked for fear of causing a thunderstorm. In Shropshire the nickname "mother-die" gave a stark warning to children as to what might happen if they dared to pick it.

FOLK MEDICINE: In North America and Europe, rosebay willowherb was used as a remedy for asthma, whooping cough and skin rashes, as it was soothing and antimicrobial. It was once the favourite herb of American doctors to treat dysentery, cholera and typhoid, while an infusion of the leaf was recommended for heavy periods, uterine bleeding and yeast infections.

Gerard also pointed to its usefulness as a pest control and in the treatment of nosebleeds:

> "The smoke of the burned herb driveth away serpents and killeth flies and gnats in the house and all nature of venomous beasts [...] being also put into the nostrils, it stopeth the bleeding of the nose."

Dried leaves can be made into a tea to ease diarrhoea, while the cooled infusion can be used as a mouthwash for ulcers and a gargle for sore throats.

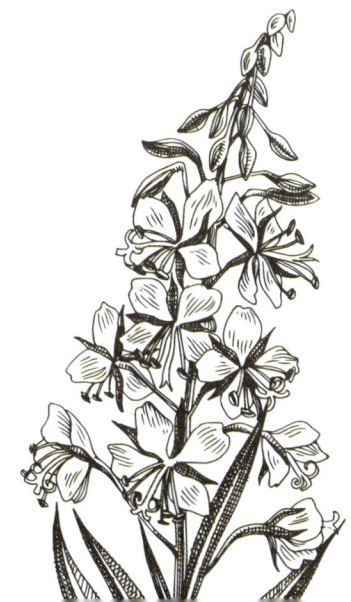

ROSEBAY WILLOWHERB JAM

I have always been a fan of making my own preserves – so much tastier than shop-bought and you can control the amount of sugar to suit your taste.

Rosebay willowherb flowers make the most delightful pretty-pink jam with a floral and fruity flavour. Spread generously onto scones for the perfect addition to afternoon tea.

Gather your flowers away from the pollution of busy roads on a dry day.

Makes a few jars

INGREDIENTS

Enough willowherb flowers to fill a 500 ml jug

500 ml boiling water

Juice of one organic lemon

400 g jam sugar (with added pectin)

EQUIPMENT NEEDED

Heatproof bowl or jug

Saucepan

Muslin or fine strainer

Small plate, placed in freezer

Jars with lids

METHOD

Place your flowers in a heatproof bowl or jug.

Pour over the boiling water.

Allow to cool, cover and refrigerate overnight.

Strain the liquid into a saucepan using a muslin or fine strainer, add the lemon juice and watch the colour change as if by magic!

Bring to a rolling boil for 2 minutes.

Add the jam sugar and stir until dissolved.

Bring back up to the boil for another 5 minutes.

When set, carefully pour the jam into hot, sterilized jars and seal with a lid.

Refrigerate once open and consume within a year.

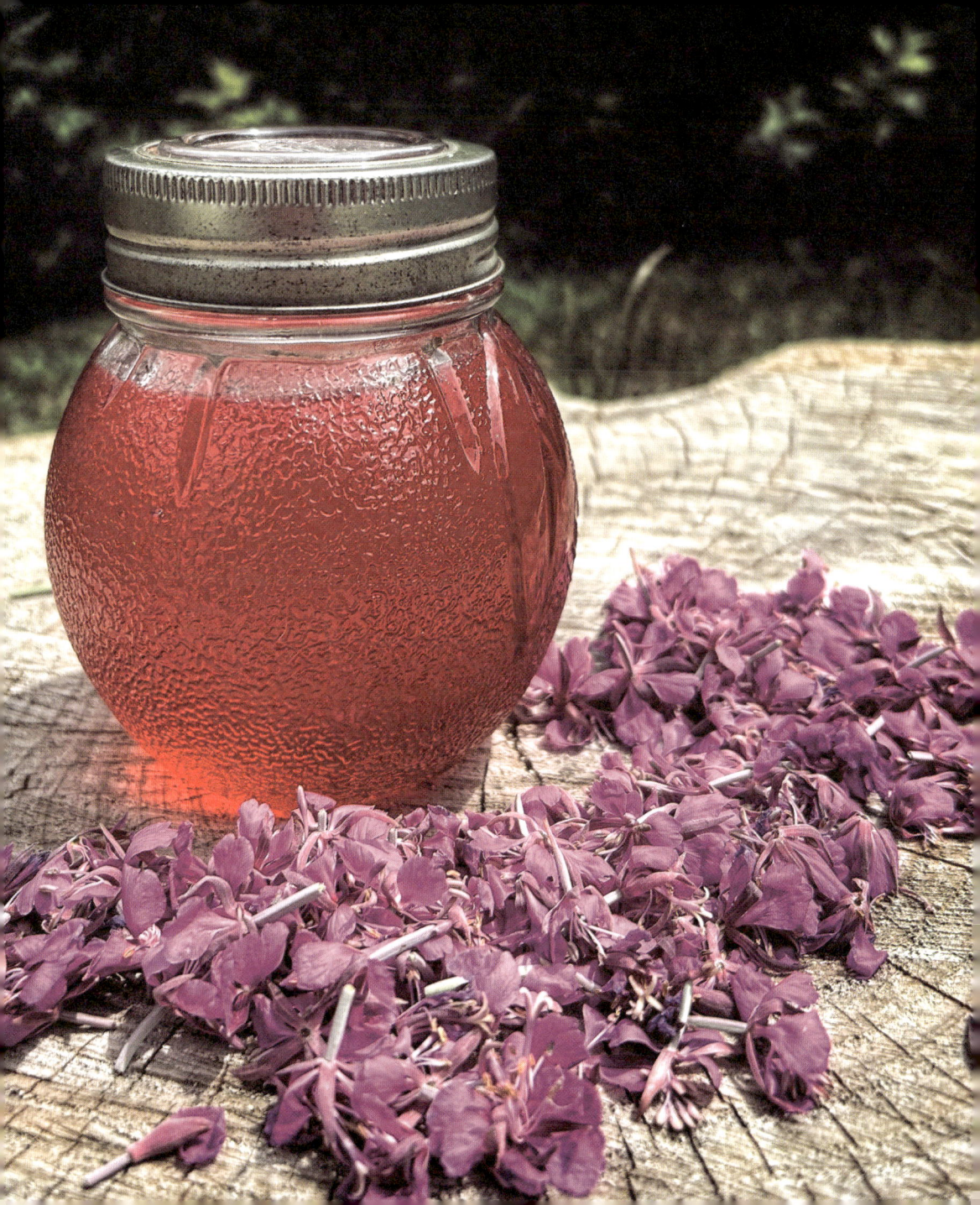

SEA HOLLY

Alternative names: Sea hulver, eryngo, star thistle

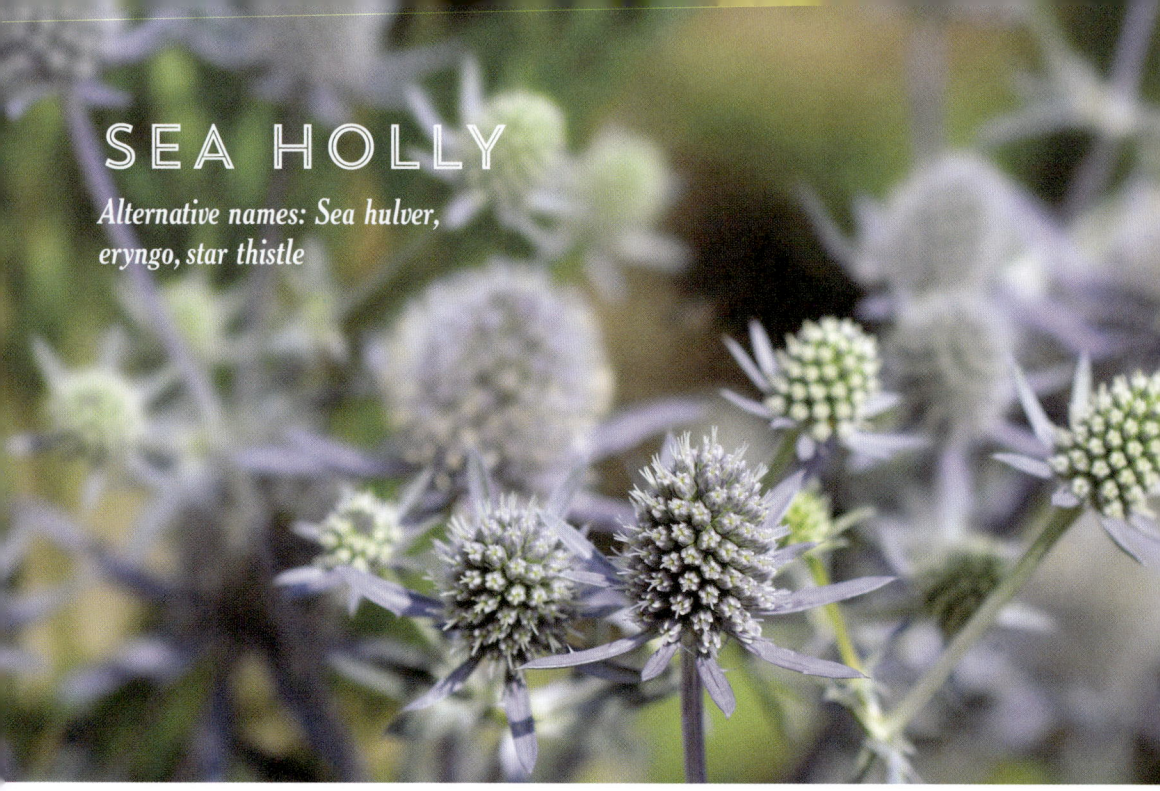

HOW TO IDENTIFY: With spiky holly-like silver leaves, sea holly is perfectly adapted to live along the coastline and sand dunes. Their waxy cuticles ensure that they retain water and survive even the roughest of coastal conditions. Topped with teasel-like blue flowers from July to September, sea holly is common along Welsh, English and Irish shorelines but is less common in Scotland and the far north of England.

HISTORY: In the seventeenth and eighteenth centuries, the historic Essex city of Colchester was famous for its candied eryngo root (sea holly). So much so that it was referenced by William Shakespeare in his play *The Merry Wives of Windsor* for its apparent aphrodisiac qualities, clearly valued by Falstaff before his liaison with Mistress Ford: "hail kissing-comfits and snow eryngoes; let there come a tempest of provocation..."

Also recommended to ease coughs and colds, the boiled and roasted roots were said to resemble parsnips or chestnuts in flavour. The roots were peeled, boiled, and cut into slivers which were then twisted together and candied with sugar, orange-blossom water or rose water, then left by the fire to dry out fully.

Gerard wrote that the candied roots *"are exceeding good to be given unto old and aged people that are consumed and withered with age [...] nourishing and restoring the aged, and amending the defects of nature in the younger".*

FOLKLORE: The striking blue colour of the flowers has long had associations with heaven and the spiritual world. In medieval times it was used as a symbol of the chastity and purity of the Virgin Mary.

Perhaps because of this virtue, folklore tells us that sea holly was often used for protection against evil spirits, faeries and witches. Carrying sea holly with you on a journey would keep you safe and bring you good fortune. It also had the power to stop couples from arguing if you placed it between them.

In Greek lore, it had a different quality. The philosopher Plutarch wrote some advice for goatherds trying to control their flock: *"They report of the sea holly, if one goat taketh it into her mouth, it causeth her first to stand still, and afterwards the whole flock, until such time as the goatherd takes it from her."*

FOLK MEDICINE: Historically, many ailments, from cramps to jaundice, have been treated using sea holly. Gerard tells us that the plant is *"good for those that be liver-sick, and for such as are bitten with any venomous beast: they ease cramps, convulsions, and the falling sickness [epilepsy], and bring down the terms [bring on menses]".*

Culpeper lists quite a few other uses: *"kernels of the throat, commonly called the king's evil [tuberculosis] [...] the roots be bruised and boiled in old hog's grease [...] and applied to broken bones, thorns & not only draw them forth, but heal up the place again, gathering new flesh where it was consumed."*

In addition, Culpeper used sea holly for snake bites, abscesses in the ears, melancholy of the heart, stiff necks, obstructions of the liver and spleen, and pains of the loins.

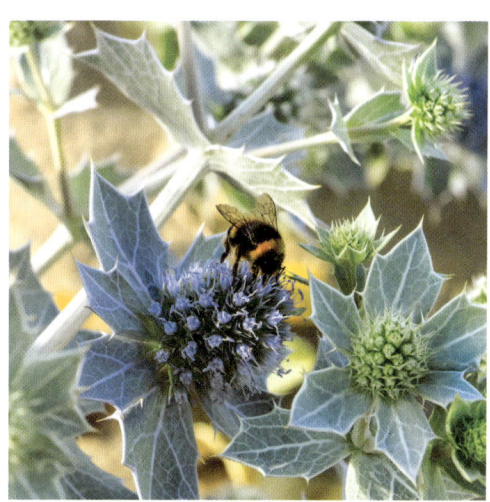

SHEPHERD'S PURSE

Alternative names: Lady's purses, hen and chickens, pick-pocket-to-London, shepherd's bag, witch's pouches, mother's heart

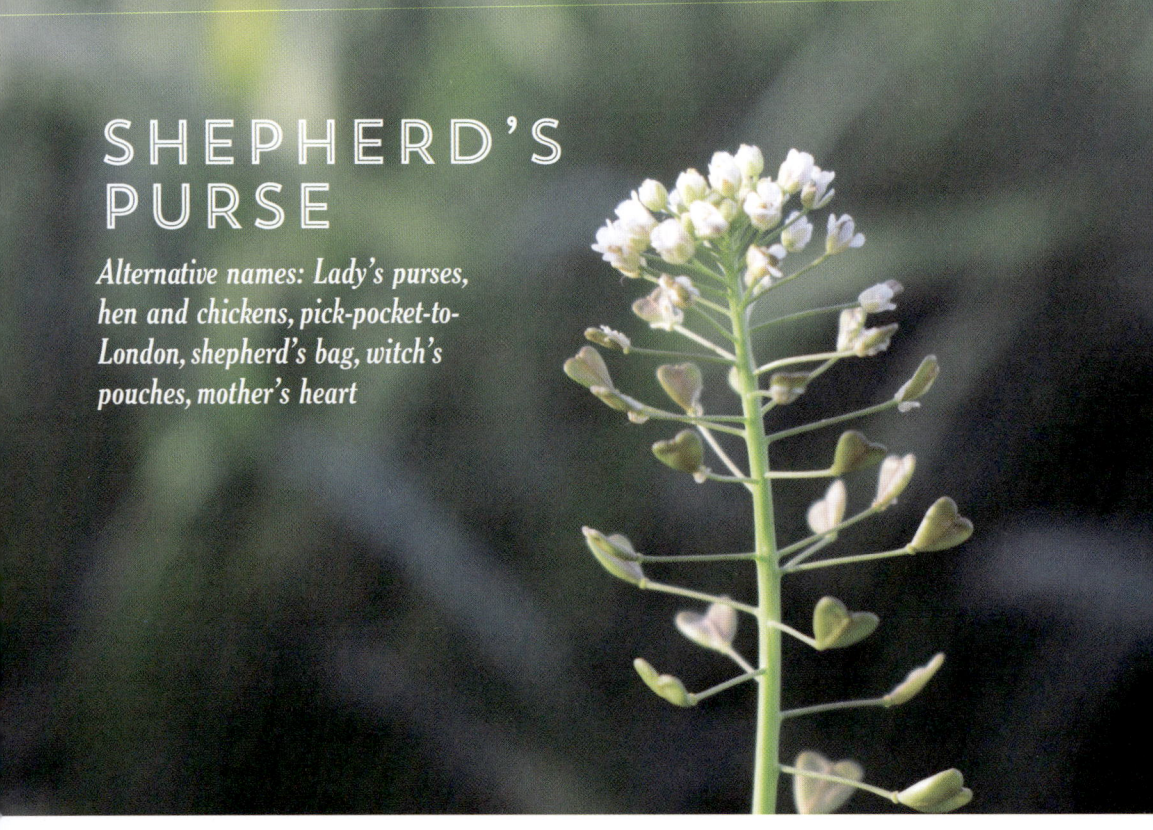

HOW TO IDENTIFY: The most recognizable features of shepherd's purse are its green heart-shaped seedpods, which are held out on thin stalks resembling little medieval purses. Clusters of small white flowers can be seen all year round in woodlands and on farmland.

HISTORY: William Coles wrote in his book *Adam in Eden*: "It is called Shepherd's purse or Scrip [wallet] from the likeness of the seed hath with that kind of leathearne bag, wherein Shepherds carry their Victualls [food and drink] into the field."

In Ireland the plant is known as *clappedepouch*, referring to the pouches hung on long poles used historically by beggars suffering from Hansen's disease (leprosy). Relying on the charity of passersby, lepers would ring a bell or "clapper" to signal their arrival.

In the bird kingdom, chaffinches are particularly fond of the seeds of shepherd's purse, while chickens fed on the seed are said to produce stronger-tasting eggs with darker yolks.

FOLKLORE: European folklore cautions children not to break open the tiny purses or they would break their mother's heart, causing her to die. Should you be brave enough to break open a "purse", however, the colour of the seeds is very important. Yellow seeds indicate that you will be rich, but if the seeds are still green, be prepared for poverty.

Once used as a protective charm against bleeding, it was also thought that if you ate seeds from the first three shepherd's purse plants that you saw in the spring you would be safe from any diseases for the following year.

In some parts of Europe, it was thought that carrying a sprig of the plant could prevent someone from getting lost. It was also a symbol of fertility and sometimes used in love potions.

FOLK MEDICINE: Shepherd's purse has been used as a remedy for both man and beast for centuries. This old recipe hails from the Isle of Man:

"A cure for scour in cattle and diarrhoea in human beings. When a young calf was bought from the mart, she always gave it some of the tea made from shepherd's purse, and it would be better within the hour."

Shepherd's purse has long had an important role to play in the control of bleeding, especially during heavy menstrual periods and nosebleeds. Gerard noted that *"Shepherd's Purse stayeth bleeding in any part of the body, whether the juice or the decoction thereof be drunk, or whether it be used poultice-wise, or in bath, or any other way else."*

Culpeper agreed: *"It helps all fluxes of blood, either caused by inward or outward wounds; as also flux of the belly, and bloody flux, spitting blood, and bloody urine, stops the terms in women."*

It was still used for this purpose by herbalists during World War One when all other plants used to stem bleeding were no longer available.

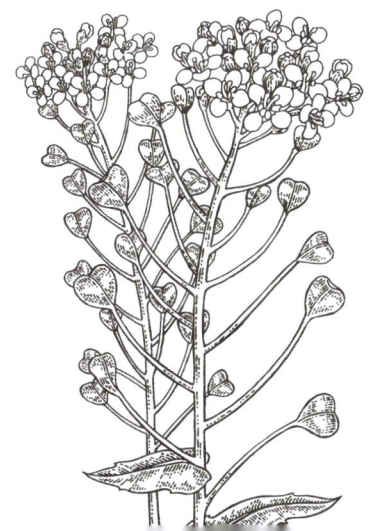

SILVERWEED

Alternative names: Goose tansy, silvery cinquefoil, trailing tansy, prince's feather, traveller's ease

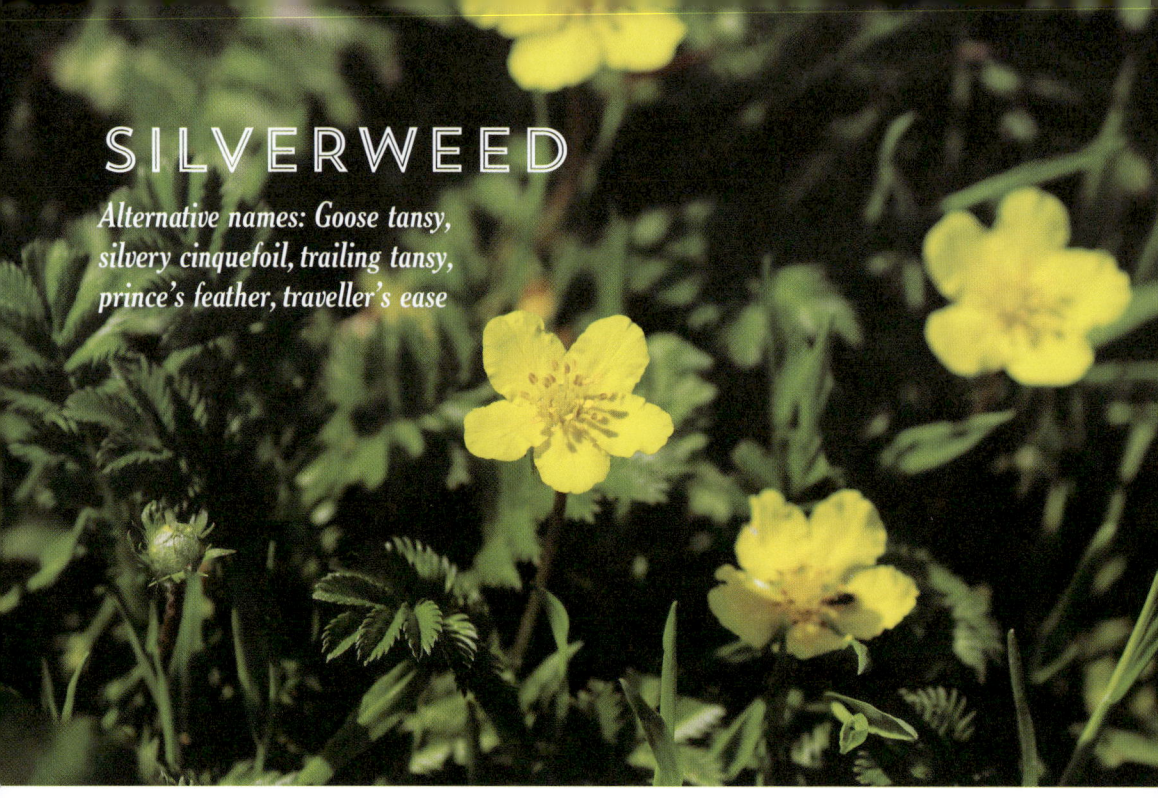

HOW TO IDENTIFY: Silverweed is not a fussy plant and can be found happily growing in a variety of habitats. As the name suggests, the leaves are silvery in colour on the underside, feathery and incredibly soft. Silverweed creeps across the soil, sending out red runners. Five-petalled yellow flowers appear between June and August.

HISTORY: Roman soldiers stationed in Britain put the silky-soft leaves of silverweed or "traveller's ease" into their boots as comfortable padding, to prevent sore feet and help absorb sweat on long marches.

With its high starch content, silverweed was once much-valued as a "hardship food". When the foliage dies back in the autumn, the creeping red roots begin to swell to form plump little nodules, which can be cooked and eaten like potatoes. Known as *brisgein* in the Scottish Highlands, silverweed tubers were considered to be palatable and nutritious, and were roasted, boiled or ground into meal for bread and porridge until the early twentieth century.

Other "hardship foods" included pignuts, dock leaves, dandelion, red clover, sea anemones and snails. Thankfully silverweed was prolific, as Gerard says: *"It groweth in moist places near unto highways and running brooks everywhere."*

FOLKLORE: There are many different beliefs about the origins and uses of silverweed.

It is known as *richette* in France as the plant is "rich" in both silver and gold colours. This richness extends to the divine, for legend has it that as Christ was growing up in Palestine he walked on the soft, yellow-flowering plants that grew on the dusty roads, leading them to be called "the footsteps of Our Lord".

Silverweed is said to flourish in the gardens of witches; however, conflicting folklore relates that historically silverweed has been used to keep witches away. In some modern pagan and Wiccan traditions, silverweed is still used in spiritual and magical practices. It is said to be associated with the element of water and is used in rituals for healing, protection and purification.

FOLK MEDICINE: Medieval ladies foraged for silverweed to improve their skin and complexions.

Gerard advises: *"The distilled water taketh away freckles, spots, pimples in the face and sun-burning; but the herb laid to infuse or steep in white wine is far better: but the best of all is to steep it in strong white wine vinegar, the face being often bathed or washed therewith."*

For bruises he recommends silverweed should be *"boiled in water and salt and drunk, dissolveth clotted and congealed blood in such as are hurt or bruised with falling from some high place".*

Culpeper adds: *"A strong infusion of the leaves stops the immoderate bleeding of the piles, and, sweetened with a little honey, it is an excellent gargle for sore throats."*

An infusion of silverweed was also used to increase urine flow, heal mouth ulcers, as a remedy for tetanus, to protect gums and teeth from scurvy and to fix loose teeth.

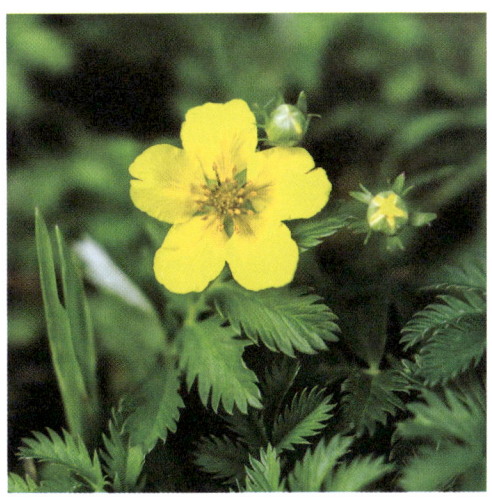

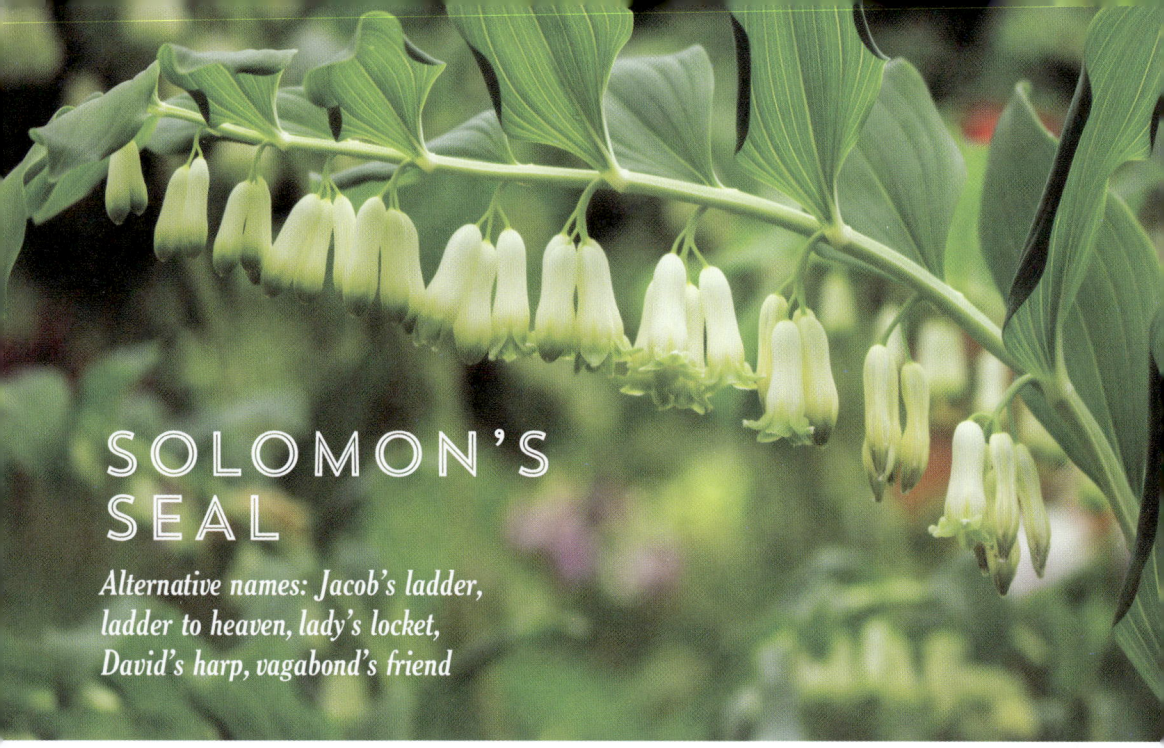

SOLOMON'S SEAL

Alternative names: Jacob's ladder, ladder to heaven, lady's locket, David's harp, vagabond's friend

HOW TO IDENTIFY: This British native wildflower can now only really be found flowering wild in the woodlands of Northumbria and southern Scotland, from May to June. Solomon's seal has distinctive arching stems from which hang clusters of green-tipped bell-like flowers. Waxy leaves grow in pairs along the stems and the flowers are followed by black berries in the autumn months.

HISTORY: Solomon's seal is a difficult plant to find, mainly due to climate change and the destruction of suitable habitats. You would be unlikely to find Solomon's seal growing wild anywhere south of Northumbria today, but it wasn't always so. In the seventeenth century, Gerard recounts discovering that it *"grows naturally wild in Somersetshire, upon the North side of a place called Mendip, in the parish of Shepton Mallet: also in Kent by a village called Crayford, upon Rough or Row hill: also in Odiham Park in Hampshire; in Bradford's Wood, near to a town in Wiltshire four miles from Bath; in a wood near to a village called Horsley, five miles from Guildford in Surrey, and in divers other places. That sort of Solomon's Seal with broad leaves groweth in certain woods in Yorkshire called Clapdale woods, three miles from a village named Settle."

FOLKLORE: There are many theories as to how Solomon's seal was given its name. One idea is that if the root was cut lengthways it was said to reveal Hebrew characters put there by Solomon, whereas Gerard believed that it was due to the healing and "sealing" powers of the root for open wounds and broken bones *"being stamped and laid thereon"*.

History tells us that King Solomon was a wise and protective king and that Solomon's seal echoes these attributes. To use Solomon's seal for protection, the root should be cut into four pieces and placed in each corner of the house. Alternatively hang a sachet of the herb in your home or sprinkle an infusion of Solomon's seal all over the house, to drive out any negative energy that may be present.

Poets and artists needing inspiration would inhale the vapours that arose when brewing the flowers, while psychics would make incense from the root and burn it to enhance their spiritual abilities.

FOLK MEDICINE: As mentioned before, Gerard recommended Solomon's seal for its healing powers. Controversially – remember that his writings are over 400 years old – he says:

"... applied, taketh away in one night, or two at the most, any bruise, black or blue spots gotten by falls or women's wilfulness, in stumbling upon their hasty husbands' fists, or such like."

Culpeper, as well as using Solomon's seal for bruises and broken bones, advised that it could be used as a beauty treatment:

"The distilled water of the whole plant, used to the face, or other parts of the skin, cleanses it from morphew, freckles, spots, or marks whatsoever, leaving the place fresh, fair, and lovely; for which purpose it is much used by the Italian dames."

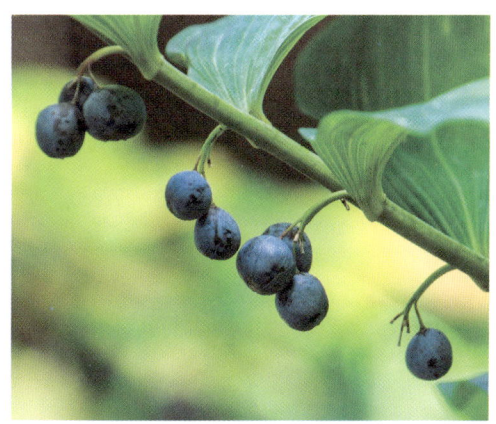

SPINDLE

Alternative names: Burning bush, dog timber, foulrush, pegwood, pincushion shrub, skewer wood, witchwood

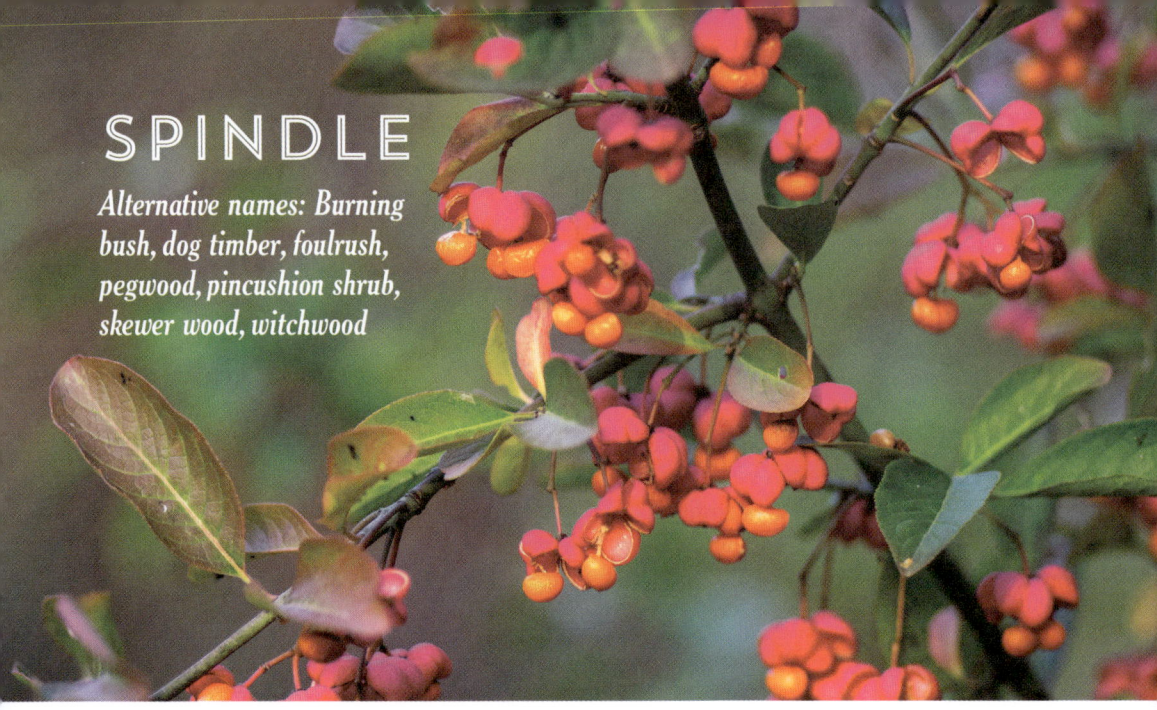

HOW TO IDENTIFY: Spindle is a deciduous shrub, which, given the right soil conditions, can grow up to 5 m (16 ft) tall and can be found in hedgerows and on the edges of forests. The spindle has very thin, straight twigs; the leaves are shiny and oval, turning red in the autumn with a serrated edge; and flowers are yellowish-green with four quite separate petals. The best time to see spindles is the autumn as the flowers turn into beautiful pink fruits with a bright orange seed at the centre.

No part of the spindle should be eaten as, although the berries are enjoyed by birds, mice and foxes, they are poisonous to us.

HISTORY: Spindle is another of our native indicators of ancient woodland, along with ferns, bluebells, primroses and other species.

So valued was the spindle in medieval Ireland that if you unlawfully damaged one you could be fined a yearling heifer, or more serious damage would cost you a two year old heifer.

The name gives us a clue to its first use: its hard, straight twigs were perfect as spindles on spinning wheels when making yarn and thread. Other uses included toothpicks, butcher's skewers for meat, knitting needles, wooden pegs for shoemaking, bird cages, bobbins for lace making and in the construction of harps. Artists loved to use charcoal made from spindle twigs as it was of very high quality. It was also used for pipe stems, pegs for shoes and even gunpowder. Spindle had so many uses, no wonder it was protected by law.

FOLKLORE: Spindle had a few ominous associations. It was believed that if the spindle flowered earlier in the year than it should, it was a stern warning to everyone that the plague was imminent.

In another negative conviction, the spindle berries themselves were believed not only to be poisonous to the person but also poisonous to the spirit. Some were prepared to risk their sanity or even death, believing that if they ate the berries they would be able to communicate with the dead.

However, the plant was known for more positive connections too. To attract wealth, carrying a spindle twig or some berries in your pocket would create a psychic shield around you to protect you from negative energies or forces.

FOLK MEDICINE: Spindle fruits were baked, powdered and sprinkled on the heads of schoolchildren and cattle to kill their nits, lice or mange. Leaves were boiled up to treat dogs for fleas, and country folk sprinkled powdered leaves around their houses as a natural insecticide.

Gerard documented spindle's toxicity: *"This shrub is hurtful to all things [...] namely to goats: [...] the fruit hereof killeth; so doth the leaves and fruit destroy goats especially, unless they scour as well upwards as downwards: if three or four of these fruits be given to a man they purge both by vomit and stool."*

The dried root bark of spindle is known as "wahoo bark". Considering that it is a cure for constipation, this seems a very fitting name.

Do not ingest any part of this poisonous plant.

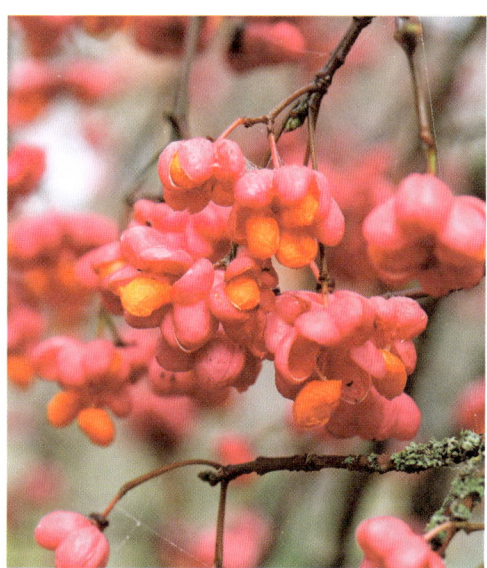

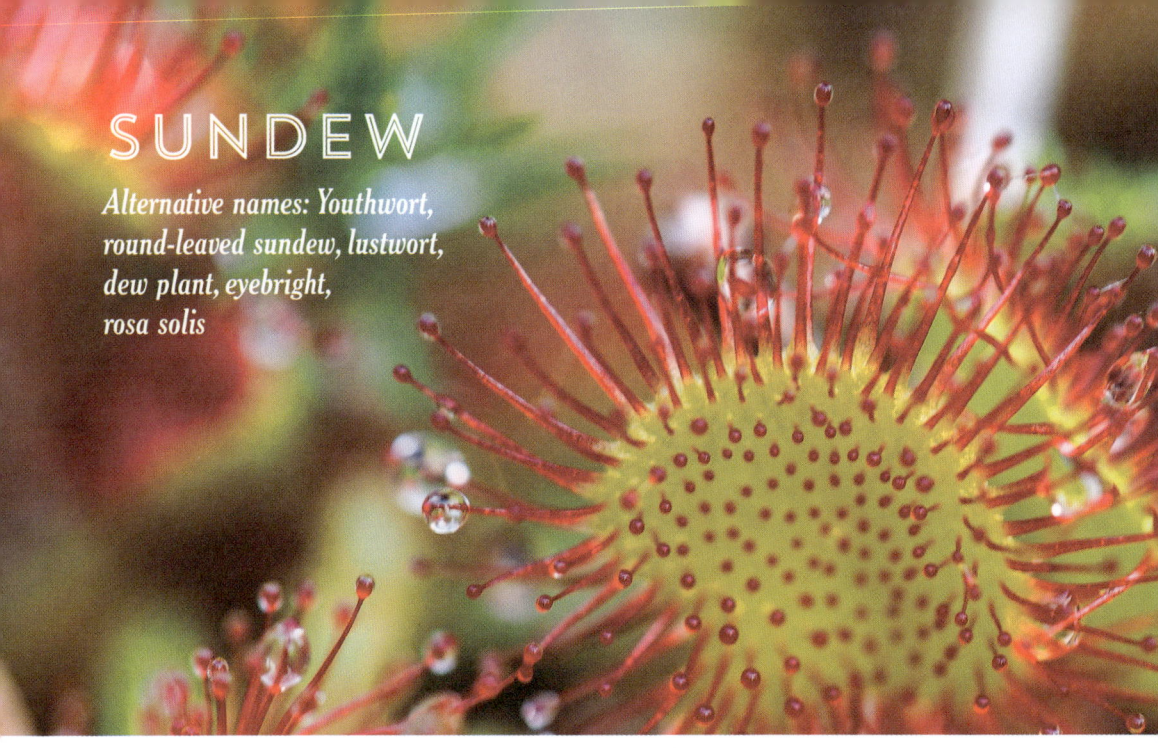

SUNDEW

Alternative names: Youthwort, round-leaved sundew, lustwort, dew plant, eyebright, rosa solis

HOW TO IDENTIFY: What an otherworldly plant sundew is! Living in peaty moors, wetlands and acidic bog pools, this fascinating insectivorous plant lies in wait for unsuspecting insects attracted to its hairy spoon-like leaves. Hair-like filaments tipped with glittering sticky droplets curl around and trap their prey, completely engulfing the insect and eventually digesting it. The sundew's insect-eating behaviour is an adaptation to the nutrient-poor soils it grows in. Sundew is a low-growing plant with very small white flowers which can be seen from June to August.

HISTORY: Sundew is a perfect example of nature providing a unique means of survival in the hostile, nutrient-lacking environment in which this plant thrives. Sundew has an amazing ability to catch and slowly digest insects, providing it with all the nutrients it needs without competition from other species.

Meanwhile, sundew has proven its usefulness for pigmentation. Ever since the Iron Age, people have been mixing sundew with ammonia (from urine) to make yellow hair dye, while purple dye can be extracted from the roots. Early settlers to the United

States managed to extract red liquid from sundews to be used as ink.

Fast-forward to the nineteenth century, and the renowned naturalist Charles Darwin became an avid admirer of sundew after noticing the large number of insects caught by the plant while he was walking on a heath in Sussex. In a letter to a friend dated 1860, he wrote that *"at the present moment, I care more about Drosera [sundew] than the origin of all the species in the world."*

It was also used in cheese making. The "juice" of the sundew is very bitter to the taste and on some farms in Scandinavia it was, and still is, used as a substitute for rennet to curdle the milk when making cheese.

FOLKLORE: It has been hinted that sundew, also known as "youthwort", could indeed be the legendary "elixir of life" sought-after by medieval alchemists. The glistening "dew" of the sundew was believed to be a source of youth and virility, and was used to make anti-ageing potions. After all, the sundew always looks glowing and moist, even on the hottest of days.

The undoubted ability of sundew to attract its prey also led to its use in love charms and love magic.

FOLK MEDICINE: Distilled with wine, sundew is said to have profound aphrodisiac properties. Gerard affirmed this by noting the effect that sundew had on sheep!

"Sheep and other cattle, if they do but only taste of it, are provoked to lust [and] Cattle of the female kind are stirred up to lust by eating even of a small quantity."

Gerard shared his recipe for making use of sundew's aphrodisiac properties ourselves:

"Lay the leaves of Rosa Solis [dew of the sun] in the spirit of wine, aiding thereto cinnamon, cloves, mace, ginger, nutmegs, sugar, and a few grains of musk suffering it so to stand in a glass close stopped from the air, and set in the sun by the space of ten days, then strain the same, and keep it for your use."

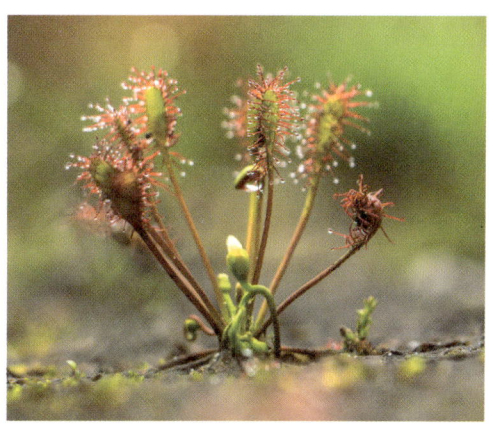

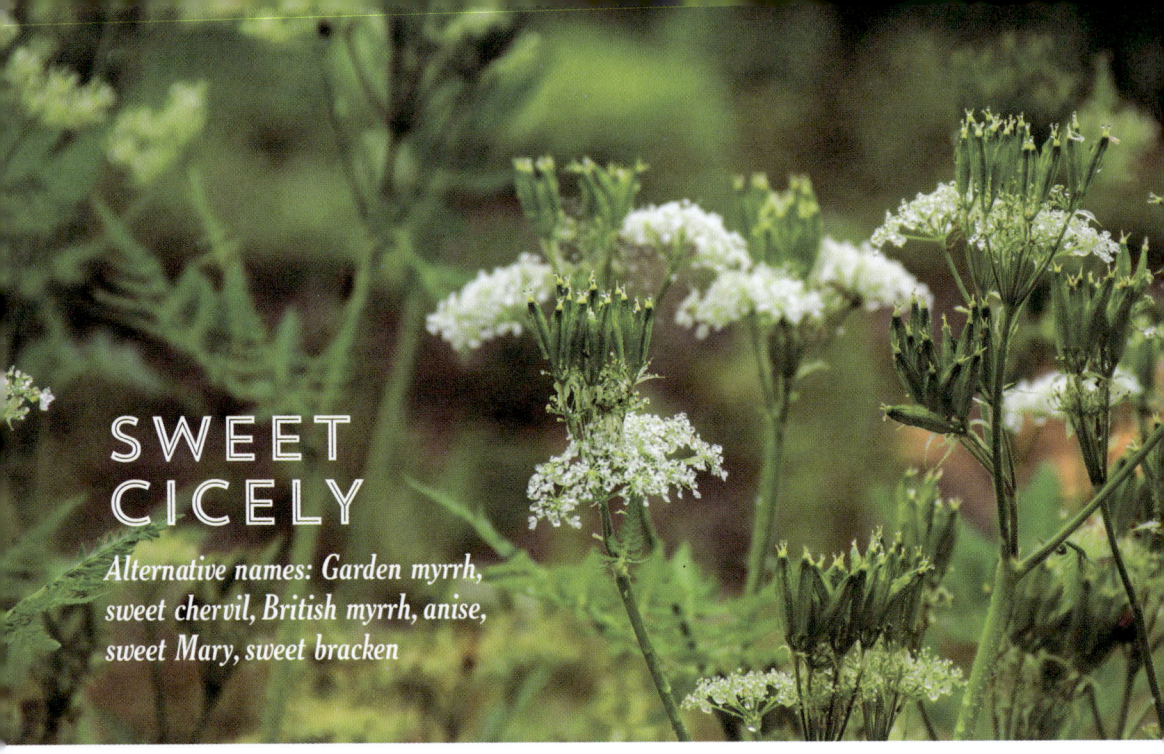

SWEET CICELY

Alternative names: Garden myrrh, sweet chervil, British myrrh, anise, sweet Mary, sweet bracken

HOW TO IDENTIFY: Widespread throughout Britain and Ireland but most common in northern England and Scotland, sweet cicely can usually be found on riverbanks and near streams. This tall plant with light green fern-like leaves has white flowers that form an umbrella shape from April to June and have a distinct smell of aniseed or liquorice when crushed.

HISTORY: All parts of the plant are edible: leaves, seeds and roots. Historically, sweet cicely was cultivated as a salad and medicinal herb, and used as a "strewing" herb to make medieval floors smell just a little sweeter.

In the fifteenth century, sweet cicely was used in Scandinavia to produce the spirit Akvavit, and in the eighteenth century by Carthusian monks to make their bright green liqueur, Chartreuse.

Sweet cicely seeds are particularly useful to add sweetness when cooking acidic dishes such as rhubarb, helping to reduce the amount of sugar needed. The roots can be candied while the young leaves can be added to salads or soups, or infused to make a delicious tea.

Gerard adds, *"It is used very much among the Dutch people in a kind of loblolly or hot-pot which they do eat, called Warmus."*

Sweet cicely leaves or juice from the pounded seeds were rubbed onto oak floors or furniture to give it a beautiful shine – it must have smelled wonderful too. In addition, the lovely white flowers are rich in nectar and highly valuable to bees and other beneficial insects.

FOLKLORE: Very little folklore exists surrounding sweet cicely. The flowers and leaves dried and added into incense are believed to bring happiness and joy, especially when burned at Beltane and midsummer. A tea of the leaf or flower is also taken at midsummer celebrations, possibly as an aid to digestion after all the festivities and feasting.

FOLK MEDICINE: Gerard gives us all a little hope for the future if we eat sweet cicely root, as it is *"very good for old people that are dull and without courage; it rejoiceth and comforteth the heart, and increaseth their lust and strength."*

It seems that Gerard enjoyed the aniseed taste of the leaves and seeds in a salad and regards them as *"exceedingly good, wholesome and pleasant"*, as well as recommending that the *"root drunk in wine is a remedy against the bitings of the venomous spiders".*

Culpeper concentrates more on the plant's abilities to relieve bruising: *"[Sweet cicely] is a certain remedy to dissolve congealed or clotted blood in the body, or that which is clotted by bruises, falls, &c […] bruised [leaves] and applied, dissolveth swellings in any part, or the marks of congealed blood by bruises or blows."* He recommended that the candied roots of sweet cicely should be eaten to prevent being infected by the great plague of the seventeenth century.

Finally, Grieve tells us that sweet cicely is *"useful in coughs and flatulence"* and *"a valuable tonic for girls from 15 to 18 years".*

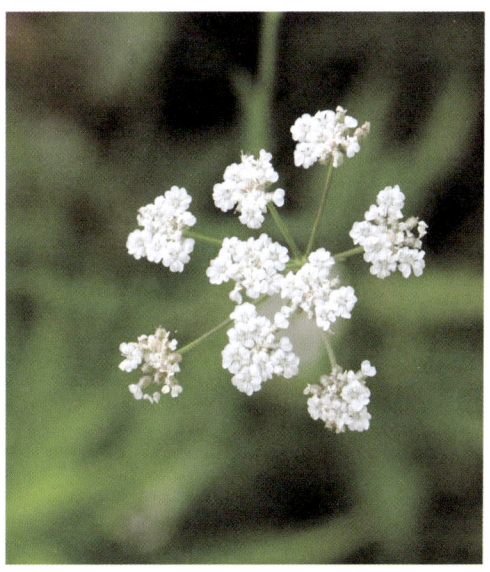

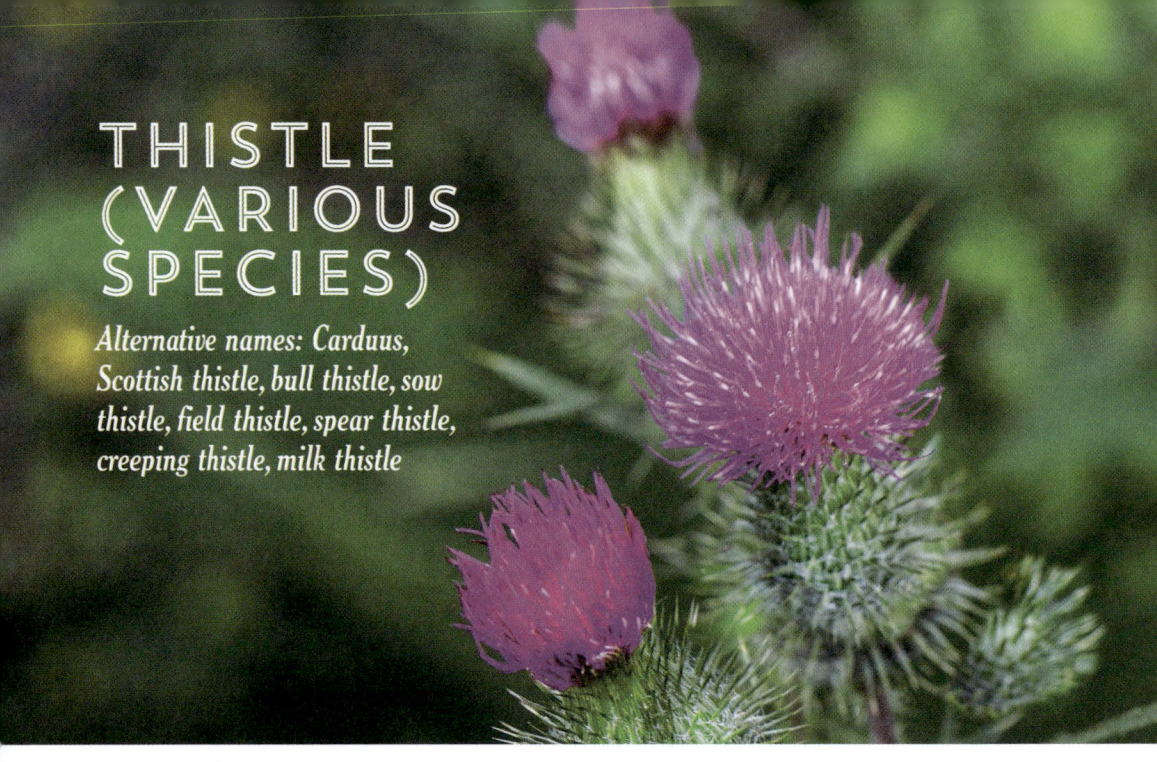

THISTLE (VARIOUS SPECIES)

Alternative names: Carduus, Scottish thistle, bull thistle, sow thistle, field thistle, spear thistle, creeping thistle, milk thistle

HOW TO IDENTIFY: The different varieties of thistle generally share the same characteristics – sharp, prickly leaves and stems, and fluffy pink or purple flower heads which appear on top of a spiny ball. Thistles can grow up to 1 m (3 ft) tall and they flourish in disturbed ground and roadside verges.

HISTORY: The thistle family boasts numerous members but possibly one of the most famous is the Scottish thistle, emblem of Scotland since the reign of the thirteenth-century king, Alexander the Third. Legend tells us that in 1263, an invading Norse army was attempting to ambush an encampment housing the sleeping Scottish clansmen. In an attempt to attack silently, the Norsemen removed their footwear. Unfortunately, one of the Vikings stepped on a thistle and cried out loudly in pain. This woke the clansmen and alerted them to the impending invasion, leading to victory for Scotland and the thistle being adopted as the national flower.

The thistle symbolized devotion, strength, determination, resilience and courage. It first appeared on a silver coin during the reign of King James III of Scotland and continued to feature on coins until 2008.

FOLKLORE: As with many spiky plants, thistles are believed to possess protective powers that can ward off negative energies and evil spirits. Thistle was often used in rituals to bless and protect a new home and its residents from misfortune.

In the Bible, thistles sprang up in the Garden of Eden after Adam and Eve had been ejected:

> *"Adam's sin resulted in God cursing the ground he was called to work. Instead of good things like food and flowers, the garden was now going to produce thorns and thistles, making work unnecessarily difficult [...] From this point forward, labour for men and women was going to be painful, time-consuming, frustrating, stressful, sweaty, and full of relational conflict."*

Thistles have long been associated with magic: wearing a shirt made from thistle fibres will break any spells that have been cast against you; wizards would always choose the tallest thistle to fashion into walking sticks and magic wands; and thistles planted by your front door will drive out evil and prevent negative energy from entering.

FOLK MEDICINE: Gerard suggests using thistles in the treatment of *"bodies drawn backwards"*. Sadly, I have failed to come up with a modern comparison for that particular malady.

Culpeper categorized each species of thistle separately. Among the uses were cures for *"pestilent fevers"*, *"rickets"*, *"venereal disease"* and for a *"crick in the neck"*.

Milk thistle, he notes, is believed to help new mothers: *"It is chiefly used now for nursing mothers, the warm infusion scarcely ever failing to procure a proper supply of milk. It is considered one of the best medicines which can be used for the purpose."*

Milk thistle also contains silymarin, an active ingredient said to promote hair growth, which explains why medieval Brits and Pliny the Elder believed it was a cure for baldness.

The list of possible cures continues. During the Early Modern Period (1500–1780), thistles were believed to be able to cure jaundice, headaches, vertigo and even cancerous sores.

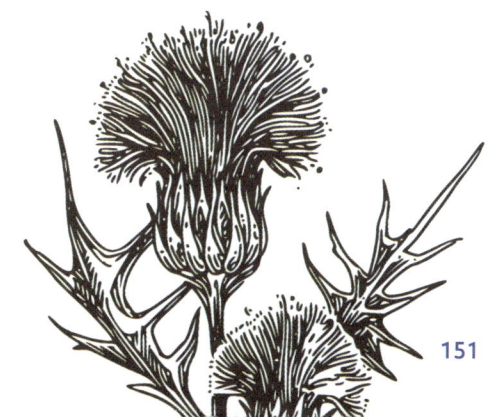

THREE-CORNERED LEEK

Alternative names: Three-cornered garlic, angled onion, wild leeks, white bluebells, stinking onion

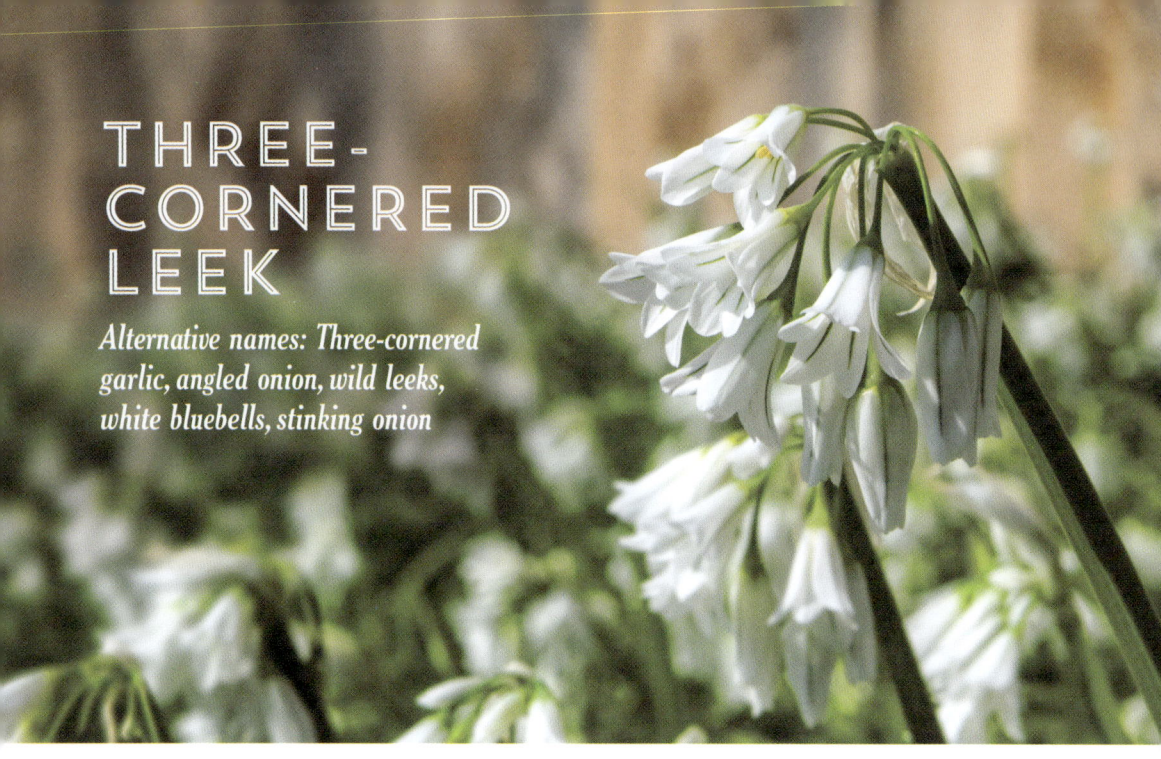

HOW TO IDENTIFY: An invasive species brought into the UK from the Mediterranean, it is illegal to deliberately introduce this plant into the wild. Many have sneaked out of private gardens and can be found growing outside garden walls and fences, making them fair game for foragers. You must not dig up the bulbs without permission, though.

As the name implies, three-cornered leek is easily identified by its triangular stalk and characteristic smell of onions, garlic or chives. Long, thin leaves emerge from the ground in late winter, followed in the spring by "three-cornered" flowering stems. The flowers resemble white bluebells with a distinctive green vein down the petals, and the entire plant smells of onions.

HISTORY: The three-cornered leek was introduced to botanical gardens in the UK from Spain and Portugal in the eighteenth century when many exotic and non-native species were prized by collectors. Interestingly, the seeds of three-cornered leek have been found to be spread naturally by ants and other insects that like to eat the natural wrapping that occurs around the seeds, meaning that they are partly responsible for their rapid spread.

All parts of the plant are edible. In Sicily they are traditionally eaten in a mixed salad with olives and cheese – sounds delicious!

FOLKLORE: In Greek mythology the three-cornered leek was associated with the goddess Persephone, who was believed to have turned the plant into a flower to represent the rebirth of spring. It was also used for its power to purify and cleanse during religious ceremonies held by the ancient Romans.

Along with garlic, three-cornered leek has been used as a plant for protection: growing these plants around your home was believed to ward off evil spirits and bring peace to the household. In some cultures, the white flowers are seen as symbols of peace and purity. The gift of a bouquet featuring three-cornered leeks was seen to be a peace offering and given generously as a representation of new beginnings.

FOLK MEDICINE: Being from the same family as garlic and onions, three-cornered leek possesses pretty much the same health benefits as its better-known cousins.

The bulb is believed to be the most active part of the plant, with cholesterol and blood pressure lowering properties. They are high in iron, potassium, vitamins A, C and K, and antioxidants, as well as being anti-inflammatory and a tonic for the digestion.

It is well worth taking the time to forage as three-cornered leek can be used as a substitute for wild garlic in any recipe.

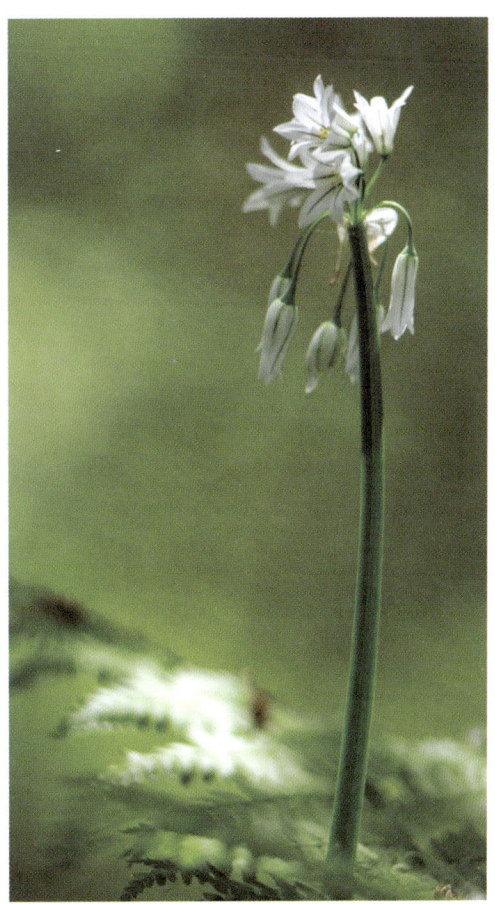

THREE-CORNERED LEEK AND CHEESE SCONES

This versatile recipe can be made with three-cornered leeks, wild garlic or even spring onions – whichever is in season.

Scones are always best baked and eaten warm on the same day, with a generous slather of butter. I also quite like to make a savoury version of a cream tea by serving these scones topped with cream cheese and homemade caramelized onion chutney.

If by some miracle you happen to have any scones left over, just pop them in the freezer for a maximum of three months, to be enjoyed another day.

I've included plant-based, dairy-free and gluten-free alternatives too.

Makes approx. eight scones

INGREDIENTS

225 g self-raising flour (gluten-free if desired)

1 tsp baking powder

Pinch of salt

½ tsp mustard powder

55 g cold cubed butter, or 3 tbsp vegetable oil

50 g washed and chopped three-cornered leek leaves and stems

100 g strong cheese, grated, or plant-based cheddar

150 ml milk, or milk alternative

Extra grated cheese for topping

EQUIPMENT NEEDED

Grater

Sieve

Mixing bowl

Knife

Scone cutter

Pastry brush

Baking tray lined with non-stick paper

Wire cooling rack

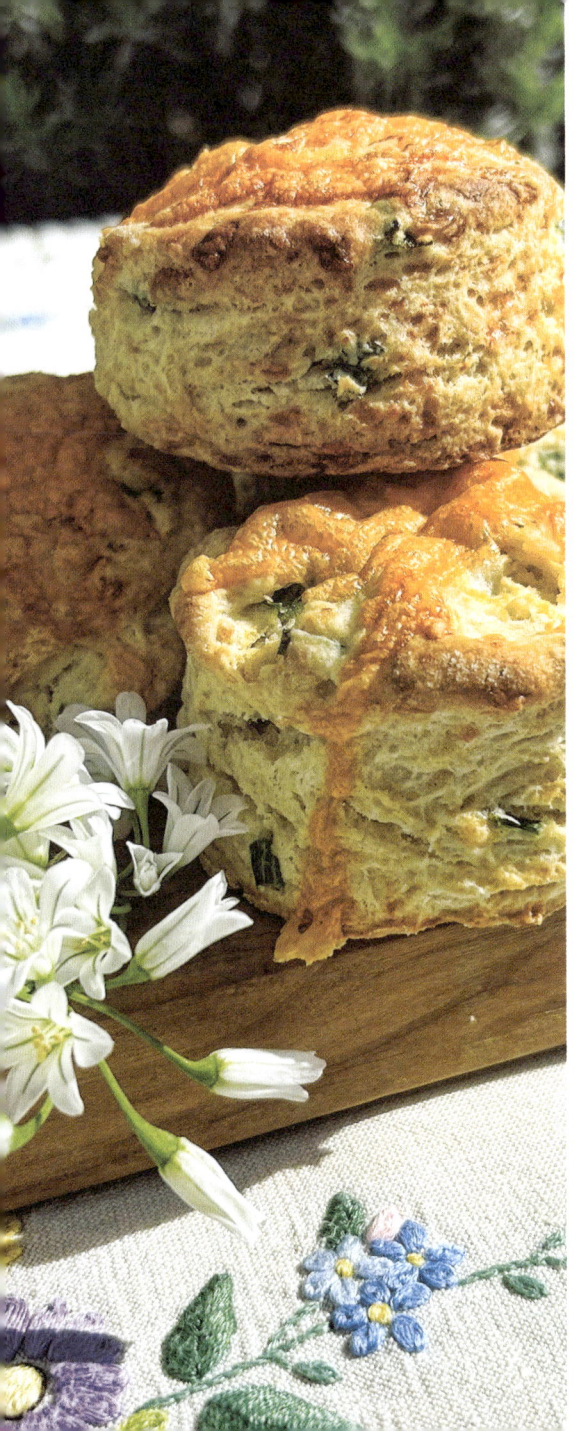

METHOD

Preheat oven to 200°C (390°F).

Sift the flour, baking powder, salt and mustard powder into a large mixing bowl.

Add the cold butter or veg oil.

Using the tips of your fingers, rub the ingredients together to form a fine crumble mixture.

Mix in the chopped three-cornered leek and grated cheese.

Make a well in the centre and pour in most of the milk.

Use a knife to combine the ingredients until a soft dough is formed, adding more milk as needed.

Turn the dough out on a floured surface and simply pat to a thickness of about 2.5 cm (1 in.).

Use a 5 cm (2 in.) cutter to stamp out rounds and place them on the baking sheet.

Carefully gather up the rest of the dough and cut out more rounds.

Brush the tops of the scones with milk and top with a little more grated cheese.

Bake for 12–15 minutes until well risen and golden.

Cool on a wire rack.

Three-cornered leek is toxic for dogs.

TOADFLAX

Alternative names: Bacon and eggs, bread and butter, brideweed, calf's snout, dead men's bones, shoes and stockings

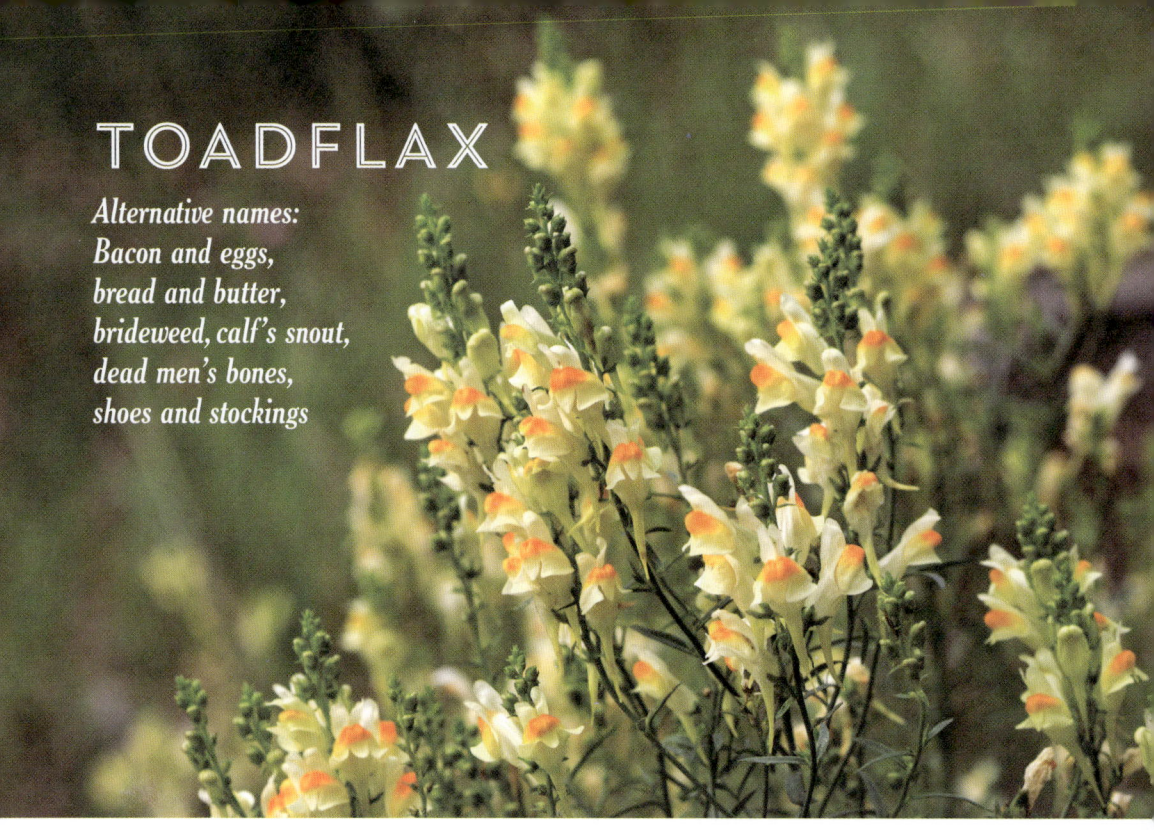

HOW TO IDENTIFY: Look out for the yellow and orange snapdragon-like flowers of toadflax along hedgerows, grassland and verges from June to November. The flower stems grow to about 90 cm (35 in.) tall, with long, slender leaves growing all the way up, and with creeping roots it can quickly create dense carpets of foliage. Toadflax provides an important food source for honeybees, white-tailed and buff-tailed bumblebees, common carder bees and various fly species.

HISTORY: Toadflax has grown in the UK for well over 400,000 years, with seeds having been identified in Suffolk dating from the Hoxnian Interglacial Period, making it well and truly a native plant for definite.

Toadflax was believed to have been introduced to the US from Wales in the seventeenth century by Welsh Quakers who went to settle in Delaware. Plagued by insects, the settlers were desperate to grow toadflax as it could be made into the most effective balm to ease insect bites.

Toadflax was also boiled in milk which was then placed around the homestead to poison the swarms of flies that were a constant nuisance.

Having used it for centuries to make yellow dye for their textiles, German immigrants to the US, especially the Mennonites, were delighted to find that toadflax was already well established.

FOLKLORE: Ancient Celtic people believed that toadflax was a "fae flower"; where it grew, hidden treasure would be waiting to be discovered. However, this bounty was closely guarded by the fae and anyone who disturbed their treasure would be subject to the wrath of the faery folk.

Toadflax is a plant of protection; a Scottish superstition states that walking around toadflax three times can break even the most powerful spell cast against you.

Some say that toadflax flowers look like little toads, while others say that toads have been known to shelter underneath the plants and this is how it got its name.

FOLK MEDICINE: Historically, toadflax seems to have been most useful for many ailments. Gerard observes:

"The decoction of Toad-Flax taketh away the yellowness and deformity of the skin, being washed and bathed therewith [...] The same drunken, openeth the stoppings of the liver and spleen, and is singular good against the jaundice which is of long continuance."

Culpeper adds other uses:

"The juice of the herb, or the distilled water, dropped into the eyes, is a certain remedy for all heat, inflammation and redness in them [...] The same juice or water also cleanses the skin wonderfully of all sorts of deformity, as leprosy, morphew, scurf [flaky skin], wheals, pimples, or spots, applied of itself, or used with some powder of lupines [lupins]."

And, according to Grieve:

"A cooling ointment is made from the fresh plant — the whole herb is chopped and boiled in lard until crisp, then strained. The result is a fine green ointment, a good application for piles, sores, ulcers and skin eruptions."

TORMENTIL

Alternative names: Bloodroot, biscuits, flesh and blood, ewe daisy, English sarsaparilla

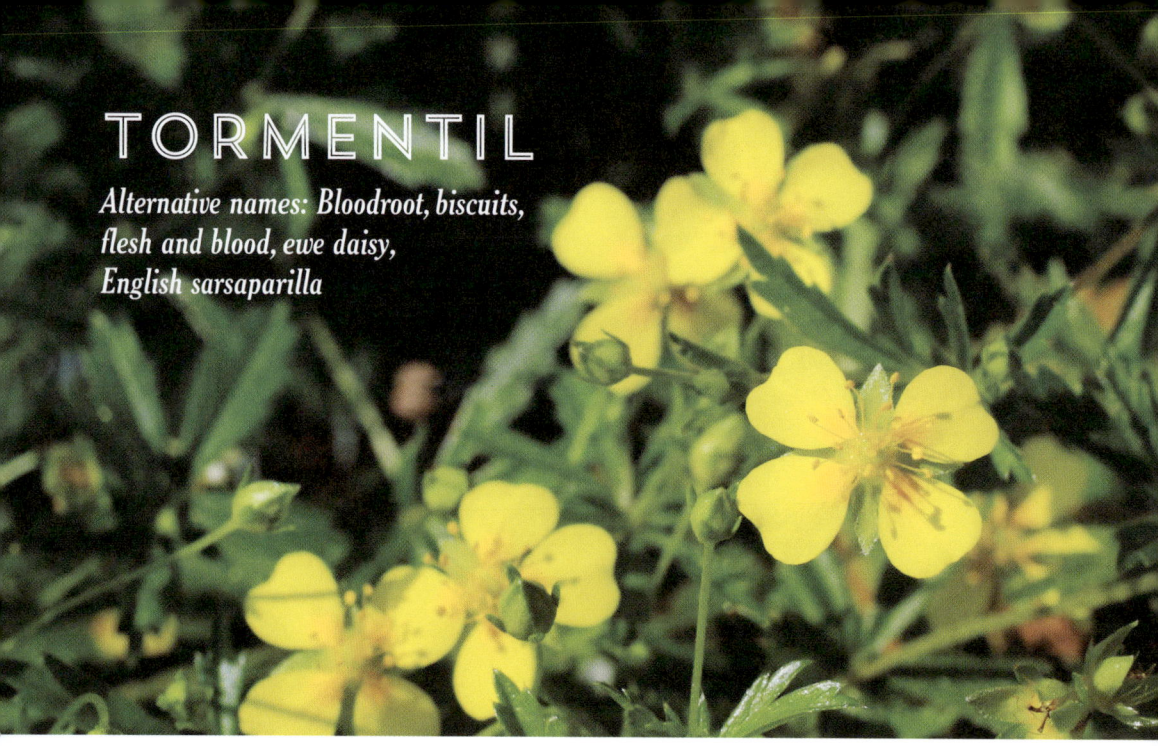

HOW TO IDENTIFY: The yellow buttercup-like flowers of the tormentil appear on acid grasslands and roadside verges from May to September. This creeping perennial grows low to the ground with glossy, deeply lobed leaves that are silvery underneath.

HISTORY: Many of the Scottish islands have been without trees since Viking times, making it difficult to source oak bark for leather tanning – to tan the skins of lambs, calves, seals and cows to make shoes and other leather goods. For many centuries the resourceful islanders have used tormentil root, or "red roots", which grow in abundance on the islands. This could be used in place of oak bark to produce a deep red dye, while adding dock to the process gave a pale yellow colour to the hide. It was a very laborious process to make the dye and it could take one person, usually a woman, a whole day just to dig up enough of the small roots for a single infusion.

Fishermen in the Highlands and islands would also use tormentil's red dye to make their nets tougher and last longer. Artists still use a pigment made from the plant called "tormentil red", while in Bavaria tormentil root is brewed into a dark red liqueur called Blutwurz.

FOLKLORE: Carrying tormentil with you was believed to attract love, while giving an infusion to your partner would also assure fidelity. Should your partner leave and you desperately wanted them back, the burning of tormentil at midnight on a Friday would unsettle them so much that they would return to you.

Psychic mediums drank the infusion to protect themselves against permanent possession by spirits, while tormentil root was hung in houses to drive away evil.

FOLK MEDICINE: Author Alexander Carmichael travelled the Highlands of Scotland, gathering miscellaneous lore. In his book *Carmina Gadelica*, published in 1900, he relates a tale about a faery encounter on the Isle of Barra. A man from the fishing and crofting hamlet of Bruernish on the east coast of Barra was out foraging for tormentil when he heard a faery woman singing a song while grinding corn with her quern (a hand mill). She sang that not only was the plant good for tanning leather, but also that it was a good cure for diarrhoea.

Culpeper agrees: *"Tormentil is excellent to stay all kinds of fluxes of blood or humours in man or woman, whether at nose, mouth or belly."*

He recommends tormentil taken with *"Venice treacle"*, which was an incredible honey-based concoction containing over 70 herbs and other ingredients, including viper flesh, cinnamon, wine and opium fermented over many years. It was as a remedy for plague, fever or measles.

Meanwhile, as well as effectively treating humans, milk infused with tormentil was an effective cure for calves with diarrhoea.

More recently, Grieve promotes tormentil as a wart remedy: *"If a piece of lint be soaked in the decoction and kept applied to warts, they will disappear."*

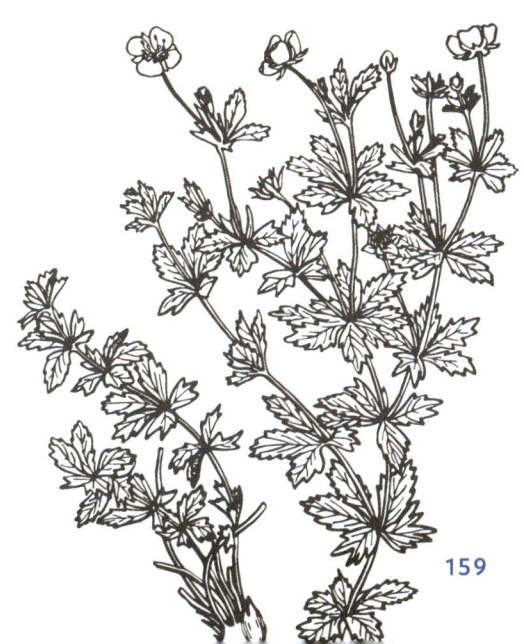

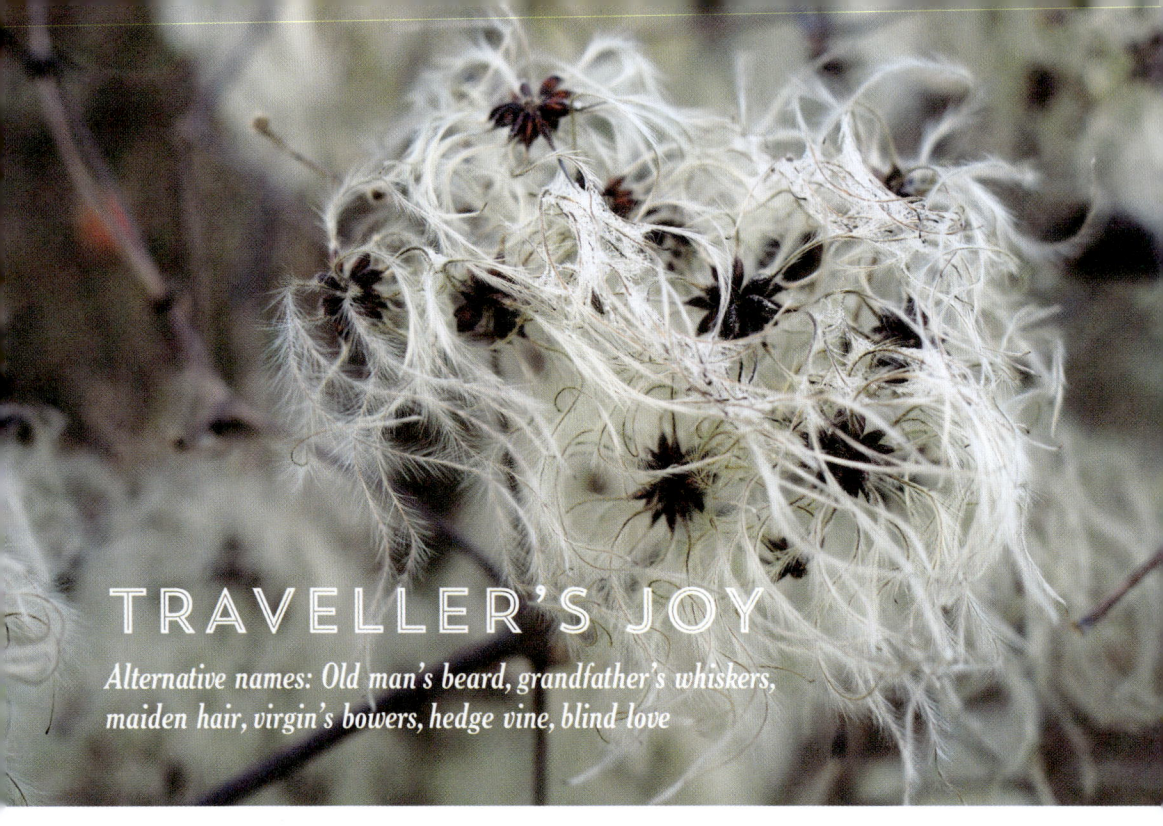

TRAVELLER'S JOY

Alternative names: Old man's beard, grandfather's whiskers, maiden hair, virgin's bowers, hedge vine, blind love

HOW TO IDENTIFY: This clematis-like climber can be seen scrambling over walls and hedgerows, producing a mass of creamy white flowers in the spring, followed by very distinctive wispy pom-pom seed heads all through autumn and into winter.

Traveller's joy likes to grow in chalky soil, making it widespread in the south of England but barely to be found in the north of Scotland.

Bees and hoverflies pollinate traveller's joy and it is an invaluable food source for the chalk carpet moth, the small waved umber moth and the small emerald butterfly, as well as hungry goldfinches.

HISTORY: The name "traveller's joy" was apparently first coined by Gerard in the seventeenth century when he was delighted by the way it *"maketh in winter a goodly show, covering the hedges white all over with its feather-like tops".*

In a poem published in 1917, English poet Edward Thomas wrote:

"Rough, long grasses keep white with frost
At the hilltop by the finger-post
The smoke of the traveller's joy is puffed
Over hawthorn berry and hazel tuft."

Thick old stems of traveller's joy have been utilized by early Brits as rope and bindings since Neolithic times. Historically the woody stems were woven into baskets and the bottom of crab pots in Devon, while the seeds have been found in the form of jewellery, amulets and necklaces.

In Sussex, traveller's joy was known as "tom-bacca" or "boys-bacca" as young men and boys would cut short lengths of the woody stalk to smoke instead of cigarettes.

FOLKLORE: This intrusive weed often kills other species by out-competing and strangling them, which led to it being believed to be doing the "devil's work" and being regarded with suspicion. Contrarily, it was also thought to have the power to protect travellers from evil spirits and was regarded as a useful refuge or "virgin's bower" for maidens – specifically the Virgin Mary – to conceal themselves in. Traveller's joy was included in bridal bouquets to signify the "binding together" of a couple.

FOLK MEDICINE: Medieval paupers and vagrants made good use of the slightly caustic sap that could be obtained from traveller's joy. Rubbing it onto their skin would create an ulcerous appearance and gain the sympathy, and hopefully charity, of passersby.

In traditional medicine, traveller's joy was used to treat a variety of ailments, including wounds, skin irritations and respiratory issues. The leaves were applied to wounds to speed up the healing process, and the stems were used to make a tea that was believed to help with coughing and bronchial problems. A decoction of the roots and stems was used in the early twentieth century to treat itchy skin, and a decoction of the leaves to ease the symptoms of rheumatism.

Modern-day herbalists do not recommend ingesting the plant.

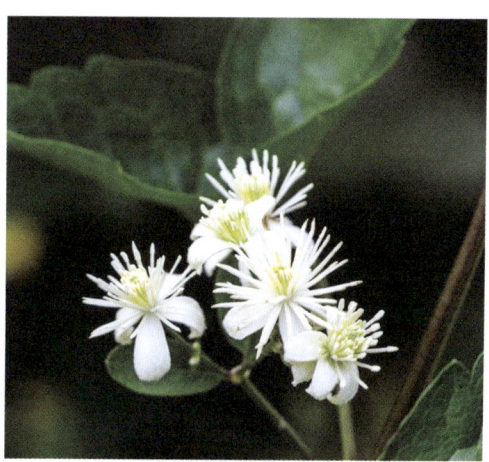

TRAVELLER'S JOY WINTER WREATH

Door wreaths date back to ancient Greece and were made from harvested plants like wheat to ensure fertile crops for the following year. Jump forward to nineteenth-century Germany, where the first recorded advent wreath was made by Lutheran priest John Hinrich Wichern, to be used as a centrepiece on a table. From then onwards, wreaths known as "welcome rings" began to be hung on front doors, usually made from holly, ivy, ribbons and pine cones.

You'll be surprised at the variety of greenery that you can forage even in the depths of winter. Keep an eye out for pretty pink spindle berries, ivy seed heads, rosehips and fir cones and of course traveller's joy, which will positively glow in the golden winter sunshine.

Makes one wreath

YOU WILL NEED

Evergreen foliage, such as ivy, holly, etc.

A moss ring or twisted willow wreath base

Traveller's joy and, honesty seed heads, berries, etc.

Binding wire or jute string

Secateurs

METHOD

Cut your evergreen foliage into similar lengths.

Gather a small handful of foliage to create your first posy. Hold the ends and bind it tightly onto your wreath base by wrapping around the base with wire or jute. Secure with a twist or knot.

Repeat the process, going the same way around the wreath base until it is completely covered in foliage posies.

Add on pieces of traveller's joy, berries, etc. using the same wiring technique.

Create a hanging loop at the top of your wreath.

Hang on your door and behold with joy!

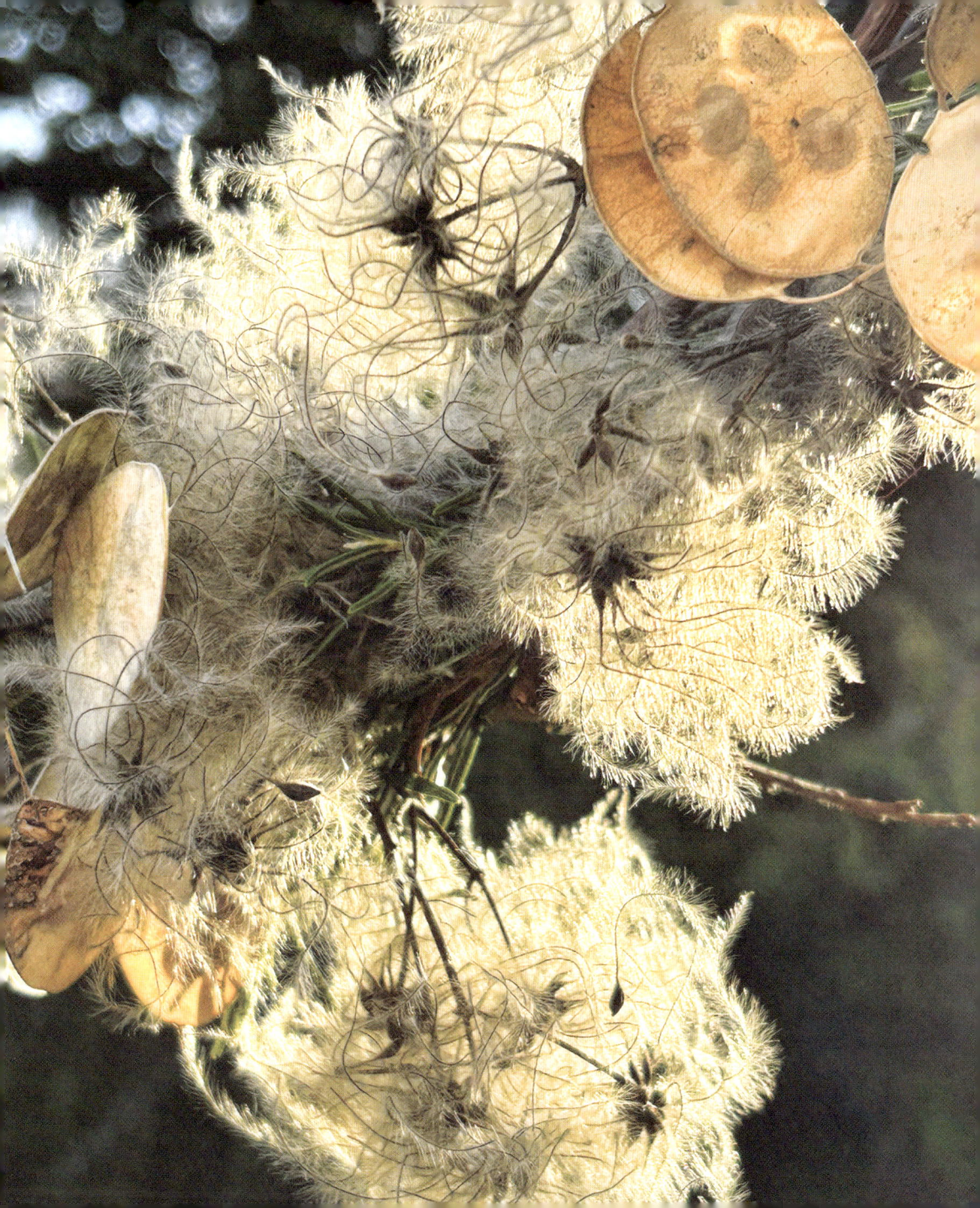

VALERIAN

Alternative names: All heal, cut finger leaf, cat's love, set well, black elder

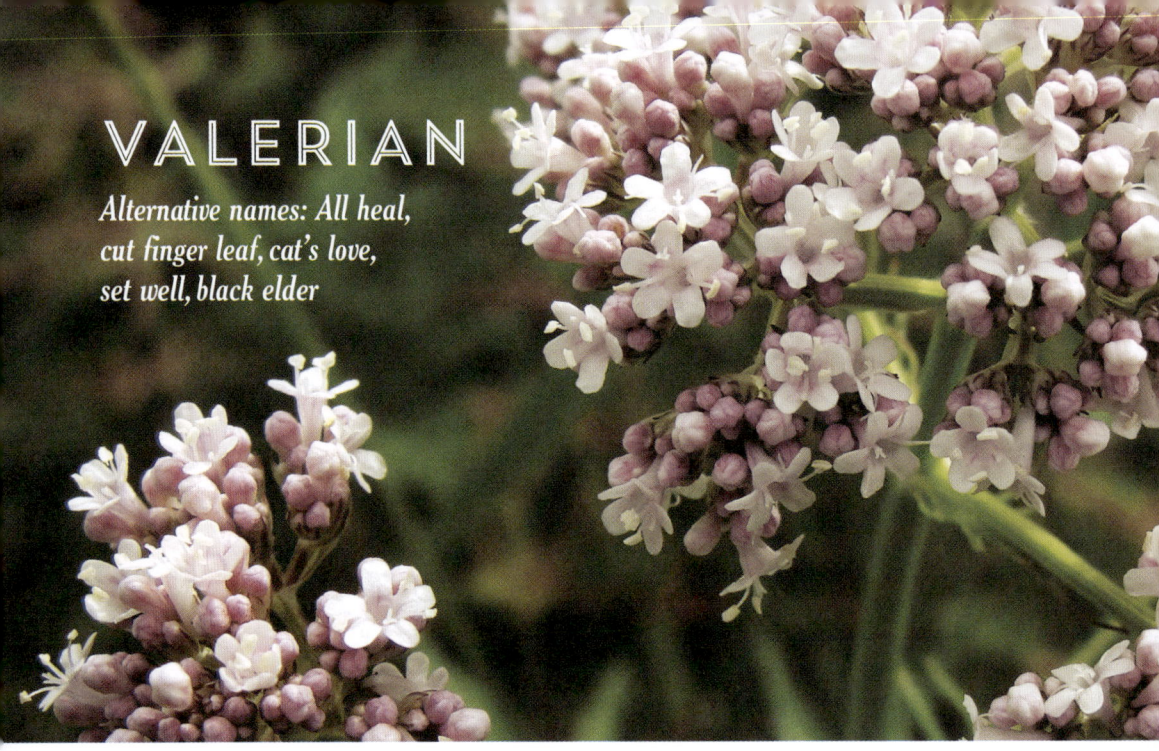

HOW TO IDENTIFY: This tall native plant produces masses of pinkish-white scented flowers that can be seen blooming from June to August. You are most likely to find it in moist, well-drained soils along riverbanks and woodland clearings. Look out for its finely divided leaves.

HISTORY: Valerian is native to Europe and has been used medicinally since the eleventh century, as shown in records written by the Ango-Saxon "leeches" (healers).

Valerian was cultivated for medicinal use in parts of England, but demand completely outstripped supply and the cost soared from 30 shillings per hundredweight to 120 shillings per hundredweight during World War One.

Known as "the Valium of the nineteenth century", valerian root was also given to shell-shocked soldiers of World War One and later prescribed to treat insomnia and nervous exhaustion in civilians during the Blitz of World War Two.

Grieve actively encouraged the use of valerian for those left at home during the war:

"During the recent war, when air-raids were a serious strain on the overwrought nerves of civilian men and women, valerian prescribed with other simple ingredients, taken in a single dose, or repeated according to the need, proved wonderfully efficacious, preventing or minimising serious results."

FOLKLORE: Cats, rats and other animals find the scent of valerian very attractive, and it is believed that the fabled Pied Piper of Hamelin carried valerian root in his pocket to lure the rats to their deaths in the river Weser. Apparently, humans find it irresistible too – love sachets containing valerian pinned to young ladies' clothing would cause men to follow them like children, or perhaps like rats?

In the bedchamber, it continued to work wonders: placed under the pillow, it not only cured insomnia and stopped nightmares but also acted as an aphrodisiac.

For the Celts, however, it had a different effect: they hung bundles of valerian in their houses to protect from lightning strikes.

FOLK MEDICINE: Culpeper wrote of how:

"The root boiled with liquorice, raisins and aniseed is good for those troubled with cough, Also, it is of special value against the plague, the decoction thereof being drunk and the root smelled. The green herb being bruised and applied to the head taketh away pain and pricking thereof."

He was well aware of valerian's benefits as a "nerve tonic": *"It is excellent against nervous affections in general, such as inveterate headaches, trembling, palpitations of the heart, vapours and hysteria complaints."*

In the Middle Ages valerian was widely used in the treatment of epilepsy and St Vitus' dance, now known as Sydenham's chorea – a disorder associated with rheumatic fever, causing the body to jerk uncontrollably.

Gerard wrote that *"No broth or medicine be worth anything if it did not contain valerian,"* and recommended its use for *"chest congestion, convulsions, bruises and falls"*. Use with care as valerian can *"purge upward and downward"*.

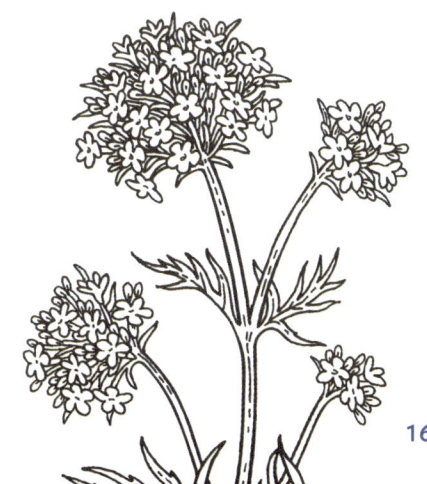

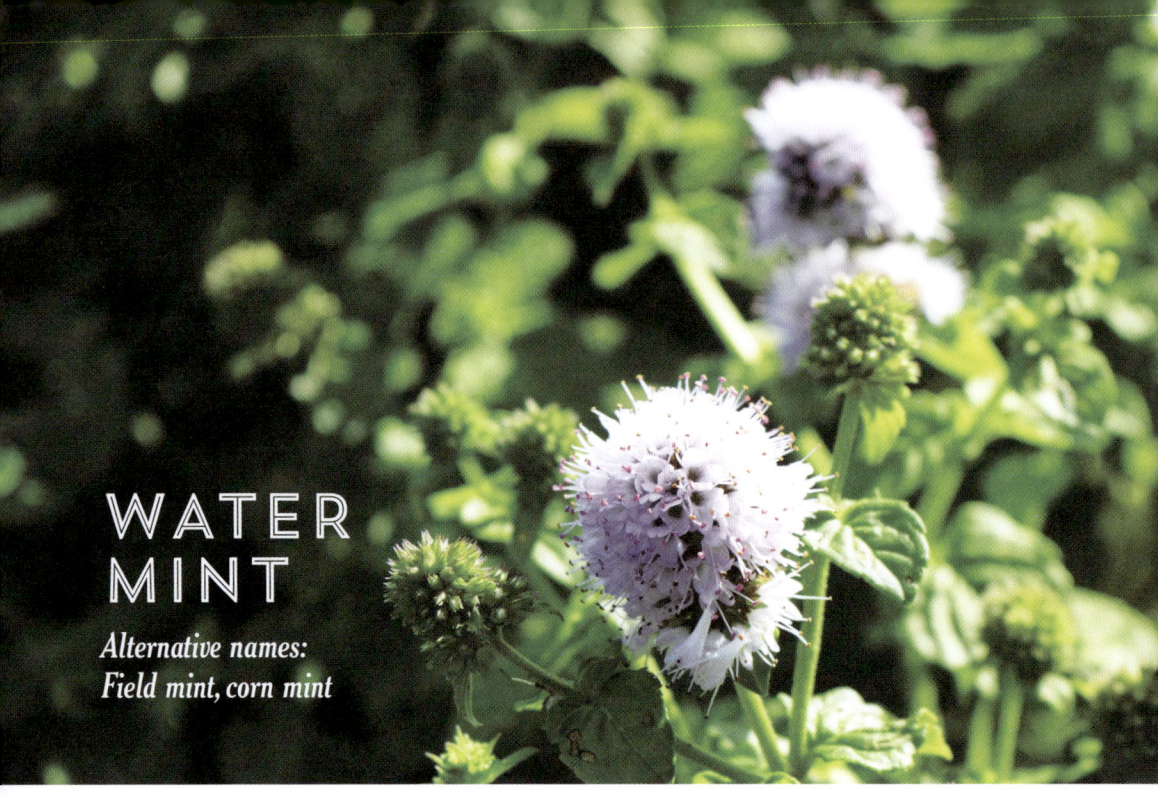

WATER MINT

Alternative names:
Field mint, corn mint

HOW TO IDENTIFY: Water mint is a UK native which prefers a damp habitat along riverbanks and boggy or flooded land. The aromatic leaves are oval with little nibbles taken out along the edges, and as with all plants in the mint family, the stem is square and covered in small hairs. The tiny, lilac flowers appear at the top of the stems from July to October.

HISTORY: In ancient Egypt, mint was deemed valuable enough to be used as a form of currency for trading and bartering, possibly resulting in the word "mint" becoming common as the word for producing money.

In the Bible's New Testament, Jesus criticizes the Pharisees for paying some tithes to the Church in mint: *"Mint and rue are plants of little value. It is easy and painless to tithe them as an offering to the divine, and their pleasant aroma may create an illusion of significance."*

Chocolate mint is a cross between peppermint and orange mint, while peppermint is a cross between water mint and spearmint. This was cultivated in the seventeenth century and became our most extensively used culinary mint.

In medieval times along with other aromatic herbs, mint was used as a "strewing" herb. Spread over floors, the herbs would release their scent, masking the more unpleasant smells of medieval life while also repelling fleas, mice and insects.

Gerard wrote that *"The savour or smell of water mint rejoiceth the heart of man…"* I have to agree with him.

FOLKLORE: Mint infused in hot water and used as a floor wash will keep away unwelcome visitors and help to return the household back to harmony after arguments.

A couple of mint leaves in your purse or wallet ensures that money will come to you, while mint in the shoes will bring good luck and remove any perceived obstacles in your way. Mint under your pillow encourages dreams of the future and will also help hay fever symptoms, while wearing a crown of mint can sharpen the brain and aid concentration.

FOLK MEDICINE: In the thirteenth-century *Compendium of Medicine*, the physician known as Gilbert of England recommends that for the *"stinking of the mouth, if there be rotten flesh, let the mouth be washed with wine that birch or mint has been soaked in [...] and let him eat marjoram, mint and parsley til they be well chewed. And let him rub well his teeth with the herbs he chewed and also his gums."*

The Roman author Pliny the Elder writes of mint: *"it prevents the recurrence of lascivious dreams".*

This differs from the view of Alexander the Great, who forbade his soldiers to diffuse peppermint oil before battle, fearing that it would stir erotic thoughts and thus lessen their desire to fight. This is echoed by Culpeper who warns that mint *"stirs up the venery [the pursuit of sexual pleasure], or bodily lust".*

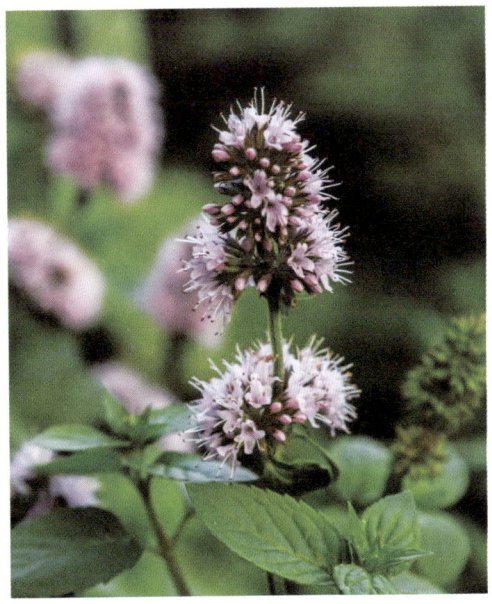

MINTY MOUTHWASH

The long list of unfamiliar ingredients in commercial mouthwash can read like a chemist's shop. Making products at home means that you can avoid harsh chemicals and regain complete control over ingredients, with the added bonus that it can save you money too.

Mint is commonly used for oral health products because menthol (found in peppermint oil) has a wonderful, cooling effect that leaves your mouth feeling clean and fresh, with the benefit of antioxidant properties. Fennel seeds and cinnamon are naturally antiseptic, helping to clear bacteria, as well as being anti-inflammatory and analgesic. Cloves fight harmful bacteria that cause gum disease and tooth decay, and can help to freshen the breath.

INGREDIENTS

Handful of fresh mint, chopped

1 tsp fennel seeds

1 cinnamon stick

2 cloves

500 ml filtered water, boiled

EQUIPMENT NEEDED

Heatproof jar or bowl with lid

Sieve

500 ml bottle with lid

METHOD

Place all ingredients into the heatproof container.

Pour over the boiled water.

Cover with a lid.

Allow to brew for 30 minutes or longer.

Sieve the mixture into a sterilized bottle.

Swoosh through the teeth for 30 seconds after meals and spit into the sink.

Use as often as needed. Keeps in the fridge for a week.

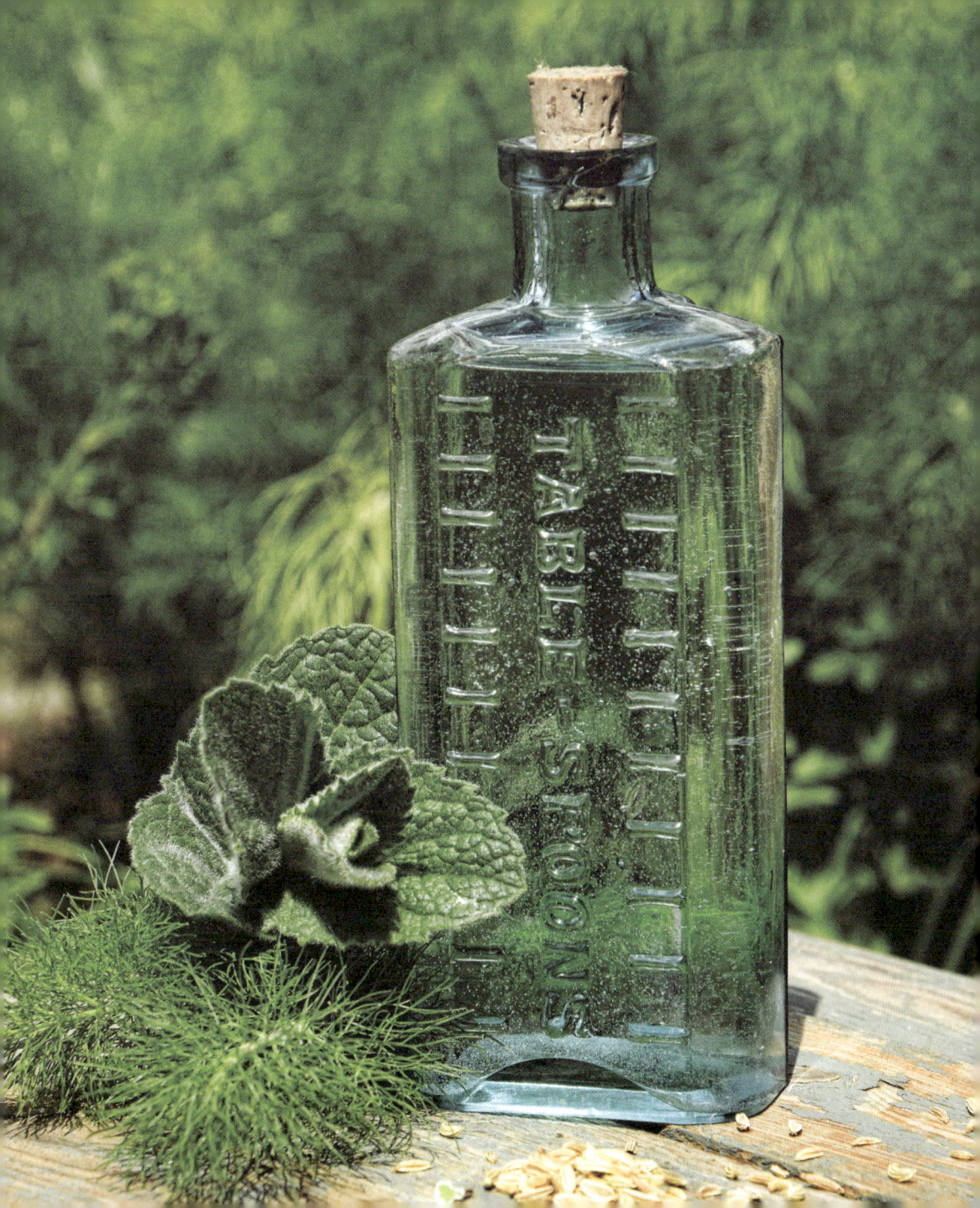

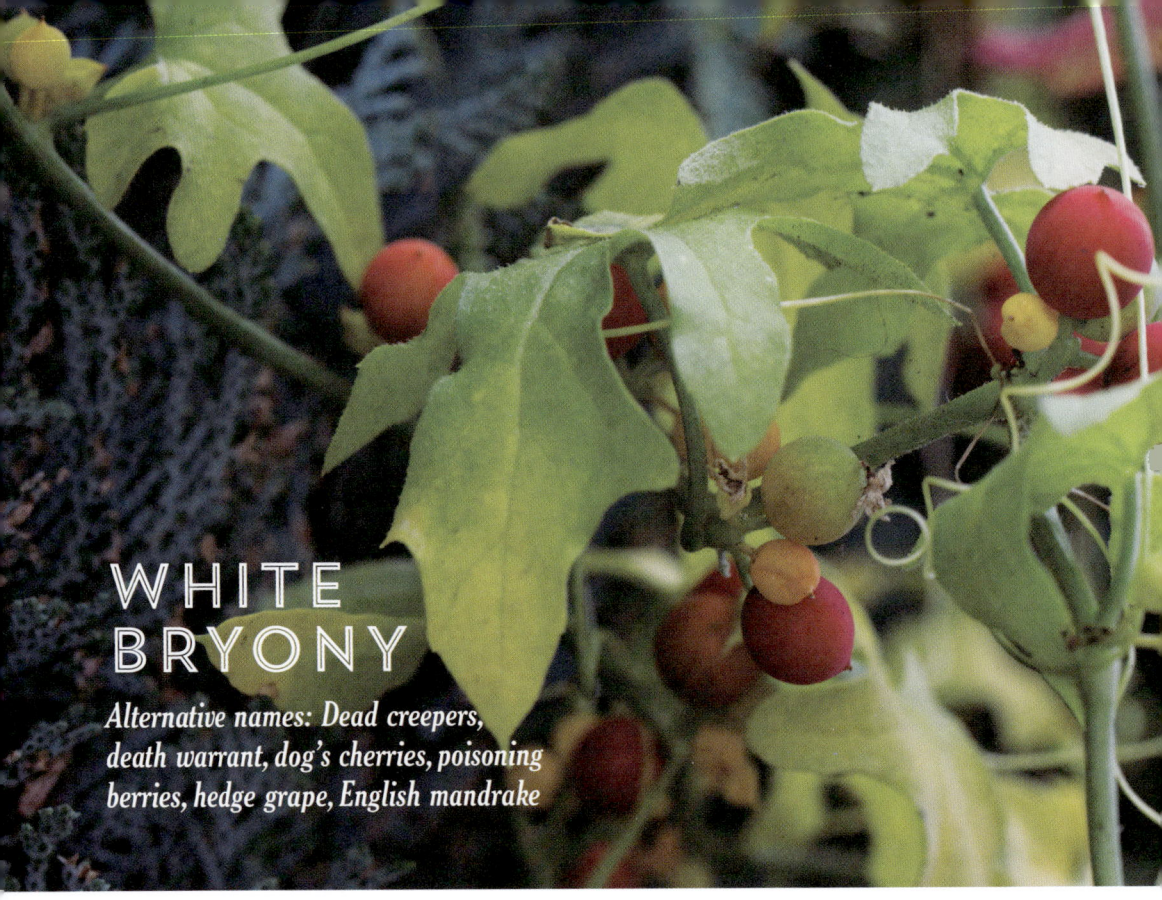

WHITE BRYONY

Alternative names: Dead creepers, death warrant, dog's cherries, poisoning berries, hedge grape, English mandrake

HOW TO IDENTIFY: White bryony likes to clamber through hedgerows and woodland edges, clinging on tight with its twisting tendrils. It produces greenish-white flowers in the summer, followed by bright red shiny berries that cascade in clusters in the autumn hedgerow. Although it is our only native species of the cucumber family, unlike cucumber, all parts of white bryony are highly toxic.

HISTORY: White bryony root was often disguised as the much more expensive mandrake root which originated from the Mediterranean and was incredibly difficult to grow. Prized as a narcotic, aphrodisiac and painkiller, mandrake was so named because its roots resembled the human form, which would supposedly scream when pulled from the earth.

Resourceful country folk realized that the roots of white bryony were very similar to mandrake root and could be carved into human form to look like mandrake. These were then buried in sand to be pulled up and sold to unsuspecting customers at an extortionate price!

The seventeenth-century English medical writer John Pechey was very unhappy with this dishonest practice: *"Jugglers and fortune-tellers make wonderful monsters of this root, which, they have hid in sand for some days, they dig up for Mandrakes; and by this imposture [deception] these knaves impose on our common people."*

FOLKLORE: White bryony has some wonderful and varied folkloric uses from all over the world. In the Balkans, it was used to not only bring wealth, but as protection for people and cattle from witches' spells. Apparently, Augustus Caesar used to wear a wreath of bryony during a thunderstorm to protect himself from lightning. And in Scandinavia, white bryony grown near the hen house was sure to keep chickens safe from birds of prey.

In Poland, witches blessed the white bryony root on Assumption Day (15 August) – a date in the Catholic Church when the Virgin Mary was "assumed" into eternal life. They then bathed the root in milk in order to be able to steal the milk from other people's cattle. Wreaths containing white bryony and other herbs such as elder, peony, nettles and thyme were burned before and after calving to cleanse the air. White bryony was also a funerary herb placed in the coffin as a pillow for the dead.

In other parts of Eastern Europe, an offering of money or bread was to be left in the soil after digging up a white bryony root. If you failed to do so, the plant might never return or you may bring illness upon yourself.

FOLK MEDICINE: The plant's toxic reputation led to it being used as a rather dangerous purge by medieval practitioners, with Gerard warning that it could *"mightily purge the belly and torment the stomach".*

This didn't stop him from prescribing the plant though:

> *"This kind of strong purgation is good for those that have the dropsy [fluid retention], the falling sickness [epilepsy], and the dizziness and swimming of the brain and head."*

All parts of white bryony are toxic.

WILD CARROT

Alternative names: Bird's nest, crow's nest, pig's parsley, devil's plague, fiddle, Queen Anne's lace, bishop's flower

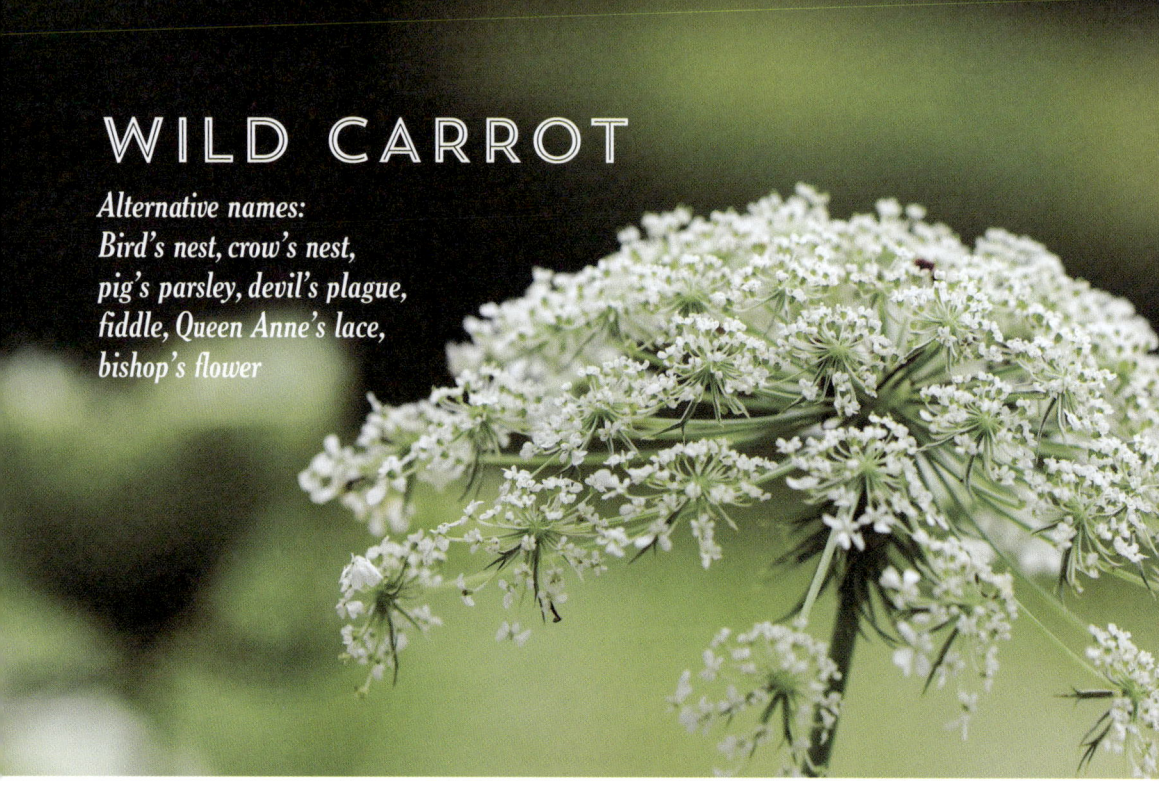

HOW TO IDENTIFY: Wild carrot likes to grow in dry, open spaces such as field margins, wasteland and along the coast. Growing to about 1.5 m (5 ft), wild carrot has feathery leaves that when rubbed have a distinctive carroty smell. Topped with white umbrella-like flowers with purple or red centres from June to September, these then turn into bird's nest shaped seed heads in autumn.

HISTORY: The wild carrot was thought to have originally come from Afghanistan and spread to Europe. The root is creamy-white rather than orange and is edible.

With its lacy flowers, wild carrot is also known as "Queen Anne's lace", supposedly because the eighteenth-century queen of Great Britain and Ireland, who was very adept at making lace, accidently pricked her finger, leaving behind a red dot in the centre of the flower.

The Sunday before the Christian festival of Michaelmas (29 September) was the traditional time for the ladies of the Scottish Hebrides to pull carrots. Considered to be a symbol of fertility, it was thought to be particularly lucky if a two-pronged carrot was pulled from the ground. Calling to her neighbours to share her good fortune she would sing:

> *"Fork joyful, joyful, joyful,*
> *Fork of great carrot to me,*
> *Endowment of carrot surpassing me,*
> *Joy of great carrot to me."*

The women tied the carrots up with three-ply red twine. Giving them to the menfolk was a sign of affection as well as being an aphrodisiac.

Wild carrot seeds have been used in the brewing of ale and the flavouring of soups, while roasted roots can be dried and ground into a powder as a coffee substitute.

FOLKLORE: Because the delicate lace-like nature of the flowers was associated with beauty, many single ladies added them to their baths in the hope of attracting true love.

When the flowers fade, a beautiful seed head forms, very similar in shape to a bird's nest. This came to symbolize safety and sanctuary in the home, just as baby birds would feel safe and secure in their nest.

Folklore tells us that the best day to collect the seeds of wild carrot is on the first windy day nearest the full moon after the bird's nest has appeared. If you rub the seed heads carefully between your hands over a white plate, the black seeds will fall onto the plate and the wind will blow all the unwanted seedpods away.

FOLK MEDICINE: Gerard reinforces the use of wild carrot seeds as an aphrodisiac: *"it also procureth bodily lust […] helpeth conception"* and *"it breaketh and dissolveth wind".*

Three centuries later, Grieve tells us that, *"An infusion of the whole herb is considered an active and valuable remedy in the treatment of dropsy [swelling in the tissues], chronic kidney diseases and affections of the bladder."*

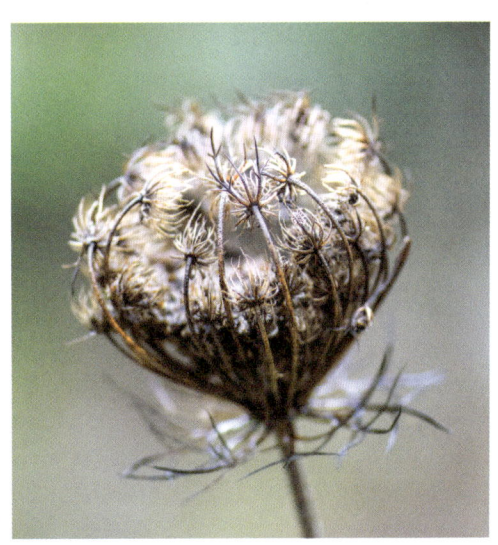

WILD GARLIC

Alternative names: Ramsons, gipsy onion, wood garlic, devil's garlic, bear garlic

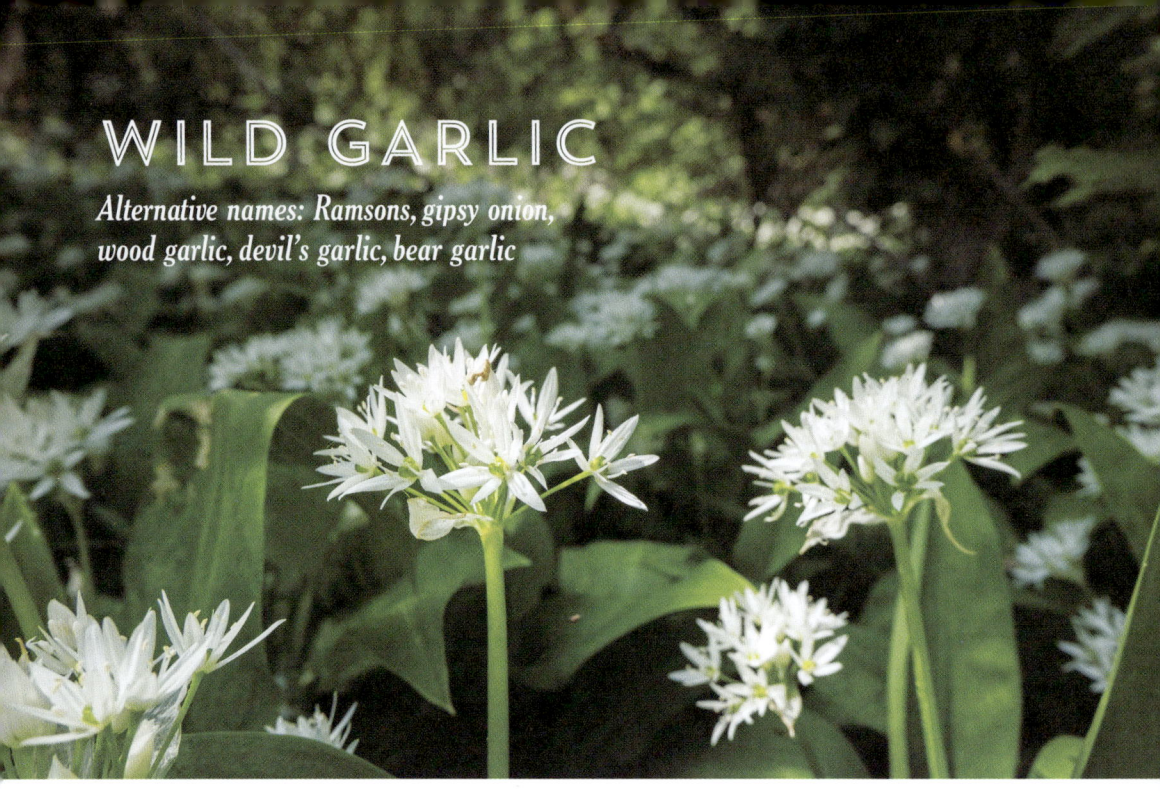

HOW TO IDENTIFY: Wild garlic grows in damp, ancient woodlands and has a distinctive garlicky smell. Be careful when foraging for wild garlic as the leaves look very similar to both lily-of-the-valley and lords and ladies, which are poisonous. Crush the leaves and sniff them for that pungent garlic smell. Its broad, spear-like leaves appear early in March, followed by a profusion of starry white flowers carpeting the woodland floor. Leaves, bulbs and flowers are all edible, adding a subtle garlic flavour to food.

HISTORY: Wild garlic leaves have often been used as fodder and cows that are fed on the leaves produce milk with a slightly garlicky flavour, which is lovely for garlic butter.

Wild garlic, along with wood anemone, wood spurge, small-leaved lime and guelder rose are all indicators of ancient woodland. The wild garlic you forage may well be the ancestor of plants that were used by early Britons in the same place hundreds of years ago.

While it is illegal to dig up the bulbs, it is permitted to gather the leaves with the consent of the landowner.

FOLKLORE: The plant's common name of "bear garlic" comes from the belief that bears, as well as wild boar and badgers, ate wild garlic to regain their strength after winter hibernation.

Wild garlic was planted in the thatch of Irish cottages to ward off faeries and bring good luck. Soldiers heading to battle and athletes about to compete chewed a piece of wild garlic to give them enough strength for victory.

FOLK MEDICINE: Rich in antioxidants and immune-boosting powers, wild garlic is considered to be a "cure-all". With all the same medicinal benefits as cultivated garlic, it's no wonder that this magical plant was so valuable to early Britons. Wild garlic cleanses the blood and intestines, improves intestinal flora and helps with acne and eczema, as well as boosting the body's immune system. Romany people are known to call it "the fountain of youth".

It has also been made into poultices to treat bad knees and mixed with lard to be rubbed into the soles of the feet as a treatment for bronchitis. Culpeper prescribed wild garlic both externally and internally: "*It wonderfully opens the lungs, and gives relief to asthmas, and is a good diuretic.*"

In other uses, an infusion was drunk to strengthen the blood, infected wounds could be cured by a poultice, and the strong smell of the leaves was used to repel insects.

In the spring, the bulbs can be dug up (with permission), covered in dark brown sugar and rum, and then left until the winter where the resultant liquid can be used as a remedy for coughs and colds. And in Ireland, people carried wild garlic in their pockets to guard against the Spanish flu epidemic of 1918.

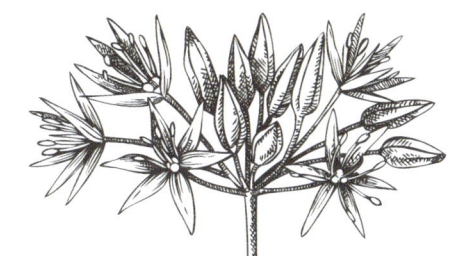

WILD GARLIC SALT AND PEPPER SEASONING

This vibrantly green, three ingredient salt is super easy to make, yet packs a real flavour punch and is a great way to preserve the flavour of spring to use all year round. Scatter a pinch into salads, over barbecue meat and vegetables, and as a finishing salt on practically everything.

Forage for wild garlic before it comes into flower – the young leaves are the tastiest. Don't pick from beside busy roads, dog-walking areas or places that may have been sprayed with pesticides.

This recipe makes enough for you to generously gift to friends and keep plenty for yourself.

Makes approx. 475 g seasoning

INGREDIENTS

50 g wild garlic leaves

400 g sea salt crystals

2 tbsp freshly cracked black pepper

EQUIPMENT NEEDED

Food processor

Baking paper

Flat baking tray

Small jars

METHOD

Add the wild garlic to the food processor with 100 g of the sea salt.

Pulse until you have a thick paste.

Add the paste to the rest of the sea salt along with the pepper.

Stir until combined.

Line the baking tray with baking paper and spread out your green mixture to an even thickness.

Leave somewhere warm to dry overnight; an airing cupboard is ideal.

When your seasoning is completely dry, crumble it into clean jars, label and store in a cool, dry place.

Keeps for about six to nine months.

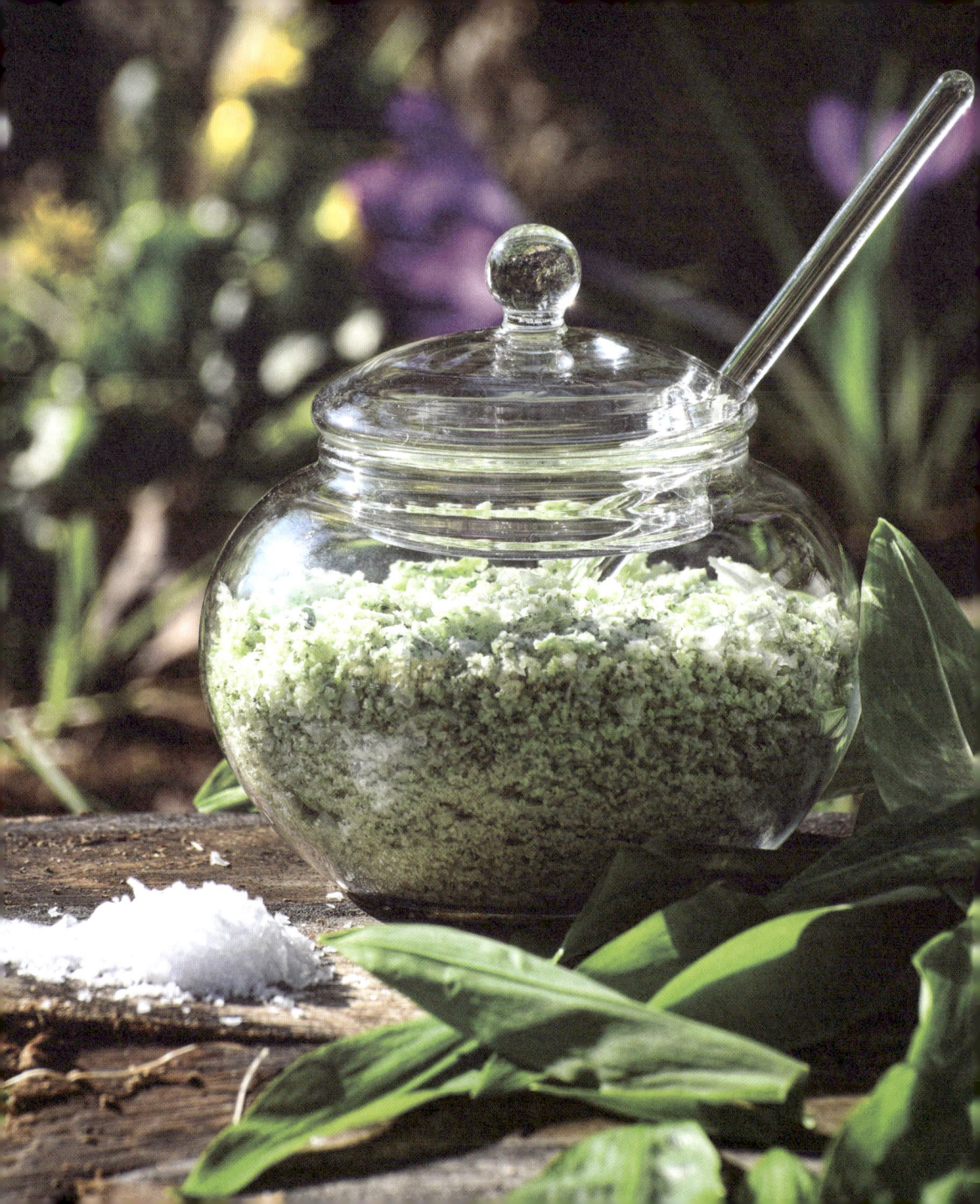

WILD MARJORAM

Alternative names: Mountain mint, sweet marjoram, sweet oregano, joy of the mountain

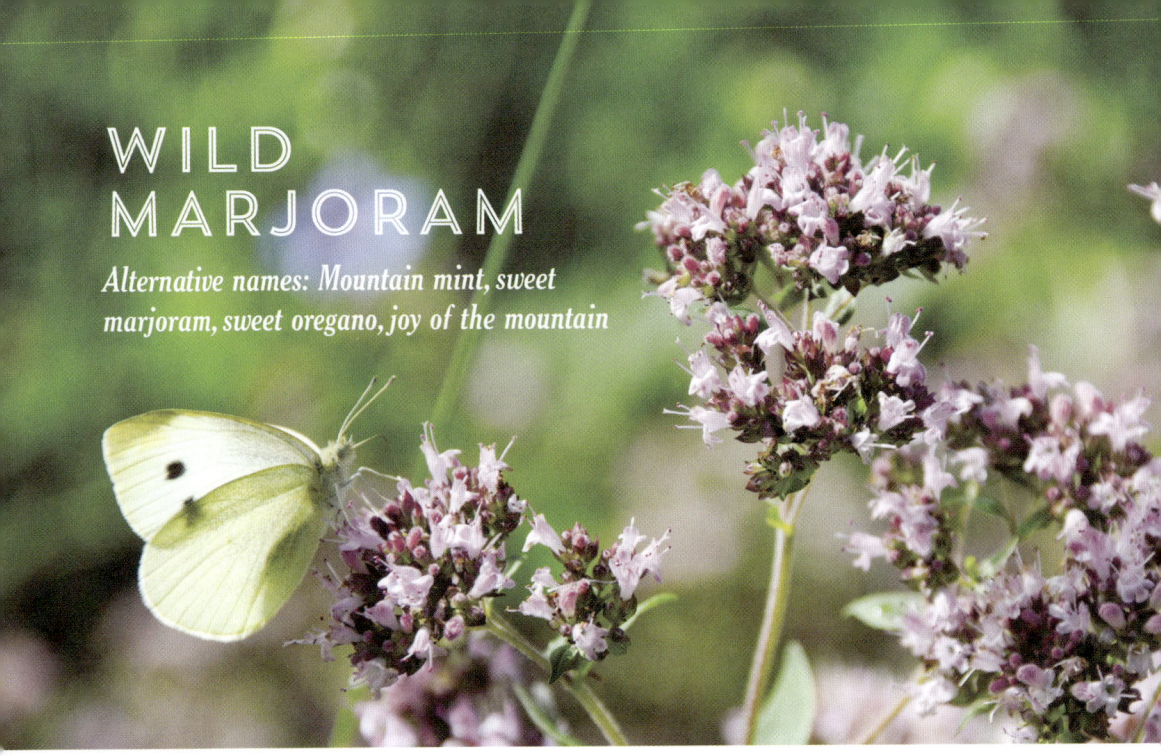

HOW TO IDENTIFY: Wild marjoram can be found flowering on limestone and chalk grasslands from June to September. It has soft, fuzzy leaves which produce a slightly minty smell when crushed, and tiny clusters of pink flowers.

HISTORY: Wild marjoram is actually a native British wildflower and did not, as you may expect, arrive from Mediterranean shores, although it is the same species and has the same culinary uses as its cultivated cousin oregano but with a slightly different scent.

In the Middle Ages, before hops were widely used in the making of a beer called "gruit", wild marjoram and herbs such as wood sage and ground ivy were used in the brewing process.

Prized for its fragrance, the sweet-scented herb was often used as a "strewing herb" to keep medieval dwellings smelling sweet. Wild marjoram was also scrubbed over wooden floors and furniture to release the sweet-smelling oils and produce a wonderful shine. It was used as an early perfume – seventeenth-century herbalist John Parkinson recounts how *"sweet margerome"* served to keep the body fragrant before the introduction of scents from abroad.

According to Culpeper, *"Marjoram is much used in all odiferous waters, pouders, etc that are used for ornament or delight."*

Marjoram flowers were used to dye wool purple and linen reddish-brown. And in Ancient Rome, marjoram was combined with lavender and rosemary to protect linens from moths and other destructive insects.

FOLKLORE: In the Victorian language of flowers, both marjoram and oregano signified joy and happiness. In some interpretations, oregano meant substance as well and sweet marjoram could symbolize blushes, maidenly innocence, consolation, kindness, courtesy or distrust. In a similar vein, wild marjoram planted on a grave not only guaranteed a happy afterlife but also ensured that the deceased would sleep peacefully and undisturbed.

To ensure good luck and protection from negative energies, place leaves of wild marjoram in every room of your house, replacing them every month to renew their potency. Carrying sprigs of marjoram around with you will have the same cleansing benefits. In other protective lore, wild marjoram and wild thyme laid alongside milk in a dairy will prevent it being turned sour by thunder.

Incorporating wild marjoram into charms or sachets will attract love, enhance fertility and keep love alive in a partnership. It will also help you to deal with grief and sorrow.

FOLK MEDICINE: In medieval times, wild marjoram was very much in common use. Says Gerard: *"Marjoram is a remedy against cold diseases of the brain and head, being taken any way to your best liking; put up into the nostrils it provoketh sneezing, and draweth forth much baggage phlegm."* He recommends that marjoram is chewed to ease the pain of toothache, cramps, convulsions and stomach aches.

Culpeper continues that wild marjoram *"helps the bitings of venomous beasts, and helps such as have poisoned themselves by eating hemlock, henbane, or opium".* In addition, *"The juice being dropped into the ears, helps deafness, pain and noise in the ears."*

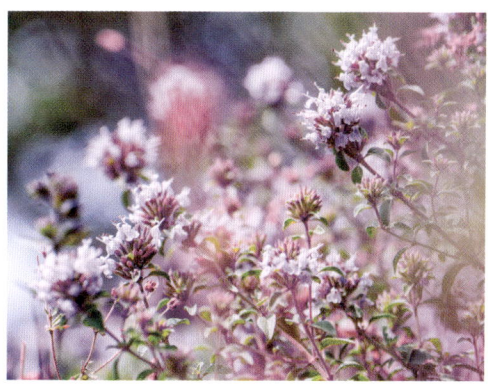

SOOTHING MARJORAM AND ROSE FACIAL COMPRESS

Wild marjoram has wonderful naturally occurring anti-inflammatory, antioxidant, antibacterial and anti-fungal properties, perfect to help soothe and calm irritated skin.

Marjoram is believed to be of benefit with conditions such as rosacea, dermatitis, eczema, psoriasis and acne, and may help to increase the skin's production of collagen to slow down the signs of ageing.

The addition of rose essential oil will help to hydrate and brighten dull skin, reduce redness and make your compress smell amazing.

Using a cold compress can reduce puffiness, tighten the pores and improve circulation as well as being a great way to wake up your skin in the morning.

Makes one small jar of compress

INGREDIENTS

4 tbsp chopped organic marjoram leaves or 2 tbsp of dried

350 ml filtered water

3 drops of rose essential oil

EQUIPMENT NEEDED

Saucepan

Jar with lid

Organic linen or unbleached cotton cloth

METHOD

Add marjoram to a pan of boiling water and pop a lid on.

Boil for 5 minutes.

Take off the heat, allow to infuse and cool to room temperature.

Strain the liquid into a clean jar.

Add the rose essential oil, put on the lid and shake.

Pop into the fridge until cold.

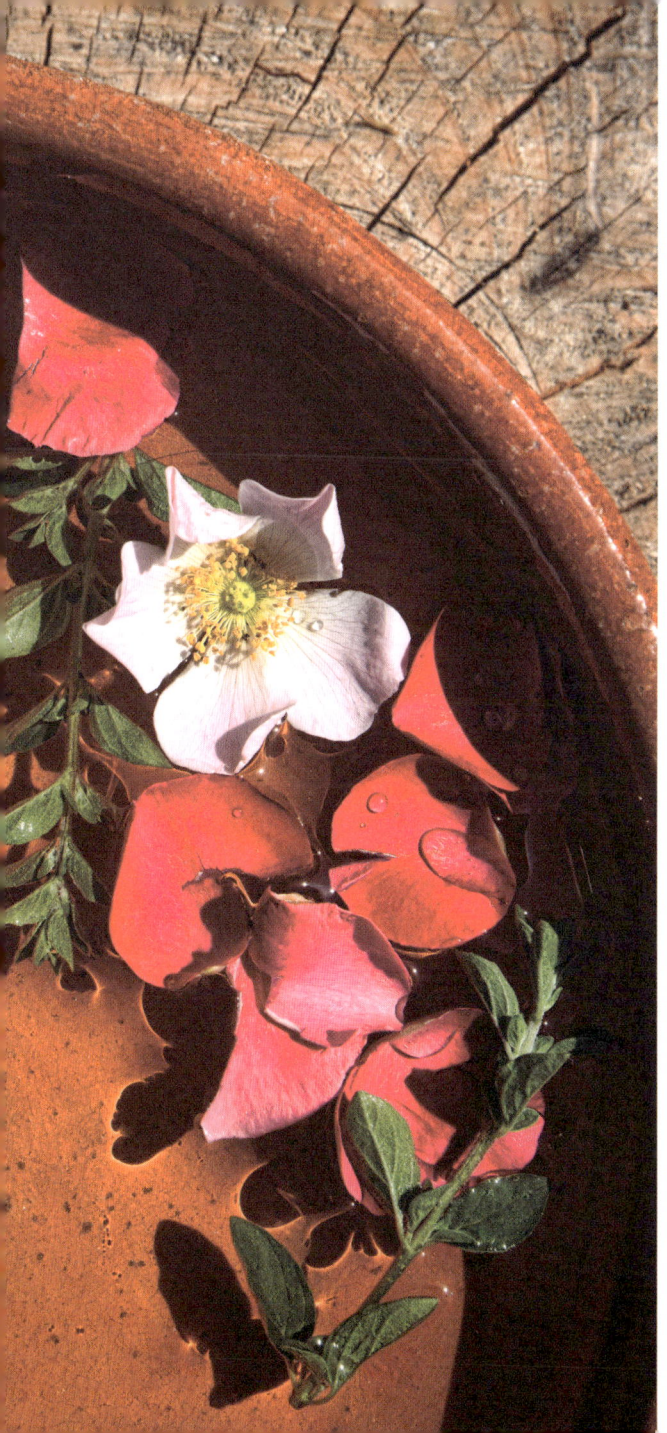

TO USE

Make sure that your face is clean and make-up free.

Soak a cloth in the cold infusion; squeeze out the excess.

Place cloth over your face, patting it gently into every contour, avoiding your eyes.

Lie back and relax for 20 minutes, refreshing your cloth as needed.

Do not rinse off.

Repeat daily, using a clean cloth every time.

Keep the infusion in the fridge, where it should last about a week.

Can also be used topically on problem areas several times a day.

Always do a patch test.

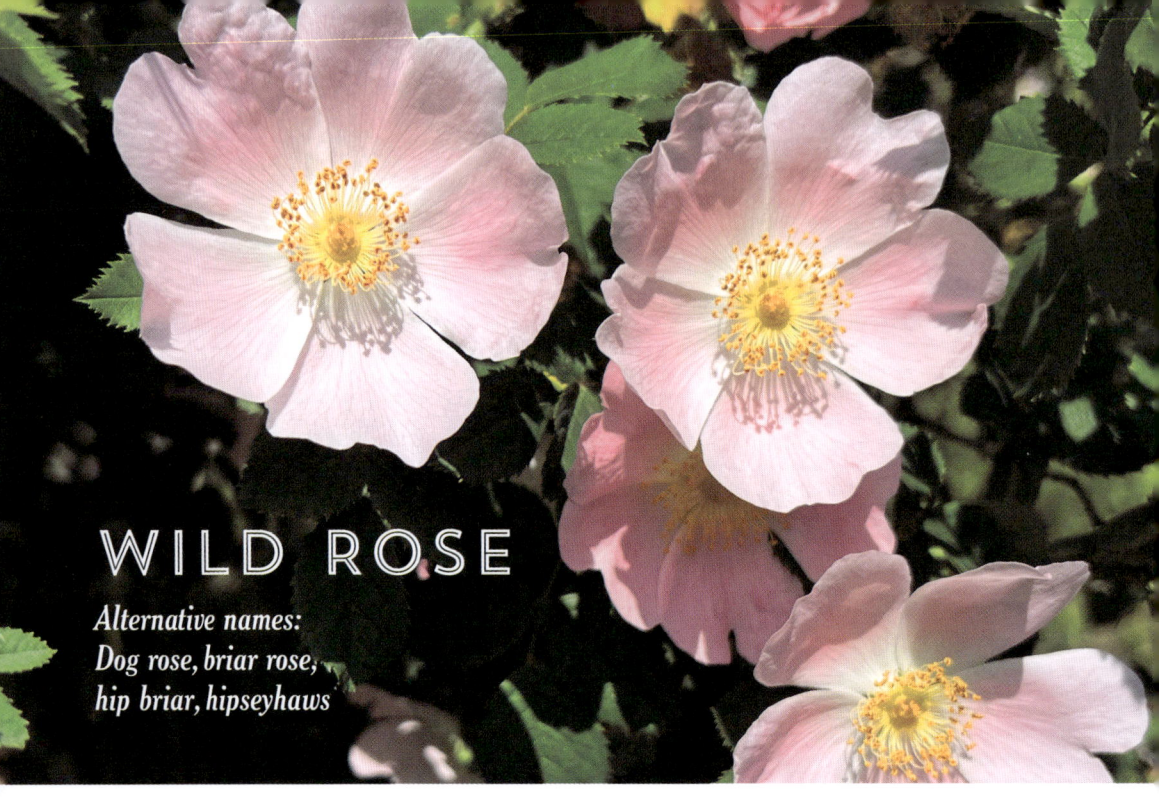

WILD ROSE

*Alternative names:
Dog rose, briar rose,
hip briar, hipseyhaws*

HOW TO IDENTIFY: A distinctive, rambling, sturdy shrub that likes to scramble through country hedgerows, the tall, arching stems are covered in curved thorns with dark green, oval-toothed leaves. It produces delicate five-petalled flowers in pink or white from June to July, followed by bright red hips, which light up the autumn hedgerows.

HISTORY: Wild roses were a common sight in Gerard's sixteenth-century England. He writes that they *"groweth very plentifully in a field as you go from a village in Essex, called Grays unto Horndon on the Hill".*

And they seem to have had many uses, *"for even children with great delight eat the berries thereof when they be ripe, make chains and other pretty gewgaws [trinkets] of the fruit: cooks and gentlewomen make tarts and such like dishes for pleasure thereof".*

Rosehips contain 40 times more vitamin C than oranges, as well as vitamins A, B and K. During World War Two, when citrus fruits were in short supply, rosehips were an important dietary supplement for

British infants. Women's Institutes, schools, Brownies and Cubs, amongst other groups, were all tasked with going out foraging into the hedgerows to collect this precious hip. It was considered your "patriotic duty" to gather rosehips and, by the end of the war, over 2,000 tons had been collected to be made into syrup. Del Rosa paid 3 d (3 pence) for every pound (454 g) in weight of rosehips collected, which they then made into syrup to be distributed to children's clinics all over the country. It was given to prevent scurvy and other related vitamin deficiencies common in infants at the time.

The fine hairs that can be found inside the hips have been used for centuries by mischievous children as "itchy seeds" to be pushed down the jumper of a poor victim. (We've all done it!)

FOLKLORE: Folklore tells us that if we carry rosehips in our pockets, we will be protected from getting piles. Schoolboys also carried rosehips in the belief that this would prevent them from getting the cane, in the days of corporal punishment. Goats with indigestion were fed young shoots of the wild rose, though how you know if a goat has indigestion is a puzzle to me!

Faeries who wish to become invisible will eat a rosehip and turn three times widdershins (anti-clockwise). To reappear, they eat another rosehip and turn three times clockwise.

FOLK MEDICINE: In traditional folk medicine, rosehips have been used as a cure for constipation due to their mild laxative effects.

Wild rose leaves were boiled together with chickweed, and the liquid dripped into sore eyes.

Insects sometimes burrow into the rosehips causing "moss galls"; these were hung inside the house to cure a child of whooping cough. Moss galls were used to treat insomnia by placing them under the sufferer's pillow, but they had to be removed in the morning or the patient might not wake up.

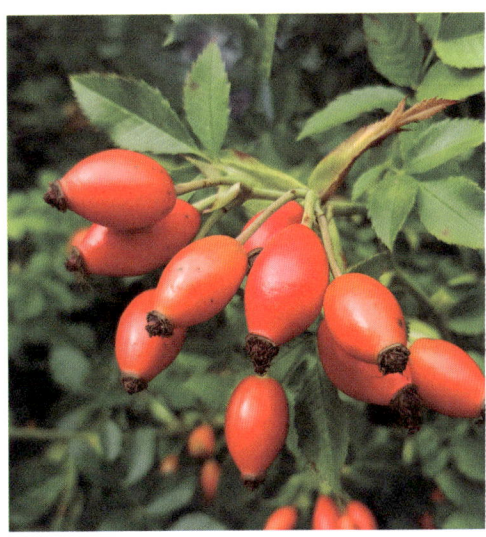

ROSEHIP UNDER-EYE OIL

The skin under our eyes is particularly thin and delicate, and is one of the first places to show signs of ageing. Rosehip oil contains fatty acids, which are incredibly nourishing and moisturizing, vitamin C to protect the skin from sun damage, and those all-important antioxidants for anti-ageing benefits.

I love to include some organic castor oil in this recipe as research is looking very positive for its effectiveness in preventing wrinkles – it can be sticky though so is best diluted with another carrier oil. Frankincense essential oil can also help to reduce under-eye puffiness and tighten the skin.

For best results this oil should be used straight from the fridge, as the cold will help to calm puffiness.

Makes a few small bottles

INGREDIENTS

70 g dried rosehips

50 ml organic castor oil

200 ml organic carrier oil

30 drops frankincense essential oil (optional)

EQUIPMENT NEEDED

Heatproof bowl

Saucepan

Sieve lined with muslin

Jug

Dark glass storage bottle

Small funnel

Small glass rollerball bottles or dropper bottle

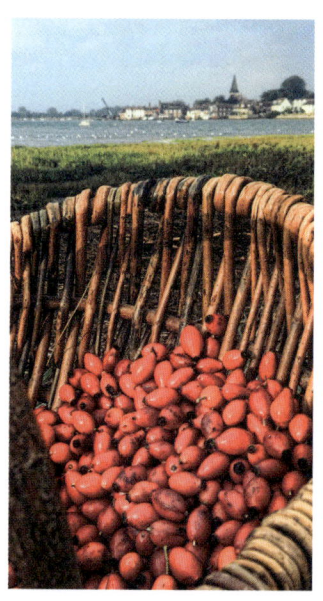

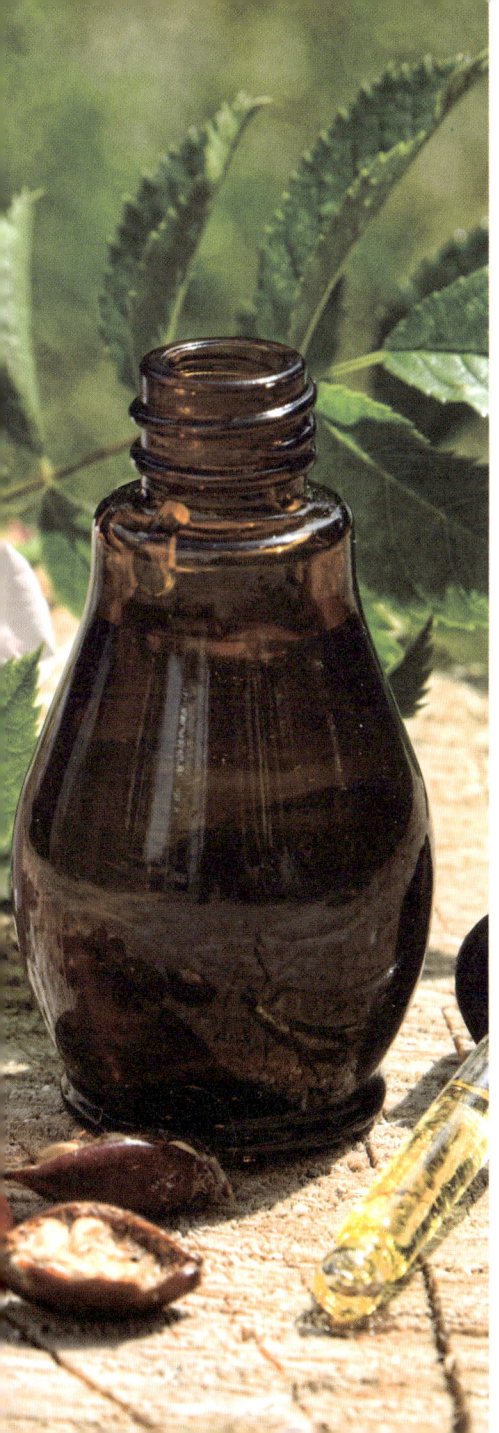

METHOD

Add the rosehips and both oils into your heatproof bowl.

Pop it on top of a saucepan of simmering water. Gently heat the oil and rosehips. This will take about 8 hours so keep topping up the water and don't leave it unattended. (Alternatively, if you have a slow cooker, you could heat your bowl in this to avoid the need to keep checking on it.) The oil will gradually take on a rich orange colour. Allow to cool.

Strain through a muslin into a clean jug, squeezing as much oil out as you can.

Add frankincense essential oil if using and mix well.

Decant your precious rosehip oil into a clean dark glass jar to protect it from sunlight and refrigerate.

Using a small funnel, fill up your rollerball/dropper bottles.

To apply, gently roll or pat the oil under your eye area without tugging the skin.

Top up your bottles as needed – a little goes a long way.

Now you also have a lovely bottle of rosehip oil to add to your bath or other home-made beauty treatments.

Always do a patch test.

WILD THYME

Alternative names: Elfin thyme, creeping thyme, breckland thyme, mother-of-thyme

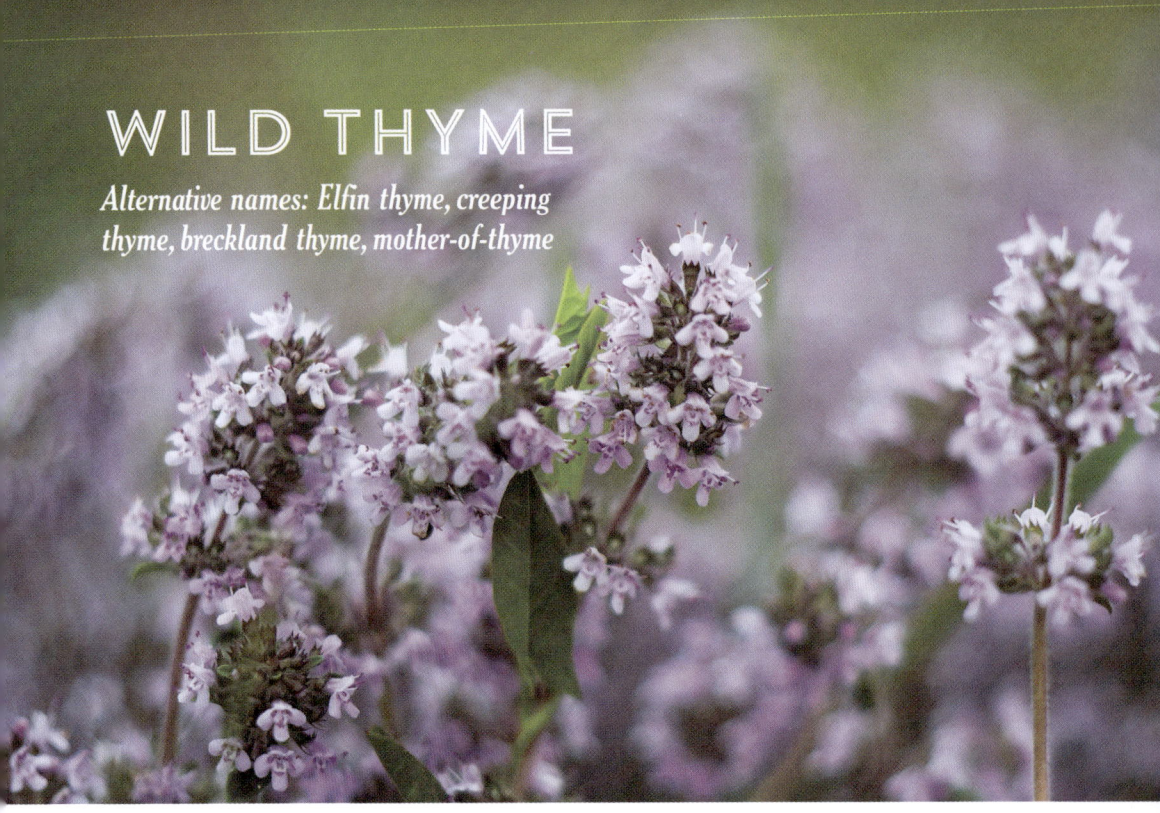

HOW TO IDENTIFY: Wild thyme is a low-growing woody herb with small aromatic leaves growing all the way along the stems. Densely packed delicate purple-pink flowers can be seen from May to July, creeping over chalk grasslands, sand dunes and rocky cliffs and beaches. Wild thyme has a strong spicy scent similar to oregano when crushed.

HISTORY: Wild thyme is one of Britain's native species, unlike varieties such as lemon thyme, which came to these shores along with the Roman invasion in the first century CE.

With other fragrant herbs, wild thyme was rubbed into the bodies of the Egyptian pharaohs as part of the mummification process. It was also believed to ease the passage of the spirit into the afterlife.

It was thought that eating thyme and even bathing in thyme would give protection from poisoning; this made it especially popular with understandably nervous Roman emperors.

It was burned in both Roman and Greek temples for purification. In addition, soldiers took strength from wild thyme: inhaling the smoke was believed to give them courage before they went into battle.

FOLKLORE: Faeries love to inhabit the twisted and knotted branches of wild thyme. It is therefore unlucky to bring thyme into the house as you will run the risk of upsetting the fae. However, thyme can be sprinkled on windowsills and doorsteps should you wish to invite the faery folk to visit, and bathing your eyes in the dew from thyme leaves before dawn on the first day of May will enable you to see your faery visitors. Patches of wild thyme were evidence that faeries had partied the night away on that very spot, and this belief led to generations of young girls camping out in the hope of glimpsing faeries. To find a lost object, leave an offering of thyme and honey in the woods on the night of the full moon and the fae will do their best to find it for you.

The Roma will never bring wild thyme into their wagons, regarding it as unlucky. They will, however, drink thyme tea outdoors with vinegar and honey to cure a cough.

Plant thyme at the beginning of a waxing moon with several coins tucked into the root ball, look after it well and, as the thyme flourishes, so will your bank balance.

FOLK MEDICINE: Plague doctors in fourteenth-century England believed that diseases were carried by "miasma" (bad air), so they wore long beak-like masks stuffed with many herbs including thyme, peppermint and rosemary to avoid becoming infected by their patients.

To quote Culpeper, thyme *"purges the body of phlegm, and is an excellent remedy for shortness of breath, it kills worms in the belly [...] gives safe and speedy delivery to women in travail [labour] and brings away the afterbirth"*.

Thyme is a natural antibiotic and antiseptic, and has been used to treat myriad ailments including coughs, colds, warts, sciatica, headaches, hay fever and hangovers. Even before bacteria and infection were properly understood, nurses in the nineteenth century were soaking bandages in a solution of thyme water.

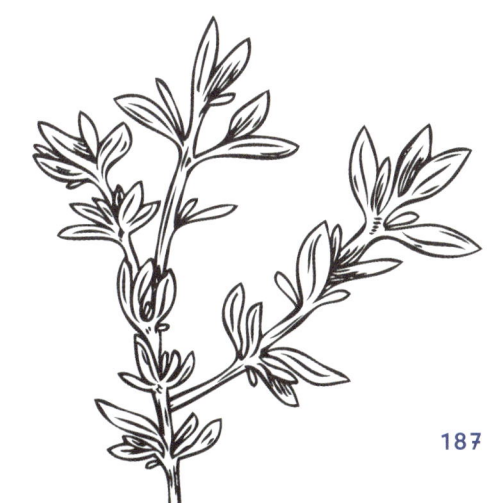

WILD THYME-INFUSED HONEY

Thyme has some amazing medicinal weapons to help ease that cough: antibacterial, anti-inflammatory and anti-viral properties all help to fight infection and soothe the throat, bringing relief in a natural form. Try to source local raw honey if you can – it hasn't been heated or processed and retains all of its beneficial nutrients and antioxidants straight from the hive.

Gather your wild thyme before it flowers as the leaves will be more potent.

Makes one 400 g jar

INGREDIENTS

400 g raw or local honey

Good handful wild or garden thyme

EQUIPMENT NEEDED

Jar

Jar label

METHOD

If your honey is set, gently heat it by putting the whole jar in some warm water. Don't overheat it; we want to retain all those healing properties and these can be destroyed by heat.

Give the thyme a little rub as you pop it into the clean jar, helping to release the oils. Cover the thyme with honey and fill to the top.

Give everything a good stir to coat the thyme leaves, trying not to make air bubbles.

Pop a lid on your jar, label and date it.

Place your wild thyme honey in a sunny spot to infuse for at least two weeks, making sure that the herb is submerged constantly.

After this time, have a taste. Does it taste of thyme? If not, it may need a little longer.

Once you're happy with the flavour, remove the thyme with a clean spoon.

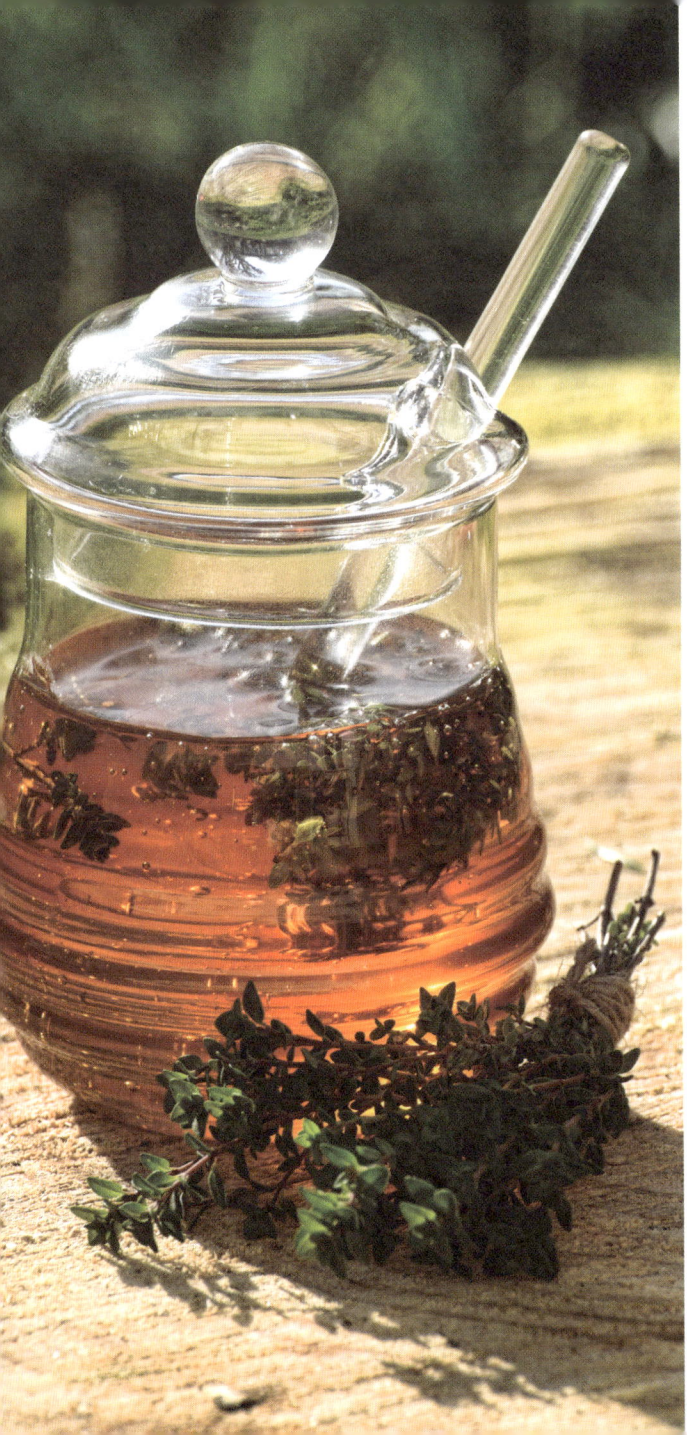

TIPS AND IDEAS FOR THYME-INFUSED HONEY

To make yourself some deliciously soothing thyme and honey tea, add a teaspoonful to a teacup and top up with hot water and a squeeze of organic lemon juice.

Transfer your thyme honey into a cool, dark place ready for cold and flu season. When needed, take the honey by the spoonful to boost immunity.

Try to consume within six months.

Honey should not be given to children under two years old.

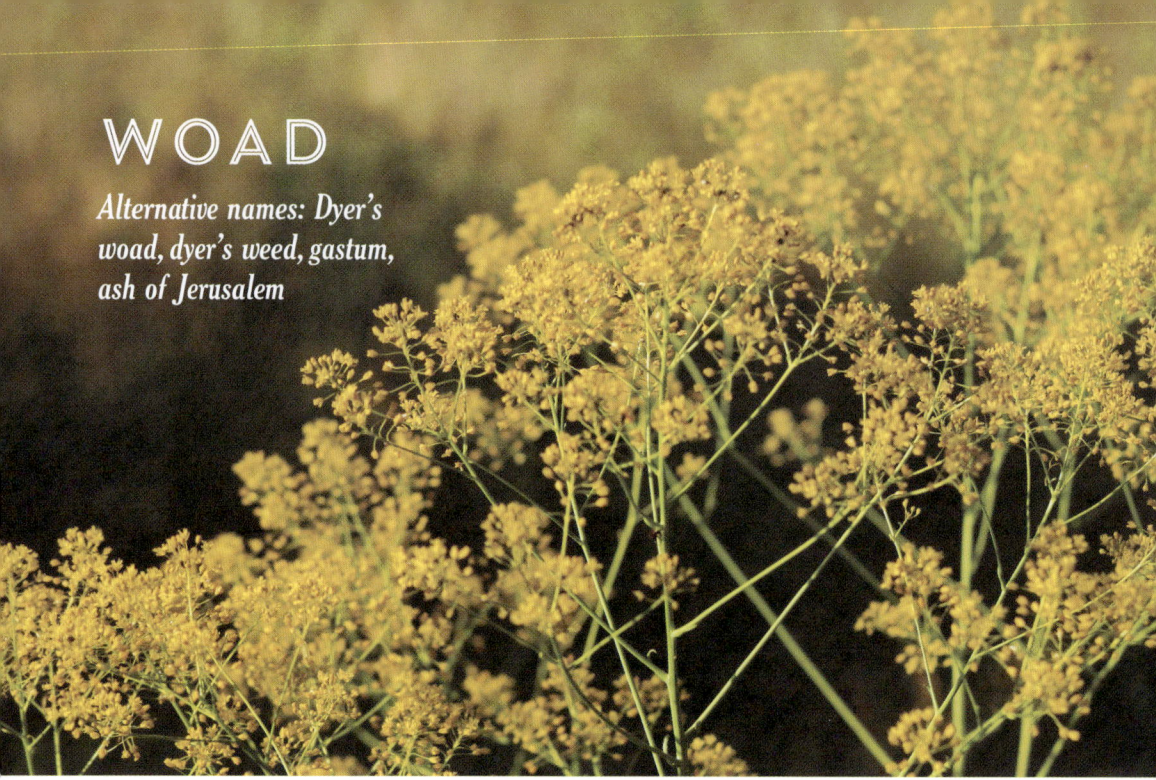

WOAD

Alternative names: Dyer's woad, dyer's weed, gastum, ash of Jerusalem

HOW TO IDENTIFY: Woad is a member of the cabbage family that grows up to 1.2 m (4 ft) tall. It is difficult to find in the UK but can sometimes grow in well-drained, sunny chalk cliff sites. The leaves are arrow-shaped, and yellow flowers hang like teardrops from July to August.

HISTORY: Originating in the Middle East and Turkey, woad spread and was used globally for hundreds of years, following the routes of human migration and finally making its way to Europe over 5,000 years ago.

Woad was used in ancient Egypt to dye cloth with which to wrap mummies, while a young girl discovered in an Iron Age tomb in Denmark was wearing a blue dress coloured by woad. If this seems surprising given its yellow flower, remember that plant dyes can come from various parts of a plant; in the case of woad, it's from the leaves. Other fabrics have been found in graves in Norway and Finland which have been dated to between the eighth and eleventh centuries CE.

By the Middle Ages woad was cultivated in France and Germany, although only the wealthy could afford the beautiful blue cloth. Wealthy German merchants gained the name *"waid Herren"* or "gentlemen of woad" and enjoyed showing off their riches to those who couldn't afford to dress in blue.

Woad was widely grown in the UK up until the sixteenth century as demand for blue cloth grew. During the reign of Queen Elizabeth I (1558–1603), when there was a real danger of famine, agricultural land previously used to grow grain had been turned over to growing woad since it was a far more profitable crop. The queen responded to the food shortage crisis by issuing a "proclamation against the sowing of woad" to prohibit the most fertile land from being used to grow the dye crop.

Right up to the 1930s, woaded cloth was used by governments to prevent uniforms from fading, but by 1932 farms in the UK had stopped growing woad commercially altogether, with indigo from India being used for blue dye instead.

FOLKLORE: Woad is associated with ancient Celtic tribes who painted their bodies with blue designs in an effort to look more terrifying during the Roman invasion in the first century CE. Warriors believed that if they were wounded in battle, the intricate patterns on their skin would protect them and help stop bleeding.

The blue tattoos were also a sign of cultural and tribal identity, and each one had a specific meaning. Some were symbols of strength, some represented Celtic gods and goddesses, and others signified connection with nature and the balance of the four elements (air, earth, wind and fire).

FOLK MEDICINE: Gerard agrees with the Celts, describing woad as *"good for wounds or ulcers in bodies of a strong constitution, as of country people, and such as are accustomed to great labour and hard coarse fare"*.

And, according to Culpeper: *"It cools inflammation, quenches St. Anthony's fire [from contaminated rye] and stays defluxion of the blood to any part of the body."*

Other historical uses have been to treat snake bites, haemorrhoids, ulcers, tumours and heartburn.

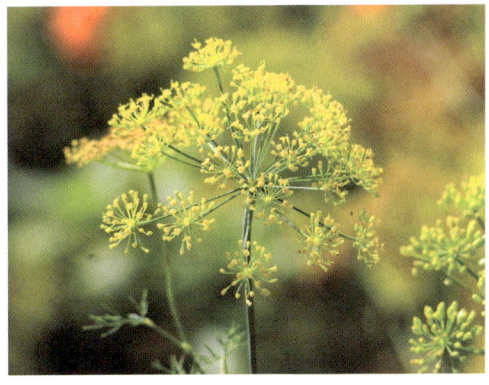

WOOD ANEMONE

Alternative names: Bread and cheese and cider, drops of snow, granny's nightcap, windflower

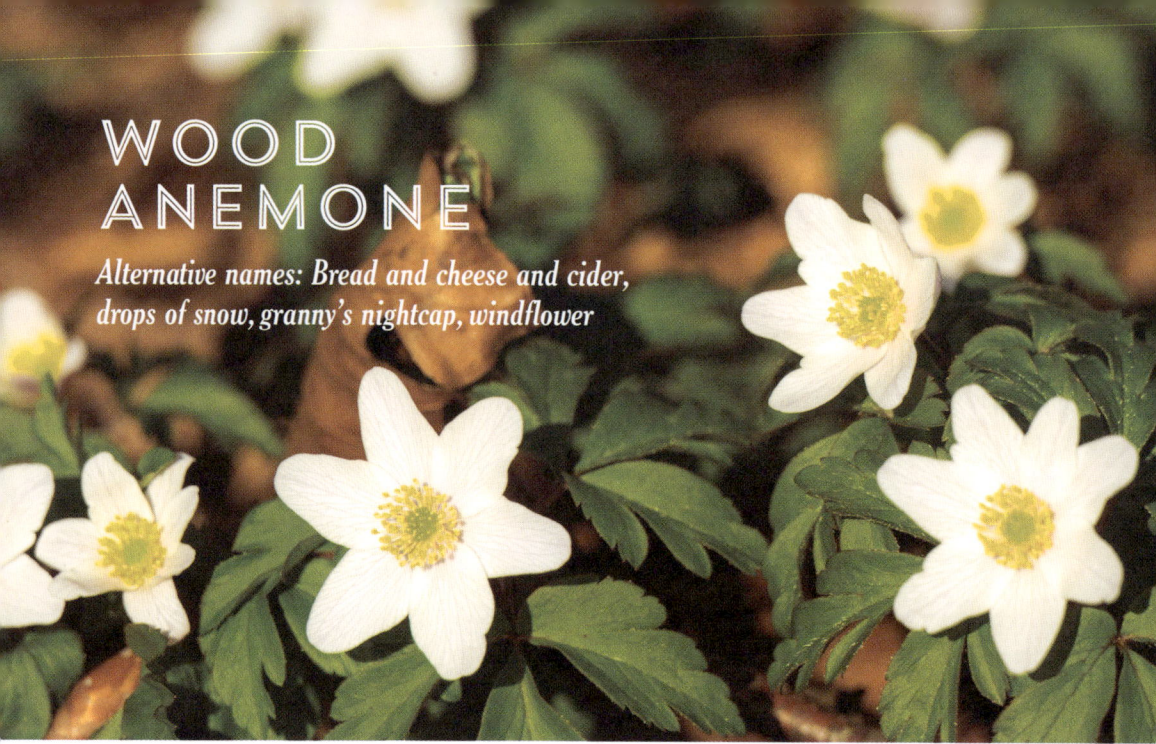

HOW TO IDENTIFY: This low-growing star-shaped flower loves to bloom in woodlands in spring before the tree canopy becomes too dense. It is easily identified by its white six- or seven-petalled flowers, blushed with a trace of pink, that grow from a rosette of three-lobed leaves.

HISTORY: Wood anemone is another of our ancient woodland indicators, with one source stating that as it relies on the spread of rhizomes, it can take a hundred years to spread just 2 m (6 ft). Grieve gives us a delightful description of wood anemones:

"In sunshine, the flower is expanded wide, but at the approach of night, it closes and droops its graceful head so that the dew may not settle on it and injure it. If rain threatens in the daytime, it does the same, receiving the drops on its back, whence they trickle harmlessly from the sepal tips. The way the sepals then fold over [...] has been likened to a tent, in which, as used fancifully to be said by country-folk, the fairies nestled for protection, having first pulled the curtains round them."

FOLKLORE: Pliny the Elder, who lived during the first century of the Roman Empire, described wood anemones as *"daughters of the wind"*, as they only open their flowers when the wind is blowing and close their petals when rain is forecast. Pliny, however, was wrong: they actually only like to open when the sun is shining.

In China, wood anemones are a symbol of both death and healing, while the Ancient Egyptians associated them with illness, believing they contaminated the air. Contrarily, in Ancient Rome, picking the first anemone was thought to be a lucky charm which could ward off fever.

The pale pink streaks on anemone petals are said to be painted by faeries in the light of the moon. When you see the wood anemone flower slowly close at dusk, be respectful and say goodnight to the faery that might be living inside. Don't forget to blow on the first flower that you see and make a wish.

In England it was considered unlucky to pick wood anemones as it would bring on a thunderstorm. If you were foolish enough to bring the flowers into the house, you risked being struck by lightning. However, in an opposite superstition, European medieval peasants went out of their way to pick the flower since carrying an anemone was believed to ward off bad luck and offer protection from pests and diseases.

In the Victorian language of flowers, anemones were said to represent fragility, anticipation and protection from evil.

FOLK MEDICINE: Culpeper claims that, *"The body being bathed with the decoction of them cures the leprosy,"* and *"The leaves being stamped, and the juice stuffed up the nose, purges the head greatly."*

In some cultures, wood anemones have been used for asthma, whooping cough, delayed menstruation, to clean infected ulcers and to ease inflammation in the eyes. Poultices made from anemone leaves were laid on the forehead to cure headaches.

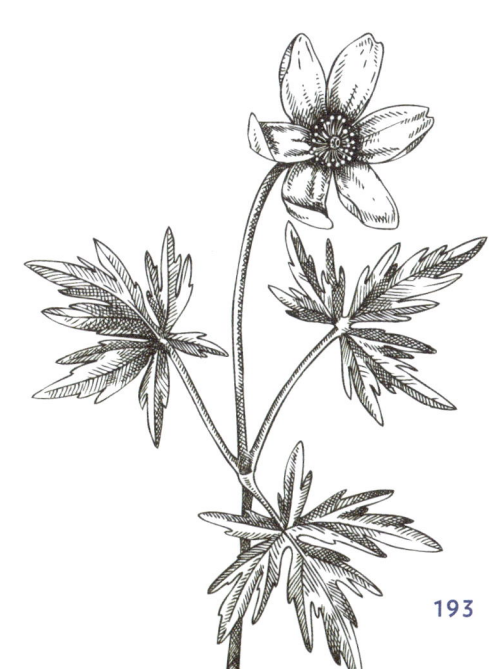

WOOD BETONY

Alternative names: Devil's plaything, bidney, purple betony, bishop's wort, common hedgenettle

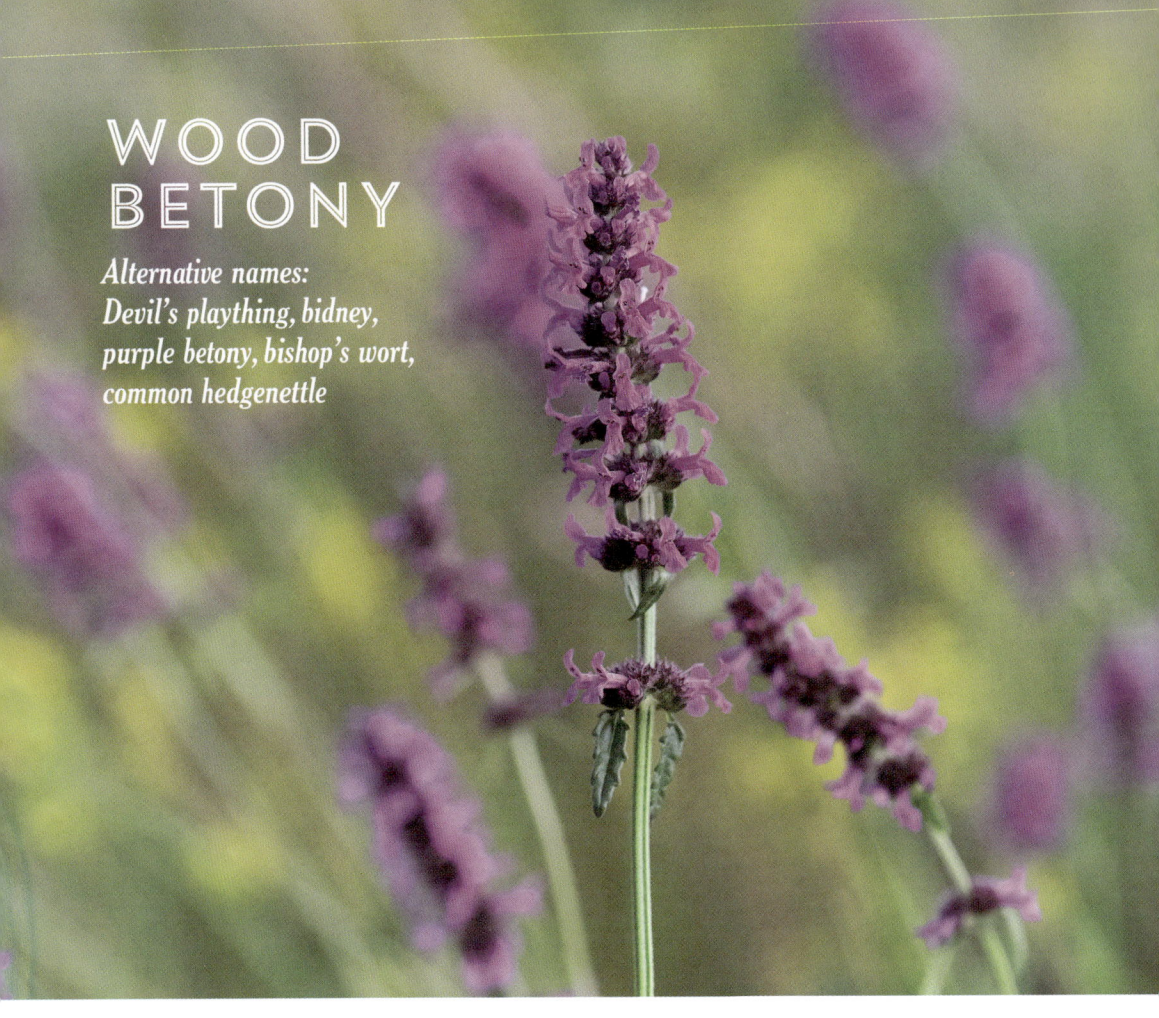

HOW TO IDENTIFY: A member of the deadnettle family, wood betony's bright magenta flowers are almost orchid-like and create striking splashes of colour from early summer well into autumn. Wood betony can be found growing in light, dry soils on sunny banks and hedgerows or at the edges of ploughed fields. The plant stands up very straight with leaves that are jagged and narrow, found mainly at the base.

HISTORY: Betony was regarded as the most precious remedy used by early European herbalists. Antonius Musa, who in 23 BCE was the physician to Emperor Augustus, wrote a book claiming that betony was a cure for no less than 47 diseases.

To demonstrate how valued betony was in the past, in the sixteenth century Gerard recommended that you should *"Sell your coat and buy betony."*

Wood betony was widely cultivated in the gardens of apothecaries and monasteries in the Middle Ages and was regarded as a panacea, for everyday use.

FOLKLORE: Traditionally, wood betony was planted in country graveyards, not only for its medicinal value, but because it was also believed to ward off evil spirits, ghosts, goblins and any other unwelcome demons.

Wood betony was added to the water used to bathe children who were alleged to be bewitched or possessed; the bathwater would wash away the bad magic.

Also used as an "amulet herb", betony tied to the arm with red wool or worn around the neck as a charm gave protection from witches, or placed under the pillow at night prevented nightmares and protected the sleeper. Superstitious people believed that the time between sunset and sunrise was when the soul needed the most protection from evil spirits.

One superstition commonly held in medieval England was that if snakes were placed inside a circle of betony, they would not stop fighting until one of them died.

FOLK MEDICINE: It was believed that wounded wild animals recognized the benefits of wood betony and would actively seek it out to heal themselves.

Traditionally, it was used to treat mental illness, headaches, indigestion, insomnia, memory loss, anxiety, nosebleeds, hangovers, chest and lung problems and gout, to name but a few.

Gerard stated that, *"It maketh a man to pisse well"*!

Culpeper sang the praises of wood betony, writing that it *"openeth obstructions both of the spleen and liver"*, as well as that it *"causes an easy and speedy delivery of women in child-birth"*.

Wild betony is still popular in English cottage gardens, where it was planted to be used as a home cure for rheumatism and general aches and pains. Betony had the added benefit that growing it around the home would protect the family from witches and goblins that come out at night.

WOODY NIGHTSHADE

Alternative names: Bittersweet, granny's nightcap, mad dog's berries, snake's food, witch flower

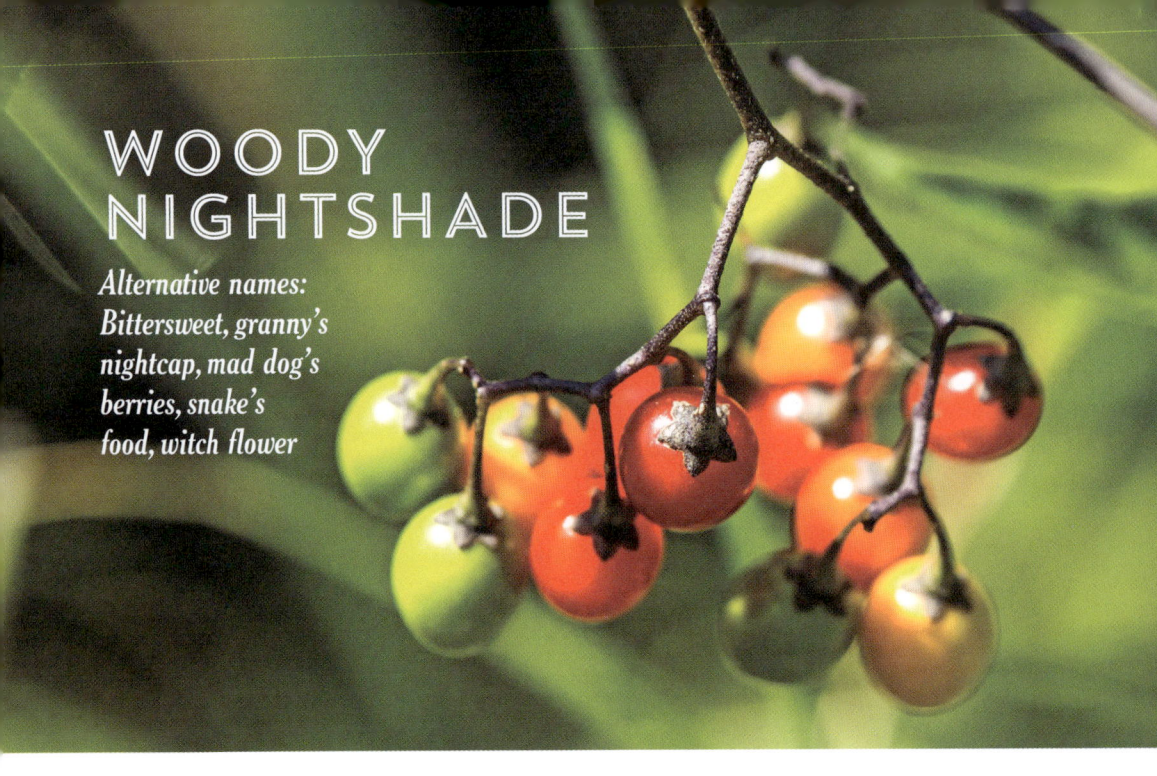

HOW TO IDENTIFY: All parts of woody nightshade are toxic and the tempting red berries can cause serious illness. Found on farmland, in hedgerows and in gardens, woody nightshade is a climbing plant dotted with attractive, deep-purple star-shaped flowers centred by protruding yellow stamens from May to September. Clusters of shiny berries appear in the autumn, much beloved by blackbirds and thrushes.

HISTORY: This woody climber has some more familiar relatives in tomatoes, peppers, potatoes and deadly nightshade, all of which have parts that should not be eaten.

The alternative name of "bittersweet" refers to the fact that as you chew the root or the stem, at first it tastes bitter and then it tastes sweet.

It was once chewed rather than smoked as a tobacco substitute in Cumbria, England, with the possibility of it making you ill perhaps adding to the experience.

In another fascinating story, a short while after Egyptologist Howard Carter found the tomb of Tutankhamun in 1925, a famous photograph was taken of the undisturbed boy king by archaeological photographer Harry Burton. The photograph clearly shows an elaborate floral and beaded collar around Tutankhamun's neck. Analysis later revealed that it was made up of willow leaves, cornflowers, pomegranate leaves and nightshade berries adorned with blue disc beads.

FOLKLORE: Woody nightshade has long associations with witchcraft and was often used as a protective herb.

Culpeper tells us that, *"It is excellently good to remove witchcraft both in men and beasts."*

Dried berries of woody nightshade were threaded into necklaces to be worn by children to protect them from being bewitched, which is presumably why Tutankhamun was buried wearing such a necklace. The same was done for cattle and to keep horses safe.

In magic, the toxic nature of woody nightshade was used in banishing spells to get rid of negative emotions and people. An unknown source counsels: *"Write the name of something, or someone that you no longer wish to have in your life on a piece of paper. Put three woody nightshade berries in the paper and wrap it up tight and pop it in a box. After three weeks remove it from the box, burn the paper and the berries and bury the ashes."*

Conversely, placing packets of the dried leaves and berries under your pillow was said to mend a broken heart.

FOLK MEDICINE: Woody nightshade is known as a useful herbal remedy to give after a fall, as Gerard explains:

"The juice is good for those that have fallen from high places, and have been thereby bruised, or dry beaten: for it is thought to dissolve blood congealed or cluttered anywhere in the entrails, and to heal the hurt places."

He also recommends it for jaundice, to help laboured breathing, to cleanse the spleen, and to *"throughly cleanseth women that are newly brought abed,"* though he doesn't elaborate on exactly what that means.

All parts of this plant could make you unwell so it's best not to put any of it in your mouth.

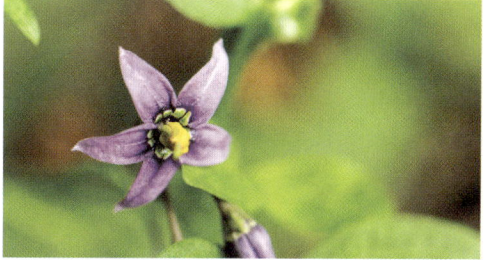

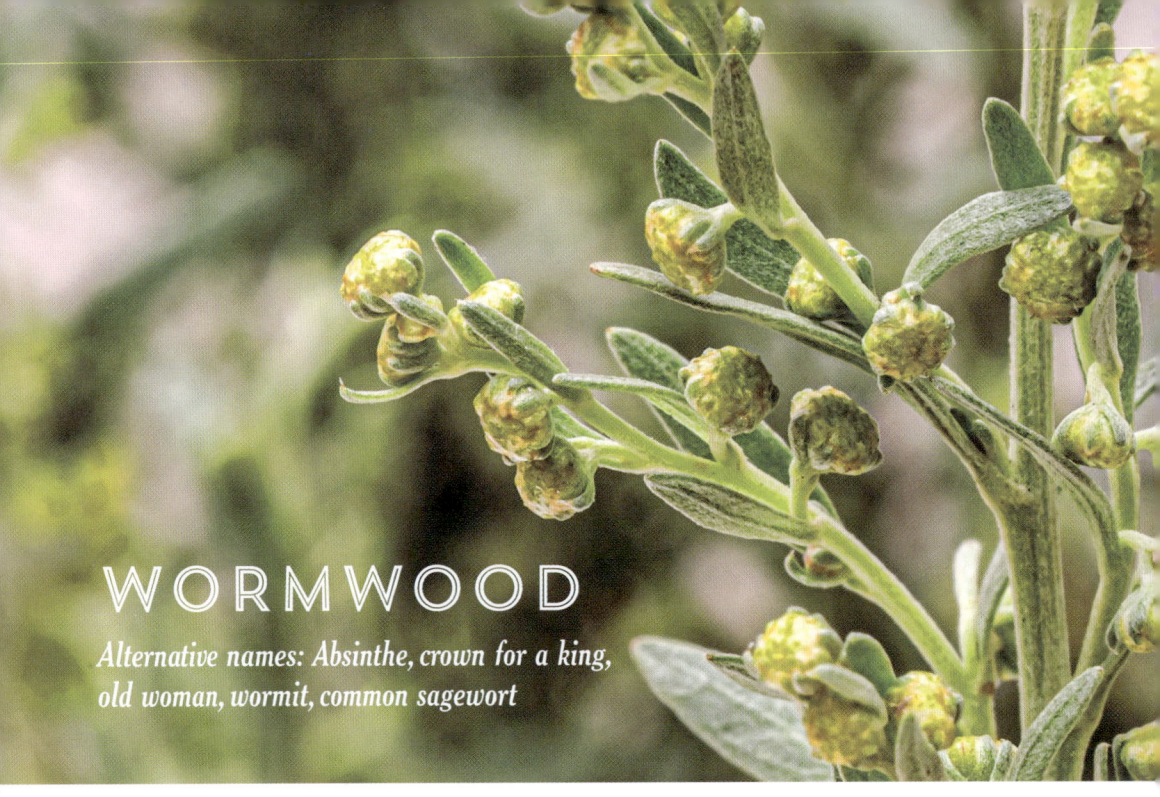

WORMWOOD

Alternative names: Absinthe, crown for a king, old woman, wormit, common sagewort

HOW TO IDENTIFY: A tall, grey, woody-stemmed plant mostly found growing in coastal areas or wasteland, wormwood has leaves that are greenish-grey on the top, white underneath and are much divided. Tiny yellow flowers can be seen from early summer until autumn.

HISTORY: Wormwood's Latin name is *Artemisia absinthium*, which gives us a clue as to its historical use. The combination of wormwood leaves and alcohol goes back to olden times, and references can be found in the Bible and in the writings of the ancient Egyptians.

For centuries wormwood-based drinks remained purely medicinal, but a war between France and Algeria in 1840 changed all that. The heat and insect infestation were so bad that the soldiers began drinking wormwood to ease fevers, deter insects and prevent dysentery. On their return to France, they brought the green drink with them as they had enjoyed it so much. Absinthe was born. By 1849 there were 26 absinthe distilleries in France, producing a whopping ten million litres a year of the aniseed-flavoured spirit.

Poets and artists such as van Gogh and Toulouse Lautrec enjoyed drinking the "green fairy". Ernest Hemingway was also a fan of absinthe and is quoted as saying, *"It's supposed to rot your brain out, but I don't believe it. It only changes the ideas."* There were many calls to ban "the green devil" as fears grew over the ill effects on mental and bodily health. France banned absinthe in the early twentieth century, only to reinstate it in 1988. It has always remained legal in the UK.

FOLKLORE: From an unknown source comes this old love charm:

"On St Luke's Day [18 October], take marigold flowers, a sprig of marjoram, thyme, and a little Wormwood; dry them before a fire, rub them to powder; then sift it through a fine piece of lawn, and simmer it over a slow fire, adding a small quantity of virgin honey, and vinegar. Anoint yourself with this when you go to bed, saying the following lines three times, and you will dream of your partner that is to be.

'St. Luke, St. Luke, be kind to me, In dreams let me my true-love see.'"

Believed to be a powerful weapon against witches and the "evil eye", a wreath made from wormwood thrown into a fire on midsummer's eve would afford protection for the coming year.

Meanwhile, burning wormwood in a graveyard is believed to bring forth the spirits of the departed and enhance psychic powers.

FOLK MEDICINE: The bitter taste of wormwood was used by new mothers to wean babies off breast milk, as referenced by Juliet's wet nurse in *Romeo and Juliet*: *"And she was weaned [...] for I had laid wormwood to my dug."*

Gerard wrote about the insect-repelling properties of wormwood: *"it keepeth garments also from the moths, it driveth away gnats, the body being anointed with the oil thereof".*

He recommends its use for choler, phlegm, indigestion, worms, wind, jaundice, shrew bites and the eating of poisonous mushrooms – quite a list!

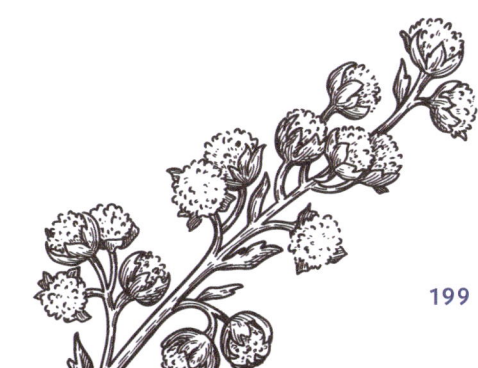

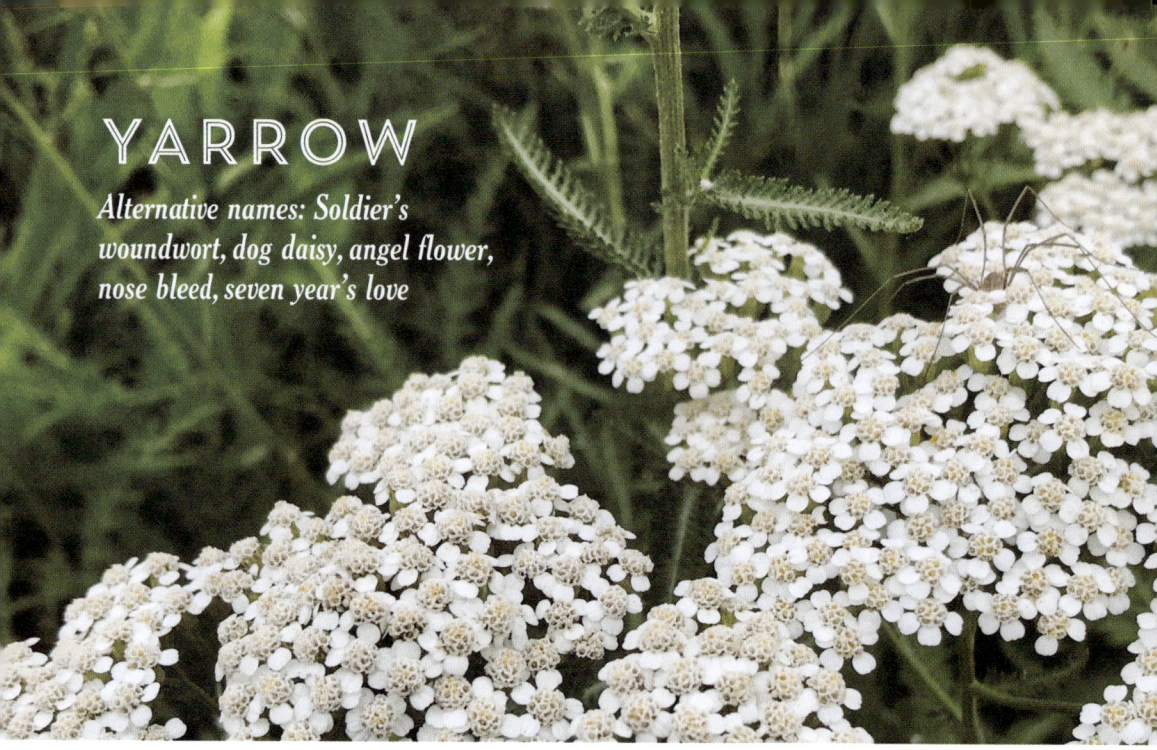

YARROW

Alternative names: Soldier's woundwort, dog daisy, angel flower, nose bleed, seven year's love

HOW TO IDENTIFY: Yarrow is found in abundance in grassland all over Britain. This ferny-leaved perennial can grow up to 1 m (3 ft) tall. The plant forms clumps that can be quite invasive with long, straight stalks and feathery leaves, with an umbrella of white or pink flowers on the top.

Crush the leaves and you will release its strong, sweet scent, similar to that of chrysanthemums.

HISTORY: The Anglo-Saxons had great respect for yarrow due to its powerful wound-healing properties. In the Middle Ages, before the widespread use of hops, yarrow was one of the many herbs used along with bog myrtle and rosemary to make "gruit" – an early form of beer.

FOLKLORE: Unmarried maidens in medieval Sussex would pick yarrow from a young man's grave by the light of the full moon and put it under their pillow saying,

"Good night fair yarrow,
Thrice goodnight to thee,
I hope before tomorrow,
My true love to see."

They would also pin it to their dresses and get as close to their potential suitors as possible. When they got home, the yarrow was placed in a drawer. If it was still fresh the next morning their love would be reciprocated. Often known as "seven year's love", yarrow was included in bridal bouquets, hung over the marriage bed and often eaten at wedding breakfasts to ensure that the newlywed couple were happy for at least seven years.

In other uses, yarrow tea was used by witches to enhance their psychic powers, and holding the plant up to the eyes would give the power of second sight.

FOLK MEDICINE: Historically, yarrow has been used to treat many ailments. The dark blue essential oil from the flowers is a good chest rub for colds and flu, and the leaves encourage clotting and can be used for nosebleeds. Leaves, stems and flowers are used to stimulate circulation, lower blood pressure and as a tonic for the blood.

An infusion of yarrow applied to the scalp will prevent baldness but unfortunately won't be able to cure it. Yarrow is also used as a treatment for snake bites, a cure for colds and flu, to give relief from toothache, and as a tea to help insomnia.

In medieval times, when headaches were believed to be caused by too much blood pressure in the head, yarrow leaves were pushed up the nostrils to cause bleeding to ease the pressure.

Gerard states that *"The leaves being put into the nose do cause it to bleed, and easeth the pain of the megrin [migraine]."*

Conversely, smelling yarrow flowers was believed to be a cure for nosebleeds.

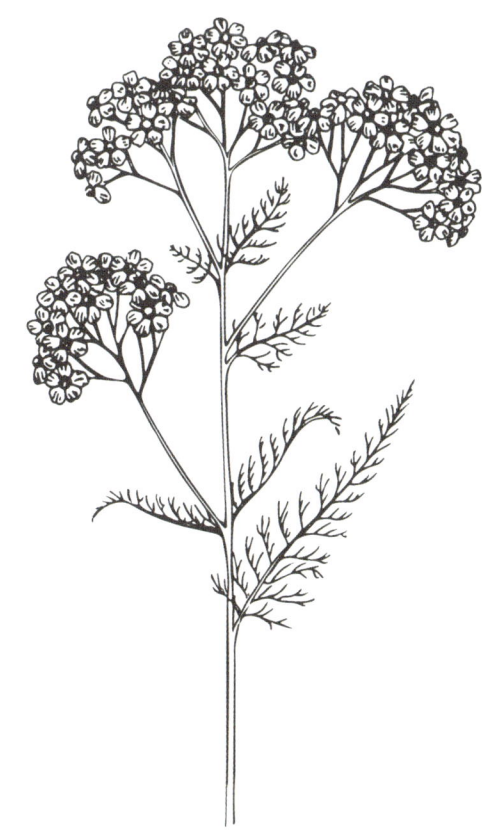

YARROW AND PLANTAIN FIRST-AID SALVE

This salve is a wonderful multi-use addition to your natural first-aid kit. Turning the healing powers of yarrow and plantain (not the banana) into a salve that you can carry around with you means that you always have something on hand for those minor scrapes and stings.

The anti-inflammatory properties of yarrow help relieve redness and itchiness. It is also antimicrobial which can speed up minor wound-healing and minimize the risk of infection. Plantain too is anti-inflammatory, helping to reduce redness and swelling, and is particularly effective at stopping the itching of insect bites and nettle stings.

The combination of these two hedgerow herbs in a salve will give you a powerful first-aid ally on foraging walks and play days in the park.

Makes a few small jars

INGREDIENTS

50 g fresh yarrow leaves, wilted for a couple of hours

50 g fresh plantain leaves, wilted for a couple of hours

200 ml carrier oil of choice (see pages 18–19)

20 g natural beeswax, or 10 g candelilla wax

20 drops lavender essential oil (optional)

EQUIPMENT NEEDED

Jar with lid

Heatproof bowl

Saucepan

Small jars or tins with lids

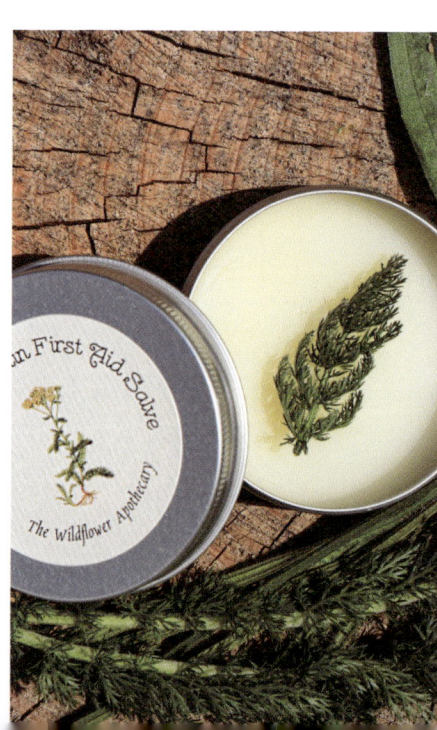

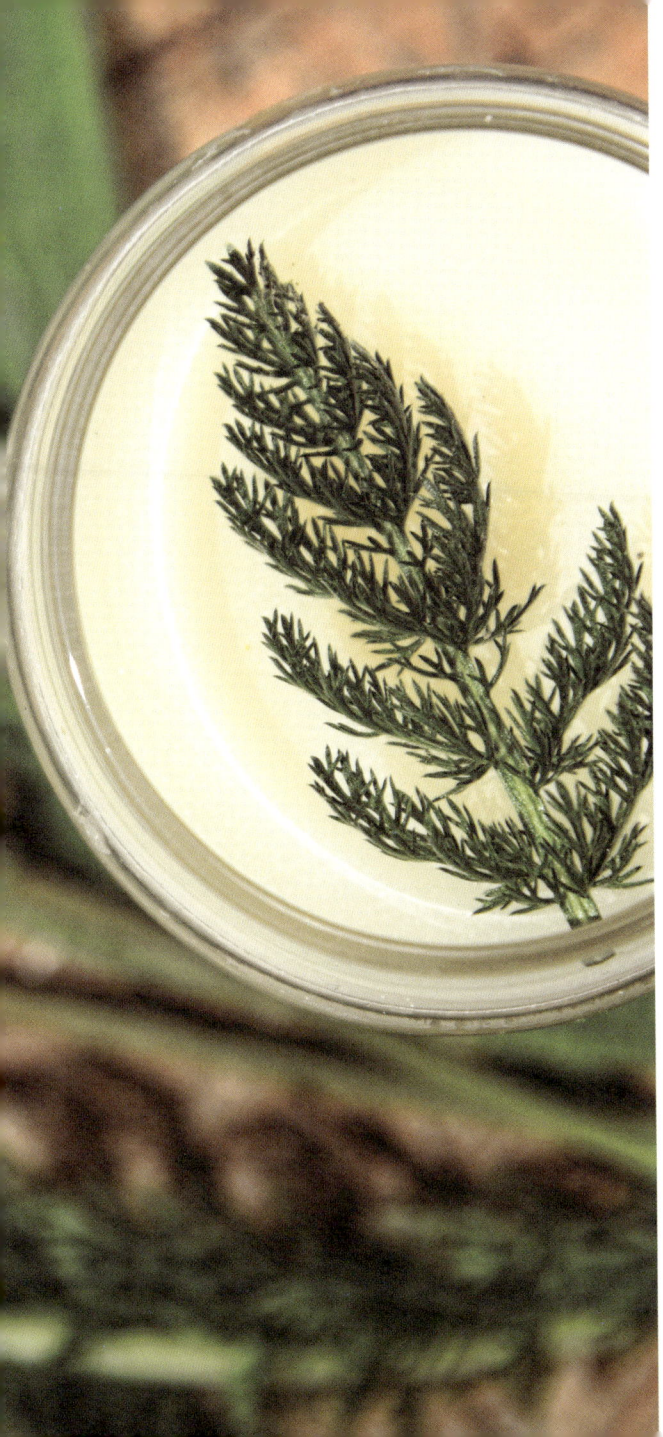

METHOD

Place your wilted yarrow and plantain in a glass jar and cover with carrier oil.

Allow to infuse in a warm spot for at least four weeks.

Strain the oil into a clean heatproof bowl and compost the herbs.

Add beeswax or candelilla wax to your bowl and place over a pan of simmering water until the beeswax has melted.

Remove from heat, add lavender oil if using, and stir. If you don't have lavender oil, lemon or peppermint essential oils both have anti-itch properties and can be substituted.

Pour the mixture into small jars or tins. The hardness of your salve will vary with the ambient temperature, so make sure it doesn't leak on hot, sunny days.

Always do a patch test.

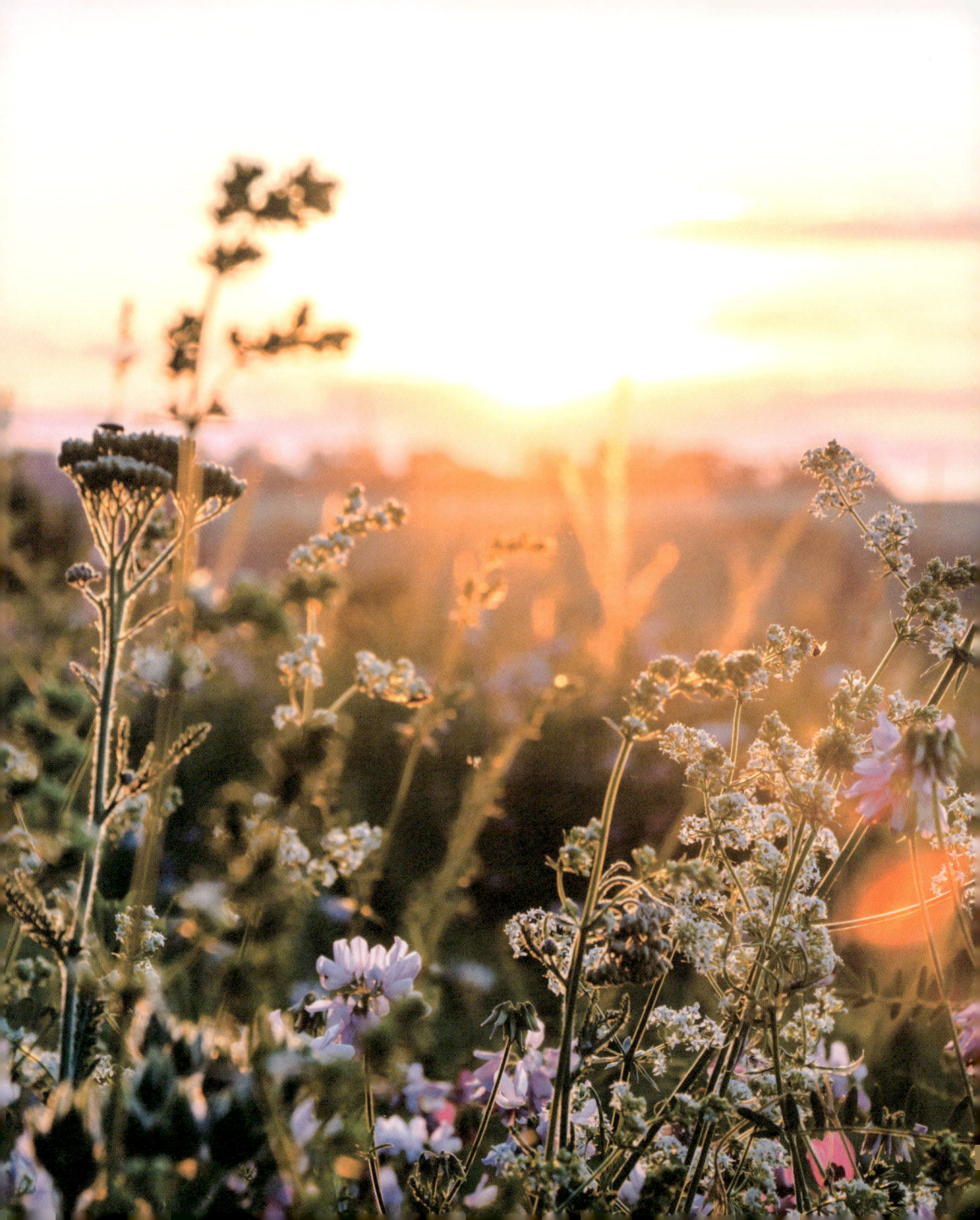

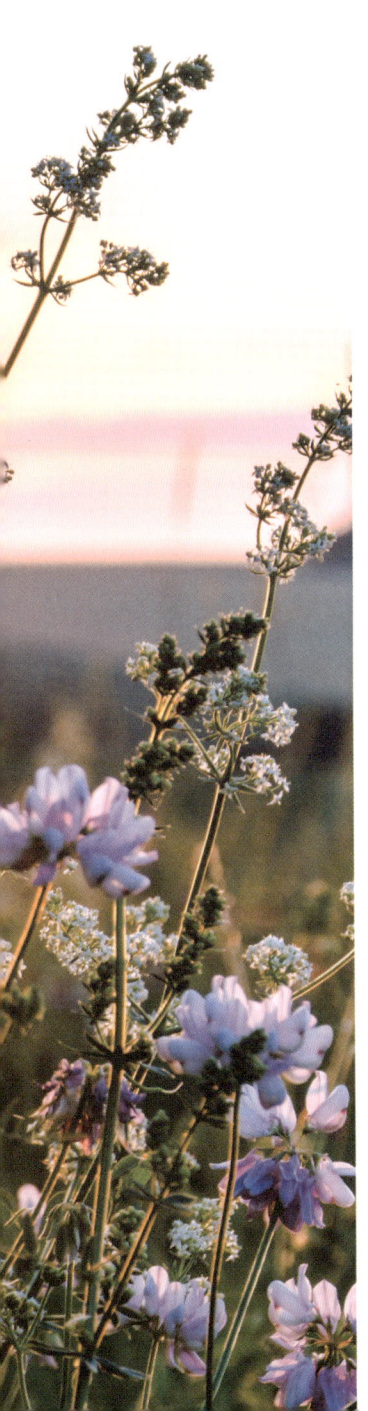

FINAL THOUGHTS

Our journey through the folklore, superstition and medicinal uses of wildflowers has taken us through hundreds, if not thousands, of years of constant use and benefits to humankind. Wildflowers have supported us in times of famine, provided cloth and dye, and given us medicines, salves and tinctures – as well as making our world a beautiful and vibrant place to live.

Wildflower meadows are also the most amazing habitat for our native wildlife, providing a source of both food and shelter from the beginning of spring right through to autumn. In one thriving meadow, you could be lucky enough to identify over 100 different species of wildflowers, all supporting a diverse mixture of insects, birds and mammals. On a summer's day, just one acre of meadow can host over three million flowers. Imagine the amount of nectar that will provide! No wonder bees love it.

Wildflowers don't just benefit our wildlife; more research is being done into the healing properties of plants for modern medicine. For example, snowdrops have been found to contain a compound called galantamine which is used in modern Alzheimer's medicines and prescribed to relieve injuries to the nervous system, and of course digitalin from foxgloves has long been an effective heart medication.

Hopefully this book has inspired you to head out into nature with fresh eyes and renewed appreciation of the vital role that wildflowers have played in our shared history.

Nurturing the natural world is of benefit to all of us. Whatever you can do, big or small, will make an impact and it needn't cost the earth, so pop on those walking boots and discover the wonderful world of our native wildflowers.

IMAGE CREDITS

Makes and recipes © Glenn Iverson; Cover and p.3 – yellow flowers © ZsuzsannaBird/Shutterstock.com; small blue flowers © Irina Boldina/Shutterstock.com; flower and bee © JeihstyZebra/Shutterstock.com; paper texture © Charunee Yodbun/Shutterstock.com; illustrations © ImHope/Shutterstock.com, Epine/Shutterstock.com and Nadezhda Molkentin/Shutterstock.com; pp.4-5 © Lois GoBe/Shutterstock.com; pp.6-7 © marilyn barbone/Shutterstock.com; p.8 © Bildagentur Zoonar GmbH/Shutterstock.com; p.9 – paper © Dmitr1ch/Shutterstock.com; photo © LN team/Shutterstock.com; p.11 © MIA Studio/Shutterstock.com; p.12 ©Sandra Standbridge/Shutterstock.com; p.14 © mspoli/Shutterstock.com; p.15 © FotoHelin/Shutterstock.com; p.21 © reflexion I nature/Shutterstock.com; p.22 left-hand image © grintan/Shutterstock.com; right-hand image © pilipphoto/Shutterstock.com; p.23 © Paladin12/Shutterstock.com; p.24 © olko1975/Shutterstock.com; p.25 © Henri Koskinen/Shutterstock.com; p.26 © Traveller70/Shutterstock.com; p.27 © Peter Groenendijk/Shutterstock.com; p.28 © Lois GoBe/Shutterstock.com; p.29 © Yevheniia Lytvynovych/Shutterstock.com; p.30 © Volodymyr Nikitenko/Shutterstock.com; p.31 © Bodor Tivadar/Shutterstock.com; p.32 © ZsuzsannaBird/Shutterstock.com; p.33 © Erkki Makkonen/Shutterstock.com; p.36 © IanRedding/Shutterstock.com; p.37 © Martin Fowler/Shutterstock.com; p.38 © aga7ta/Shutterstock.com; p.39 © Bodor Tivadar/Shutterstock.com; p.42 © Dima Brinza/Shutterstock.com; p.43 © Morphart Creation/Shutterstock.com; p.44 © Karolina Gabrys/Shutterstock.com; p.45 © Anna-Nas/Shutterstock.com; p.47 © SeonDeok OH/Shutterstock.com; p.48 © Andris Tkacenko/Shutterstock.com; p.49 © Yevheniia Lytvynovych/Shutterstock.com; p.50 © Skrypnykov Dmytro/Shutterstock.com; p.51 © KirillAm/Shutterstock.com; p.54 © Estuary Pig/Shutterstock.com; p.55 © Morphart Creation/Shutterstock.com; p.56 © Arda_ALTAY/Shutterstock.com; p.57 © Eileen Kumpf/Shutterstock.com; p.60 © mapimarf/Shutterstock.com; p.61 © SurfsUp/Shutterstock.com; p.62 © Martin Fowler/Shutterstock.com; p.63 © Martin Fowler/Shutterstock.com; p.64 © Vipul1989/Shutterstock.com; p.65 © adehoidar/Shutterstock.com; p.67 – ice cubes © Stivog/Shutterstock.com; p.68 © doolmsch/Shutterstock.com; p.69 © Analgin/Shutterstock.com; p.70 © Orest lyzhechka/Shutterstock.com; p.71 © Cat_arch_angel/Shutterstock.com; p.72 © Cornel99Sala/Shutterstock.com; p.73 © catalinatomir/Shutterstock.com; p.74 © Igor Poluchin/Shutterstock.com; p.75 © Patrusheva Yana/Shutterstock.com; p.76 © HAL-9000/Shutterstock.com; p.78 © olko1975/Shutterstock.com; p.79 © SPublishings/Shutterstock.com; p.80 © Dreamfinity Ltd/Shutterstock.com; p.81 © marineke thissen/Shutterstock.com; p.82 © Ellyy/Shutterstock.com; p.83 © Masha_tolk_art/Shutterstock.com; p.84 © doroninanatalie4/Shutterstock.com; p.85 © Lasse Johansson/Shutterstock.com; p.86 © Orest lyzhechka/Shutterstock.com; p.87 © wasilisa/Shutterstock.com; p.88 © Mariola Anna S/Shutterstock.com; p.89 © Antares_NS/Shutterstock.com; p.90 © Medvedeva Oxana/Shutterstock.com; p.91 © Lewis Pidoux/Shutterstock.com; p.92 © Zhukovskaya Elena/Shutterstock.com; p.96 © Ksenia Lada/Shutterstock.com; p.97 © Antares_NS/Shutterstock.com; p.98 © Sanna Huttunen/Shutterstock.com; p.99 © KateChe/Shutterstock.com; p.100 © Maren Winter/Shutterstock.com; p.101 © AC Rider/Shutterstock.com; p.102 © Robert Adami/Shutterstock.com; p.103 © Ekonst/Shutterstock.com; p.104 © Fabrizio Guarisco/Shutterstock.com; p.105 © zcebeci/Shutterstock.com; p.106 © Mr. Meijer/Shutterstock.com; p.107 © Sabelskaya/Shutterstock.com; p.108 © Tom Meaker/Shutterstock.com; p.109 © Martin Fowler/Shutterstock.com; p.110 © garmoncheg/Shutterstock.com; p.111 © Epine/Shutterstock.com; p.114 © AylinGuneyiPhotograpy/Shutterstock.com; p.118 © Lewis Pidoux/Shutterstock.com; p.119 © Orest lyzhechka/Shutterstock.com; p.122 © bonilook/Shutterstock.com; p.123 © Morphart Creation/Shutterstock.com; p.124 © Bolbot Visuals/Shutterstock.com; p.126 © olko1975/Shutterstock.com; p.127 © cherryyblossom/Shutterstock.com; p.128 © KariDesign/Shutterstock.com; p.132 © Ihor Hvozdetskyi/Shutterstock.com; p.133 © mart/Shutterstock.com; p.136 © Nahhana/Shutterstock.com; p.137 © agsaz/Shutterstock.com; p.138 © Asif Naseem Photographer/Shutterstock.com; p.139 © Jka/Shutterstock.com; p.140 © Kazakov Maksim/Shutterstock.com; p.141 © Lyubov_Nazarova/Shutterstock.com; p.142 © R. Knapp/Shutterstock.com; p.143 © bykot photo/Shutterstock.com; p.144 © Iva Vagnerova/Shutterstock.com; p.145 © Alex Manders/Shutterstock.com; p.146 © Nicram Sabod/Shutterstock.com; p.147 © Rudmer Zwerver/Shutterstock.com; p.148 © barmalini/Shutterstock.com; p.149 © MIROFOSS/Shutterstock.com; p.150 © JPC-PROD/Shutterstock.com; p.152 © Tom Meaker/Shutterstock.com; p.153 © Photo-Saint-Tropez/Shutterstock.com; p.156 © V. Tarasenko/Shutterstock.com; p.158 © Vankich1/Shutterstock.com; p.160 © Alice8648/Shutterstock.com; p.161 © meiningi/Shutterstock.com; p.164 © meiningi/Shutterstock.com; p.165 © goran_safarek/Shutterstock.com; p.166 © agatchen/Shutterstock.com; p.167 © olko1975/Shutterstock.com; p.170 © A.Luna/Shutterstock.com; p.172 © Wirestock Creators/Shutterstock.com; p.173 © Ian Peter Morton/Shutterstock.com; p.174 © Rejdan/Shutterstock.com; p.175 © Yevheniia Lytvynovych/Shutterstock.com; p.178 © Alis Photo/Shutterstock.com; p.179 © Den SkyLung/Shutterstock.com; p.182 © Manfred Ruckszio/Shutterstock.com; p.183 © Fabian Junge/Shutterstock.com; p.186 © Dmytro Balkhovitin/Shutterstock.com; p.187 © Sabelskaya/Shutterstock.com; p.190 © laykamars/Shutterstock.com; p.191 © meunierd/Shutterstock.com; p.192 © teddiviscious/Shutterstock.com; p.193 © Yevheniia Lytvynovych/Shutterstock.com; p.194 © Ksenia Lada/Shutterstock.com; p.196 © hjochen/Shutterstock.com; p.197 © Antoni M Lubek/Shutterstock.com; p.198 © nnattalli/Shutterstock.com; p.199 © Epine/Shutterstock.com; p.200 © Alphabetman/Shutterstock.com; p.201 © logaryphmic/Shutterstock.com; pp.204–205 © Artur Sniezhyn/Shutterstock.com; p.208 © Leszek Kobusinski/Shutterstock.com

ALSO BY CHRISTINE IVERSON

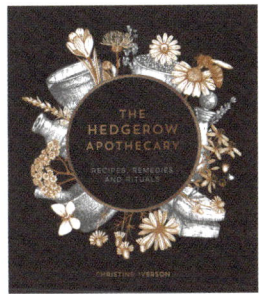

THE HEDGEROW APOTHECARY

Recipes, Remedies and Rituals

Hardback
ISBN: 978-1-78783-029-5

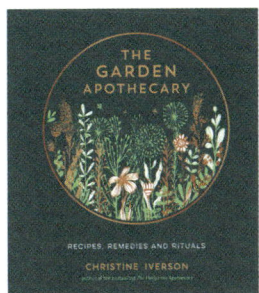

THE GARDEN APOTHECARY

Recipes, Remedies and Rituals

Hardback
ISBN: 978-1-78783-979-3

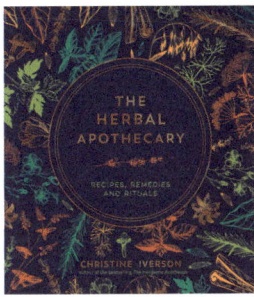

THE HERBAL APOTHECARY

Recipes, Remedies and Rituals

Hardback
ISBN: 978-1-80007-985-4

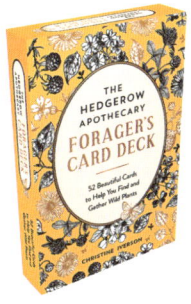

THE HEDGEROW APOTHECARY FORAGER'S CARD DECK

52 Beautiful Identification Cards and Booklet to Help You Find and Gather Wild Plants

Cards
ISBN: 978-1-83799-484-7

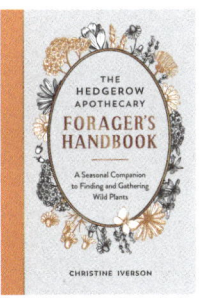

THE HEDGEROW APOTHECARY FORAGER'S HANDBOOK

A Seasonal Companion to Finding and Gathering Wild Plants

Paperback
ISBN: 978-1-80007-181-0

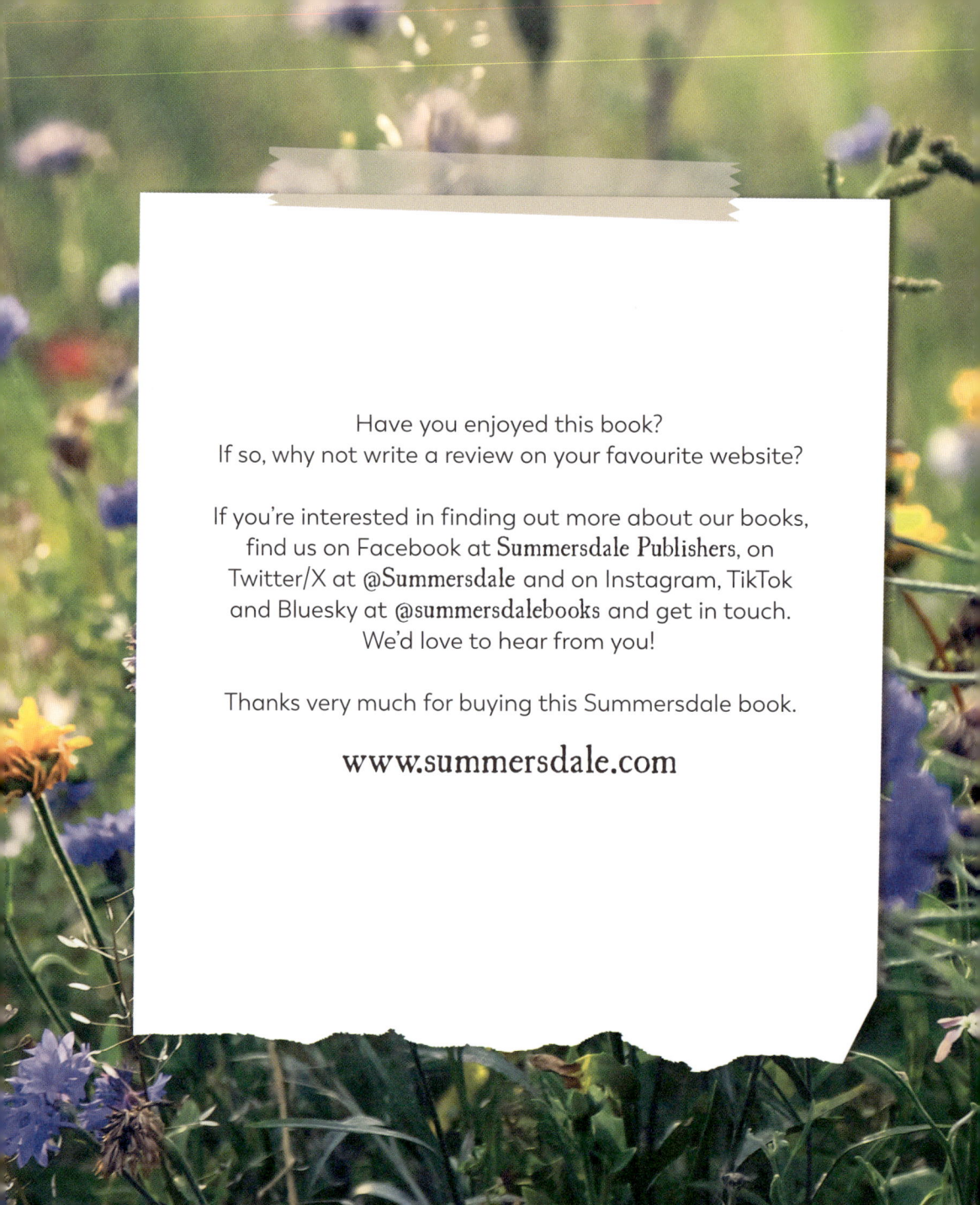

Have you enjoyed this book?
If so, why not write a review on your favourite website?

If you're interested in finding out more about our books, find us on Facebook at **Summersdale Publishers**, on Twitter/X at **@Summersdale** and on Instagram, TikTok and Bluesky at **@summersdalebooks** and get in touch. We'd love to hear from you!

Thanks very much for buying this Summersdale book.

www.summersdale.com

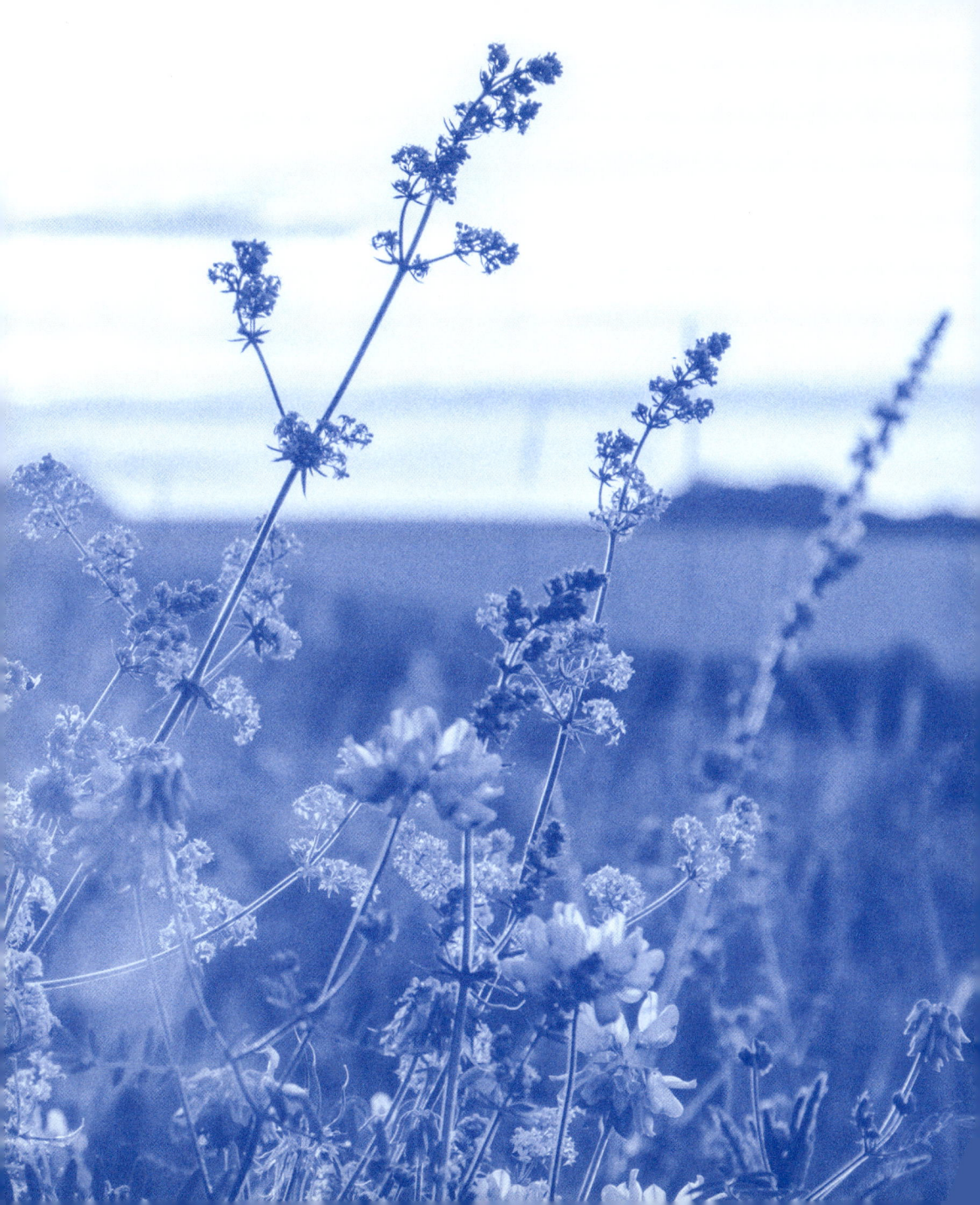

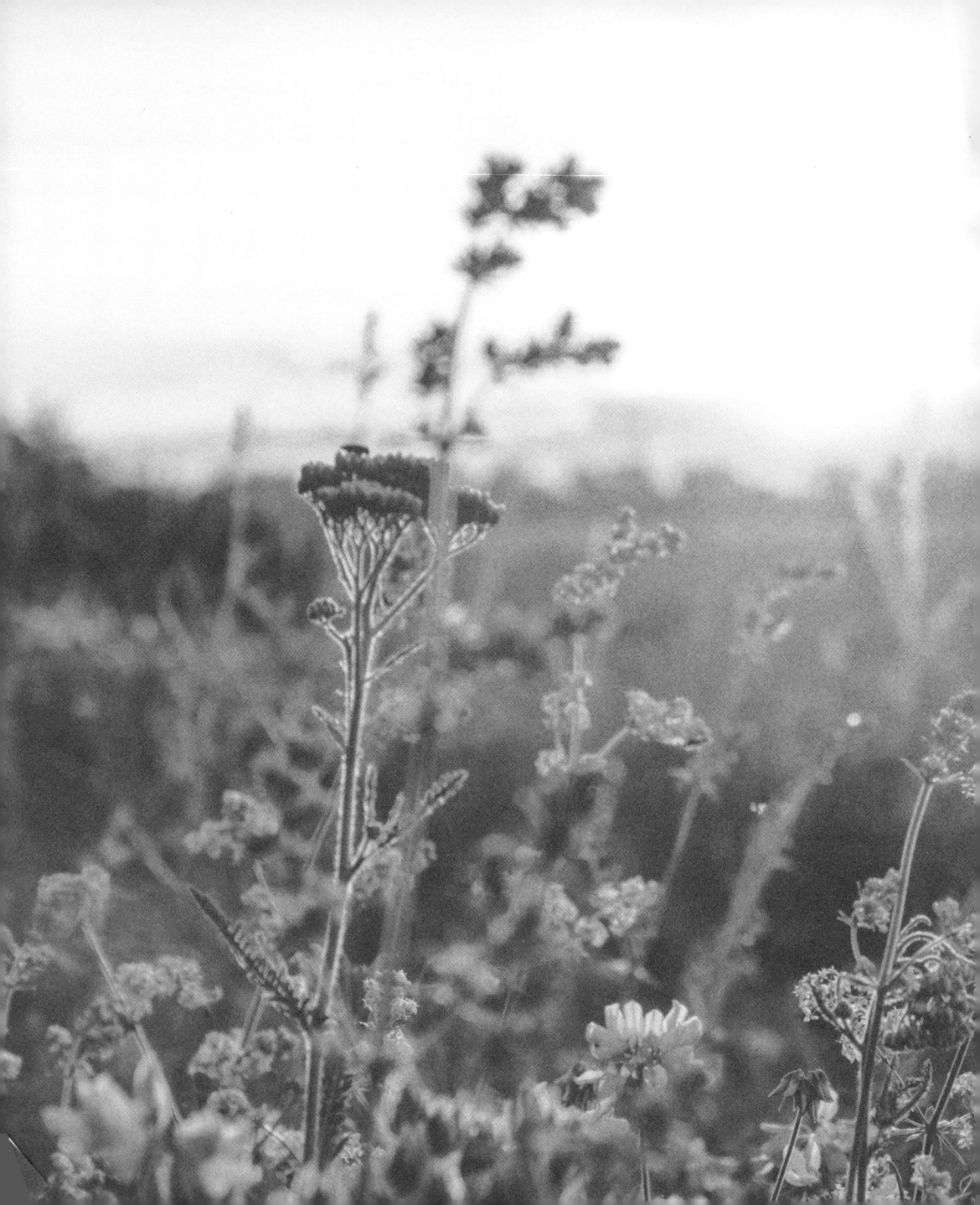